Jennie Brand-Miller and her research colleagues have done pioneering work, showing how the glycemic index can help you lose weight and improve your health. They are leading scientific authorities, and I often rely on their important findings in our research studies to help people reduce weight, control diabetes, tackle triglycerides, and return to health.

NEAL BARNARD, MD, founder and president,
Physicians for Responsible Medicine, and author of eight books, including
Dr. Neal Barnard's Program for Reversing Diabetes and *Breaking the Food Seduction*

Forget *Sugar Busters*. Forget *The Zone*. If you want the real scoop on how carbohydrates and sugar affect your body, read this book by the world's leading researchers on the subject. It is the authoritative, last word on choosing foods to control your blood sugar.

Jean Carper, bestselling author of
Miracle Cures, Stop Aging Now! and *Food: Your Miracle Medicine*

Clear, accessible, and authoritative information about the glycemic index. An exciting, new approach to preventing obesity, diabetes, and heart disease—written by internationally recognized experts in the field.

David Ludwig, MD, PhD, Director, Obesity Program,
Children's Hospital, Boston, and coauthor, *Ending the Food Fight:
Guide Your Child to a Healthy Weight in a Fast Food/Fake Food World*

The Glucose Revolution is nutrition science for the twenty-first century. Clearly written, it gives the scientific rationale for why all carbohydrates are not created equal. It is a practical guide for both professionals and patients. The food suggestions and recipes are exciting and tasty.

Richard N. Podell, MD, MPH, Clinical Professor, Department of Family
Medicine, Robert Wood Johnson Medical School, and coauthor
of *The G-Index Diet: The Missing Link That Makes Permanent Weight Loss Possible*

The New Glucose Revolution summarizes much of the recent development of dietary glycemic index and load in a highly readable format. The authors are able researchers and respected leaders in the nutrition field. Much that is discussed in this book draws directly from their years of experimental and observational research. The focus on dietary intervention and prevention strategies in everyday eating is an especially laudable feature of this book. I recommend this book most highly as an indispensable source of good nutrition.

Simin Liu, MD, MS, MPH, ScD,
Professor, Department of Epidemiology, UCLA School of Public Health

Mounting evidence indicates that refined carbohydrates and high glycemic index foods are contributing to the escalating epidemics of obesity and type 2 diabetes worldwide. This dietary pattern also appears to increase the risk of heart disease and stroke. The skyrocketing proportion of calories from added sugars and refined carbohydrates in westernized diets portends a future acceleration of these trends . . . Brand-Miller and colleagues are to be congratulated for an eminently lucid and important book that explains the science behind the glycemic index and provides tools and strategies for modifying diet to incorporate this knowledge. I strongly recommend the book to both health professionals and the general public who could use this state-of-the-art information to improve health and well-being.

Joann E. Manson, MD, DrPH, Professor of Medicine,
Harvard Medical School, and Codirector of Women's Health,
Division of Preventive Medicine, Brigham and Women's Hospital

As a coach of elite amateur and professional athletes, I know how critical the glycemic index is to sports performance. *The New Glucose Revolution* provides the serious athlete with the basic tools necessary for getting the training table right.

Joe Friel, coach, author, consultant

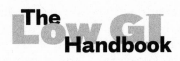

The Low GI Handbook

The Low GI Handbook

The NEW GLUCOSE *Revolution*
Guide to the Long-term Health Benefits of Low GI Eating

Jennie Brand-Miller, PhD
Thomas M. S. Wolever, MD, PhD
Kaye Foster-Powell, M Nutr & Diet
Stephen Colagiuri, MD

Da Capo
LIFE
LONG
A Member of the Perseus Books Group

Copyright © 1996, 1998, 1999, 2002, 2003, 2007, 2010 Dr. Jennie Brand-Miller, Kaye Foster-Powell, Dr. Stephen Colagiuri, Dr. Thomas M. S. Wolever.
Chapter 15 copyright © Dr. Emma Stevenson
Recipes on pages 274, 275, 276, 277, 287, 290, and 293 copyright © 2002 Lisa Lintner.

This is a completely revised edition of *The New Glucose Revolution*, published in North America by Da Capo Press in 2007 and 2003 (and in a previous edition, as *The Glucose Revolution*, in 1999). This completely revised and updated fourth edition was originally published as *The Low GI Handbook* in 2008 by Hachette Livre Australia. This edition is published in arrangement with Hachette Livre Australia.

Design and production by Eclipse Publishing Services
Set in 11-point Legacy Serif

Cataloging-in-Publication data for this book is available from the Library of Congress.

First Da Capo Press edition 2010
ISBN: 978-0-7382-1389-7

Published by Da Capo Press
A Member of the Perseus Books Group
www.dacapopress.com

Note: The information in this book is true and complete to the best of our knowledge. This book is intended only as an informative guide for those wishing to know more about health issues. In no way is this book intended to replace, countermand, or conflict with the advice given to you by your own physician. The ultimate decision concerning care should be made between you and your doctor. We strongly recommend you follow his or her advice. Information in this book is general and is offered with no guarantees on the part of the authors or Da Capo Press. The authors and publisher disclaim all liability in connection with the use of this book.

Da Capo Press books are available at special discounts for bulk purchases in the U.S. by corporations, institutions, and other organizations. For more information, please contact the Special Markets Department at the Perseus Books Group, 2300 Chestnut Street, Suite 200, Philadelphia, PA, 19103, or call (800) 810-4145, ext. 5000, or e-mail special.markets@perseusbooks.com.

10 9 8 7 6 5 4 3

Contents

Introduction

THE LOW GI HANDBOOK is the definitive guide to the long-term health benefits of low GI eating. The glycemic index (which we will often abbreviate as GI) is the universally recognized way to distinguish how different carbohydrates affect your blood glucose levels. It can help you choose both the right *amount* of carbohydrate and the right *sort* of carbohydrate every day and every meal. *Eating the best sources of carbohydrates can positively affect your health today—and over the course of your entire life.* That was the fundamental message of the original edition of this book, first published in 1996. Now, nearly fifteen years later, that message is more relevant to more people than ever before.

You probably know that your blood glucose levels rise and fall throughout the day, helping determine how you feel and how your body functions. ("Blood sugar" and "blood glucose" mean the same thing. Throughout this book we will use the term *blood glucose,* which is scientifically more precise.) Grounded in nearly thirty years of research, *The Low GI Handbook* thoroughly explains the relationship between carbohydrates and blood glucose and how the connection between the two affects your health, both immediately and later in life.

Who Can Use *The Low GI Handbook*?

Now more than ever, the glycemic index is for everybody, every day, at every meal. The GI—as well as its newer companion concept, the glycemic load—is relevant for everyone. People concerned about heart health—who are at risk for heart disease or heart attack or who have metabolic syndrome (insulin resistance syndrome, formerly known as syndrome X)—will greatly benefit by putting into practice the findings and recommendations of *The Low GI Handbook*.

So, too, will women with polycystic ovarian syndrome (PCOS) and everyone interested in controlling his or her weight.

The Low GI Handbook is essential reading for everyone with diabetes and prediabetes, offering an alternative to misguided and often counterproductive dietary restrictions. Many people with type 1 or type 2 diabetes find that despite doing all the right things, their blood glucose levels fluctuate excessively and/or remain too high. If you or someone you are caring for has diabetes, *The Low GI Handbook* will give you the knowledge and know-how to choose the right kind of carbohydrate for optimum blood glucose management.

This book is also for those who want to prevent these conditions in the first place and to improve their overall health. Particularly in the last decade, scientific research has underscored—not only to us, but to many individual experts and health authorities worldwide—that the GI has implications for everybody. It is truly a glucose revolution, in that a growing mountain of research on the GI has permanently changed the way we understand carbohydrates and their effect on our bodies.

What's New in This Edition

This new and fully revised edition, now called *The Low GI Handbook*, presents the most comprehensive, up-to-date information about the GI, including exciting new research and feedback from people whose lives have been changed by adopting a low GI diet approach.

Low GI eating . . .

. . . has science on its side. There are no strict rules or regimens to follow. It's essentially about making simple dietary changes, such as swapping one type of bread or breakfast cereal for another.

The scientific evidence to support the central role the GI can play in your health has now been firmly established. Indeed, it goes much further than we ever imagined when we began our research in the early

The Low GI Handbook helps people:

- with type 1 diabetes
- with type 2 diabetes
- with prediabetes (who may have been told they have "a touch of diabetes" or impaired glucose tolerance)
- with gestational diabetes (diabetes during pregnancy)
- with hypoglycemia, or low blood glucose
- who are overweight or obese
- who are at a normal weight but have too much fat around the middle (abdominal weight)
- with higher than desirable blood glucose levels
- with high levels of triglycerides
- with low levels of HDL cholesterol, the "good" cholesterol
- with metabolic syndrome
- with polycystic ovarian syndrome (PCOS) (irregular periods, acne, facial hair)
- with nonalcoholic fatty liver (NAFL) disease or nonalcoholic steatohepatitis (NASH)
- who want to delay or prevent age-related vision problems (such as age-related macular degeneration)
- who want to prevent all of the above and live a long and healthy life

The reason *The Low GI Handbook* can help you is simple: high blood glucose levels are a key—and undesirable—characteristic of all these conditions, with both short- and long-term adverse effects. *The Low GI Handbook* will show you why being choosy about the type of carbohydrates you eat (because their glycemic potency varies) will get you off the roller coaster and stabilize your blood glucose levels.

1980s, when the glycemic index was first developed. We share our own and other scientific findings with you—and what they mean for your long-term health and well-being.

Among the features that are new in this edition are:

- All of the very latest findings (as at time of publication) regarding the glycemic index and diabetes, heart disease, weight loss, and non-alcoholic fatty liver disease
- An introduction to and overview of glycemic load
- Insights into a woman's diet during pregnancy, gestational diabetes, diseases such as polycystic ovarian syndrome (PCOS, closely linked to insulin resistance), and celiac disease
- Real-life success stories from people who have dramatically improved their health by making the switch to low GI eating
- A clear rationale for choosing our low GI eating plan from among the many different diets that circulate today
- An extensive glossary, with more than eighty key terms, now clearly defined, all in one place
- The newest published GI values for a wide variety of recently tested foods

A Quick Guide to *The Low GI Handbook*

Part 1 presents a complete overview of the glycemic index (what it is, why it matters) and carbohydrates, specifically, why we need them and how many are right for you. We explain the importance of being choosy about the types of carbohydrates and fats you eat—no matter what the proportions of protein, fat, and carbohydrate. We also discuss "glycemic load" and when and how it should be used.

In Part 2, we explain exactly how the GI—and specifically, a low GI diet—can aid in weight control, as well as how it can help manage or prevent a variety of health conditions and concerns, including type 1 diabetes, type 2 diabetes, prediabetes, polycystic ovarian syndrome (PCOS), heart disease, metabolic syndrome, gestational diabetes, and hypoglycemia. We also discuss how the GI applies to healthy eating for children, sports performance, and exercise.

Part 3 answers fifty of the most commonly asked questions about the GI. If you've wondered about something relating to the GI, you should find the answer here.

Part 4 is your practical guide to low GI eating. We set out our ten steps to a healthy, low GI diet and explain how easy it is to make the switch to eating the right kinds of carbs and what to keep stocked in your pantry, refrigerator, and freezer, along with our quick and easy ideas for breakfast, lunch, dinner, and between-meal snacks. Part 4 also includes fifty simple and delicious recipes, including their estimated GI ratings and nutritional analysis. We also show how vegetarians and people who need to eat a gluten-free diet can enjoy the healthy benefits of low GI eating.

You'll find the actual GI values for approximately 1,300 foods in the updated tables in Part 5, the most comprehensive and authoritative list of GI values for different foods. You'll find foods listed alphabetically as well as according to types (breads, fruits, vegetables, etc.); the information includes not only the GI value and amount of carbohydrate per serving, but also their glycemic load. We've added the foods that we're often asked about—meat, fish, cheese, broccoli, avocados, and others—even though many of them don't contain carbohydrate and their glycemic load equals zero.

Finally, we end with an A-to-Z glossary of key terms we have used throughout this edition, as well as our comprehensive references section.

A note about the references section: we are scientists, medical doctors, and dietitians (to read more about us, see About the Authors, on page 384). We value the research and clinical data that form the backbone of this book and are behind every one of our recommendations. Every piece of advice we offer in this book has scientific validity. The references underscore our grounding in medical research and they're there for all of you who like to familiarize yourselves with original scientific findings and may want to trace our suggestions back to their original sources.

We make this promise to you: with *The Low GI Handbook,* you'll discover and come to understand a way of eating for lifelong health that is easy, delicious, wonderfully varied, does not depend on deprivation, and is truly satisfying on many levels.

Throughout this book, we'll dispel a number of myths about food and carbohydrates. To start you off, on the following pages, we bust the ten most common myths about food (sugar and other carbs, especially) and health.

Ten Big Myths about Food and Health Dispelled

Myth 1: Starchy foods such as potatoes and pasta are fattening.
Fact: Starchy foods are often bulky and nutritious. They fill you up and stave off hunger pangs—which means they can actually help with, rather than hinder, weight loss. The key, as with all foods, is to be choosy about the kinds of starchy foods you're eating.

Myth 2: Sugar causes diabetes.
Fact: Today, there's consensus among health researchers and scientists specializing in diabetes that sugar in food does not cause diabetes. Type 1 diabetes is an autoimmune condition triggered by unknown environmental factors. Type 2 diabetes is largely inherited, but lifestyle factors such as a lack of exercise or being overweight increase the risk of developing it. Foods that produce high blood glucose levels may increase the risk of type 2 diabetes, but sugar has a more moderate effect than many starches.

Myth 3: Sugar is the worst thing for people with diabetes.
Fact: People with diabetes used to be advised to avoid sugar at all costs. But research shows that moderate consumption of refined sugar (thirty–fifty grams or six to ten teaspoons per day) doesn't compromise blood glucose management. This means people with diabetes can choose foods that contain refined sugar or even use sensible amounts of table sugar. Saturated fat is of greater concern for people with diabetes than refined sugar.

Myth 4: All starches are slowly digested in the intestine.
Fact: Not so. Most starch, especially in cereal products, is digested in a flash, causing a sharper increase in blood glucose than many sugar-containing foods.

Myth 5: Hunger pains are inevitable if you want to lose weight.
Fact: High-carbohydrate foods, especially those with a low GI (rolled oats and pasta, for example), can keep you feeling full, often until you're ready to eat your next meal.

Myth 6: Foods high in fat are more filling.
Fact: Studies show that many high-fat foods are among the least filling. That's why, in part, it's so easy to passively overconsume high-fat foods like potato chips.

Myth 7: Sugar is fattening.
Fact: Sugar has no special fattening properties. It is no more likely to be turned into fat than any other type of carbohydrate. Apples and soft drinks have the same sugar content (10 percent to 12 percent). Yes, sugar is often present in high-calorie foods (cakes, cookies, chocolate, and ice cream, for instance). But it's the total calories in those foods, not the sugar, that's the problem.

Myth 8: Diets high in sugar are less nutritious.
Fact: Studies have shown that diets containing a moderate amount of sugar (from a range of sources, including dairy foods and fruit) often have higher levels of micronutrients, including calcium, riboflavin, and vitamin C, than low-sugar diets.

Myth 9: Sugar goes hand in hand with dietary fat.
Fact: Many foods high in fat are also high in sugar—think chocolate, full-fat ice cream, cake, cookies, and pastries. But *most* high-sugar diets are actually low in fat, and vice versa. The reason: most sources of fat in our diet are not sweet (e.g., potato chips, French fries, steak), while most sources of sugar contain no fat (e.g., soft drinks and sweetened juice drinks). Nutritionists call this the "sugar-fat seesaw."

Myth 10: Starches are best for optimum athletic performance.
Fact: In many instances, starchy foods (like potatoes or rice) are too bulky to eat in the quantities needed for active athletes. Sugars (from a range of sources, including dairy food and fruit) can help increase carbohydrate intake.

What Is the Glycemic Index?

■

1
The GI—A Brief Overview

TODAY WE KNOW that carbohydrate foods are not created equal. In fact, they can behave quite differently in our bodies. The glycemic index, or GI, is a measure of carbohydrate quality. It is a ranking that describes how much the carbohydrates (sugars and starches) in individual foods affect blood glucose levels. It is a physiologically based measure, too—a comparison of carbohydrates based on feeding real foods to real people.

Foods containing carbohydrates that break down quickly during digestion, like those in white bread, have the highest GI values. The blood glucose response is fast and high—in other words, the glucose in the bloodstream increases rapidly. We call them "fast action" carbs, or "gushers."

Foods that contain carbohydrates that break down slowly, releasing glucose gradually into the bloodstream like those in legumes, pasta, and barley, have low GI values. They can keep you feeling full longer, help you achieve and maintain a healthy weight, and provide you and your brain with more consistent energy throughout the day. They can also have a major effect on the way the body functions and whether or not you develop health problems.

For most people, under most circumstances, foods with low GI values have advantages over those with high GI values. But there are exceptions: some athletes can benefit from high GI foods during and after competition (which we explain in Chapter 15), and high GI foods are also useful in the treatment of hypoglycemia (covered in Chapter 11).

What Is the GI?

- It's a tool to help you choose the right type of carbs.
- It's a scale from 0 to 100 that reflects how fast the carbohydrates in foods hit the bloodstream.
- It's based on scientific testing of real foods in real people.
- A low GI food contains carbs that have less effect on blood glucose levels; its GI is 55 or less.
- A high GI food contains carbs that have the greatest effect on blood sugar levels; its GI is 70 or more.
- The most important thing to remember is that the GI compares foods not per 100 grams of food, but per gram of carbohydrate.

The Early Development of the Glycemic Index

The glycemic index was introduced in 1981 by Dr. David J. A. Jenkins, now a professor in the Department of Nutritional Sciences at the University of Toronto, where he is also Canada Research Chair in Nutrition and Metabolism.

Jenkins set out to determine which foods are best for people with diabetes. At the time, the diet most often recommended for people with diabetes was based on a system of carbohydrate exchanges. Each exchange, or portion of food, contained the same amount of carbohydrate. The exchange system assumed that all starchy foods produced the same effect on blood glucose levels—even though some earlier studies had suggested otherwise. Jenkins was one of the first researchers to challenge the use of exchanges and to investigate how individual foods actually affect our blood glucose levels.

Jenkins and his colleagues, who include our coauthor Dr. Thomas M. S. Wolever, tested a large number of foods that people commonly ate. Their results generated some surprises.

First, they found that the starch in foods such as bread, potatoes, and many types of rice was digested and absorbed very quickly, not slowly, as had previously been assumed.

Second, they found that the sugars in foods such as fruit, chocolate, and ice cream did not produce more rapid or prolonged rises in blood glucose, as had always been thought. The truth was that most of the sugars in foods produced quite moderate blood glucose responses, lower than that of many starches.

Because Jenkins's approach was so logical and systematic, yet also contrary to prevailing thinking and recommendations, it attracted an enormous amount of attention from other scientists and medical researchers when the original scientific paper was published in the *American Journal of Clinical Nutrition* in March 1981.

Since that time, nutrition scientists around the world, including the authors of this book, have tested the effect of many foods on blood glucose levels, thus further developing Jenkins's classification of carbohydrates based on what he had termed the glycemic index (GI). Today we know the GI values of about 2,000 different items (worldwide) that have been tested in healthy people and people with diabetes. See the detailed tables in Part 5 for the GI of many foods you'll find on your supermarket shelves.

A Growing Body of Research Supports the GI

The GI was a very controversial topic among researchers and health authorities for many years, for a variety of reasons. Initially, some criticism was justified. For example, in the early days, there was no evidence that the GI values of single foods could influence the resulting blood glucose levels of the entire meals in which they were consumed—or even that low GI foods could bring long-term benefits. There were no studies of the glycemic index's reproducibility, or of the consistency of GI values from one country to another. Many of the early studies used only healthy volunteers rather than those with relevant health conditions. What's more, there was no evidence that the results could be applied to people with diabetes.

But today, studies from major leading medical institutions and research universities around the world have repeatedly demonstrated that the glycemic index holds up in tests (in scientific terms, it is reproducible) and is a clinically proven tool in its application to weight control, diabetes, and coronary health. Studies all around the globe, including the United States, the United Kingdom, France, Italy, Sweden, Canada, and Australia, have proved the value of the GI. Moreover, diabetes organizations in many countries have endorsed the judicious use of the GI in the dietary management of diabetes.

In 2007, the International Diabetes Federation recommended in its new guidelines for "Management of Post-meal Glucose" that people with diabetes use the GI to stabilize their blood glucose levels as it "can provide an additional benefit for diabetes control beyond that of carbohydrate counting."

Health authorities in the United States have been slower to embrace the GI than many of their counterparts elsewhere in the developed world. This may be the result of a number of factors, including the fact that the earliest research into the GI was conducted outside the United States. In the diabetes realm, the American Diabetes Association (ADA) has for many years endorsed dietary recommendations premised on the idea of carbohydrate counting (which assumes that all starchy foods have the same effect on blood glucose levels).

However, in its 2006 nutrition recommendations for the management of diabetes, the ADA noted, "The use of the glycemic index/ glycemic load may provide an additional benefit over that observed when total carbohydrate is considered alone."

A new study by Professor David Jenkins, the doctor who invented the GI concept, was published in 2008 in the *Journal of the American Medical Association*. This study allocated 210 volunteers to either a low GI diet or a high cereal-fiber diet for six months. Both diets were designed to contain similar amounts of fats, proteins, carbohydrate, and dietary fiber, and the only difference was in GI (low vs. moderate). The researchers found that the best measure of blood glucose control over the longer term (hemoglobin A1c) improved more in those allocated to the low GI diet (by more than 0.33 percentage points, for those readers who like to know the details). The people in this group also showed greater improvements in the good cholesterol fraction known as HDL. In fact, the volunteers in the high cereal-fiber group suffered a fall in this good cholesterol, suggesting that they were at greater risk of heart disease and stroke at the end of the study than they were at the beginning. And there's more. A greater proportion of subjects in the low GI group were able to reduce their dose of diabetes medications. All in all, these findings provide the level of reassurance necessary to convince us (and even the skeptics!) that a low GI diet has something important to offer over that of conventional high-fiber diets.

The wind has shifted to a more positive attitude toward the GI in general—as a tool for *everyone*. Several studies have shown that a low GI diet is easier to follow than other diets—meaning you're more likely to stick with it than you would other regimes. In fact, one study from the Royal Children's Hospital Melbourne reported that children and parents found a low GI diet regimen more flexible and family-friendly than conventional diets and it "enhances quality of life in children with [type 1] diabetes."

What They Say about the GI

In recent editorials in the world's major medical journals, public health authorities had this to say about the GI:

"The clinician should consider a low GI diet to be a prudent approach to the prevention and treatment of diabetes, heart disease, and obesity."
—Associate Professor David Ludwig, *The Lancet*, March 2007

". . . the most fundamental conclusion of research into diet and disease during the last decade . . . it is the type of fat and type of carbohydrate rather than the total amount of either that influence risk of cardiovascular disease."
—Professor Walter Willet, *Journal of Internal Medicine*, May 2007

". . . it is time to shift the diet-heart paradigm away from restricted fat intake and toward reduced glycemic load. [This] should be considered a public health priority."
—Professor Frank Hu,
Journal of American College of Cardiology, July 2007

Just What Was So Revolutionary about the GI?

Before the GI came along, the nature of carbohydrates was described by their chemical structure: *simple* or *complex*. Sugars were simple, and starches found in foods like bread and potatoes were complex, only because sugars were small molecules and starches were big ones.

It was assumed that complex carbohydrates, such as starches, because of their large size, would be slowly digested and absorbed and would therefore cause only a small and gradual rise in blood glucose levels. Simple sugars, on the other hand, were assumed to

Ten Myths about the GI

Myth 1: The GI is complex and difficult to put into practice.
Fact: The GI is a ranking from 0 to 100 that allows us to instantly assess the glycemic punch of a food's carbohydrates. Putting the GI into practice is as easy as "this for that." Simply substituting high GI foods with low GI alternatives will give your overall diet a lower GI and deliver the benefits of low GI eating.

Myth 2: The GI doesn't work in mixed meals.
Fact: Dozens of studies show that the GI works perfectly in mixed meals. Compared with a high GI food, the low GI counter-part will have a lower glycemic effect, whatever accompaniments you add.

Myth 3: Carrots have a high GI.
Fact: Carrots have a low GI (41 for cooked carrots). The original value of 92 was found to be incorrect when they were retested.

Myth 4: Whole grains have a low GI. The benefits of GI are really due to fiber.
Fact: The majority of whole-grain cereal products such as whole-wheat bread and toasted bran flakes actually have a high GI. That's because the finely milled bran doesn't slow down digestion and absorption. Whole grains are good for us, but in studies in which fiber contents have been matched, low GI diets incorporating *whole* grains offer benefits over and above that of processed whole grains.

Myth 5: The GI doesn't make nutritional sense. Chocolate has a low GI but watermelon has a high GI.
Fact: The GI makes a lot of nutritional sense. Nature intended us to eat slowly digested and absorbed carbs. *Most* low GI foods are nutritious—legumes, oats, rye, quinoa, pasta, dairy, and most fruits and vegetables. You'd be hard-pressed to find a bad, low GI diet. But like anything, common sense is required. Nutritionists don't recommend jellybeans just because they are low in fat. So it is with the GI.

Myth 6: Glycemic load is more important than the GI.
Fact: Glycemic load (GL) and GI are both useful concepts. One depends on the other. Think of the GI as a "characteristic" of the carbohydrate and GL as a measure of quantity of carbohydrate

in a diet—after *adjustment* for its glycemic potency. Too much emphasis on GL, at the expense of the GI, can mean a diet with too few carbohydrates.

Myth 7: Refined and sugary foods have a high GI.
Fact: It is tempting to generalize and say refined foods are high GI and unprocessed foods are low GI, but plenty of sugary foods are low GI (soft drinks range from 55 to 60) and plenty of unprocessed foods are high GI—potatoes, brown rice, and watermelon. But it would be true to say that a diet with a lot of soft drinks and refined flour has a high glycemic load.

Myth 8: Glycemic responses are too variable to make the GI useful.
Fact: Glycemic responses are variable, but this variability can be managed. If they are too variable, then why do we recommend other strategies such as carbohydrate counting in people with diabetes? Why is the diagnosis of diabetes made on the basis of a simple glucose tolerance test? Testing the GI by the recognized method takes into account day-to-day variability within individuals and allows us to distinguish clearly between low GI foods and high GI foods. Statistically speaking, in any one person at any given meal, a low GI food will produce a lower glycemic response than a high GI food, more than nine times out of ten.

Myth 9: The GI restricts food choices.
Fact: Indeed, our experience is quite the opposite. Low GI diets open the door to nutritious meals from the world's favorite cuisines—Mediterranean, Italian, and Asian (dhals, pasta, sushi, noodles, etc.). We say that a low GI diet is the "back door" approach to a good diet. There's no need to harp on eating more fiber and less saturated fat; it comes automatically when people make nutritious, low GI choices.

Myth 10: Food manufacturers will add more fat and fructose in order to lower the GI of their foods.
Fact: In Australia, food manufacturers that have deliberately set out to formulate low GI foods have added good-quality ingredients such as intact grains, guar gum, oat bran, dried fruit, and high-amylose starches. American consumers should be looking for independent, credible endorsements of healthy low GI products.

be digested and absorbed quickly, producing a rapid increase in blood glucose.

In the early years of nutrition research, scientists had conducted simple experiments on pure solutions of starches and sugars and drawn conclusions about *all foods containing starches and sugars* from the findings. It is important to note, however, that their conclusions did not apply to real foods eaten in realistic meals. For fifty years, the conclusions from these experiments were taught to every medical and biochemistry student as "fact." These facts, and the assumptions on which they were based, were challenged by the arrival of the GI.

What research on the glycemic index showed is that the concept of simple versus complex carbohydrates tells us nothing about how the carbohydrates in food actually affect blood glucose levels in the body. The rise in blood glucose after meals cannot be predicted on the basis of a chemical structure. In other words, the old distinctions that were long made between starchy foods (complex carbohydrates) and sugary foods (simple carbohydrates) have no useful application when it comes to blood glucose levels—and all of the health issues that relate to them.

Summing up, the GI ranks the "glycemic potency" of the carbohydrates in different foods exactly as they are eaten. Many factors influence whether they will be "tricklers" or "gushers," as we discuss in Chapter 4.

Foods with a high GI value . . .

. . . contain carbohydrates that cause a dramatic rise in blood glucose levels, while foods with a low GI value contain carbohydrates that have much less of an impact.

2
Exactly How Does the GI Work?

A FOOD'S GI VALUE must be measured in people (we call this "*in vivo* testing") according to an internationally standardized method. Currently, about twenty-five facilities around the world test GI values by following the standard international testing protocol. These facilities include:

North America
- Glycemic Index Laboratories, Inc., Toronto, Canada (www.gilabs.com)

Australia and New Zealand
- The University of Sydney's Glycemic Index Research Service (SUGIRS), Sydney, Australia (www.glycemicindex.com)
- Glycaemic Index Otago, University of Otago, New Zealand (www.glycemicindex.otago.ac.nz)

U.K. and Europe
- Leatherhead Food International, Surrey, U.K. (www.lfra.co.uk)
- Oxford Brookes University, Oxford, U.K. (www.brookes.ac.uk/bms/research/nfsg/index.html)
- Hammersmith Food Research Unit, Hammersmith Hospital, London, U.K. (www.foodresearch.co.uk)
- Reading Scientific Services Limited (RSSL), Reading, U.K. (www.rssl.com)

- Biofortis, Nantes, France (www.biofortis.fr)
- NutriScience BV, Maastricht, Netherlands (www.nutriscience.nl)
- Oy Foodfiles Ltd., Kuopio, Finland (www.foodfiles.com)

You may have heard about *in vitro* (test tube) methods, but these are shortcuts that may be useful for manufacturers developing new products and may not reflect the true GI of a food.

How Scientists Measure a Food's GI Value

Here's how we test the GI of a food following the protocol set out by the International Standards Organization:

Step 1. Ten volunteers consume a fifty-gram carbohydrate portion of the reference food on three separate days (e.g., one cup of rice). Pure glucose dissolved in water is the usual reference food, and its GI is set at 100. The test is carried out in the morning after an overnight fast. The solution is consumed within ten to twelve minutes, and blood glucose levels are measured eight times over the next two hours (we use capillary testing, as it is associated with much less variability than venous testing). The findings from those three days of testing are averaged to find each person's usual response to the reference food, glucose.

Step 2. Next, we measure his or her glycemic response to a fifty-gram available carbohydrate portion of the test food (e.g., one cup of rice) once, using exactly the same two-hour testing protocol.

Step 3. Then we calculate each person's response to the test food as a percentage of his or her average response to the reference food. We do this by plotting his or her blood glucose response to the test food on a graph and comparing this with the response to the reference food; the response can be summarized as the **area under the curve**—the exact value of which is calculated using a computer program (see Figure 1).

Step 4. Finally, we average the responses of all ten volunteers to the test food; this is the GI value that we publish. If the average test food response area (i.e., the area under the curve) is only 40 percent of the reference food, then the GI of the test food is 40. Not everyone will give exactly the same number, of course, but the law of averages

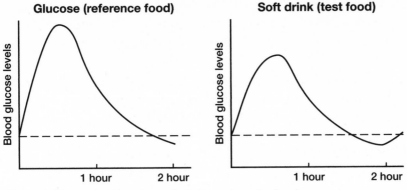

Figure 1. Measuring the glycemic index value of a food

applies. If we tested them over and over again, people would all tend to congregate around the same number.

Because each person is his or her own control, testing foods in volunteers with diabetes or prediabetes gives approximately the same GI values as testing people who don't have diabetes.

In practice, the average result in the group of ten healthy people is the published GI value of the food. *At least* 240 blood glucose assays (the technical term for the test measuring the blood glucose) will have been made to generate that number. In some labs, up to 640 assays are made. So there is nothing crude about GI testing.

For example, the GI value of bread (70) means that the overall fluctuation in blood glucose after eating an exchange of white bread will be about 70 percent of the effect of pure glucose (GI value of 100).

High, medium, or low GI . . .

- A high GI value is 70 or more.
- A medium GI value is 56–69 inclusive.
- A low GI value is 55 or less.

Note: See pages 301–302 for information on the scientific rationale behind these GI cutoff points.

A food's GI value cannot be predicted from its appearance, composition, carbohydrate content, or even the GI values of related foods. The only way to know a food's GI value is to test it, following the standardized methodology we've just described.

Unfortunately, there is no easy, inexpensive substitute test. Now, after nearly thirty years of GI testing, we and others around the world have determined the GI values for more than 2,000 foods. The values of foods available appear in Part 5 of this book, as well as in annually updated editions of *The New Glucose Revolution Shopper's Guide to GI Values* and online at our Website: www.glycemicindex.com.

Why is glucose used as the reference food? Pure glucose itself produces one of the greatest effects on blood glucose levels. GI testing has shown that *most* foods have less effect on blood glucose levels than glucose. For that reason, the GI value of pure glucose is set at 100, and every other food is ranked on a scale from 0 to 100 according to its actual effect on blood glucose levels.

(Note: A few foods have GI values of more than 100—for example, jasmine rice [GI 109]. The explanation is simple: glucose is a highly concentrated solution that tends to be held up briefly in the stomach. Jasmine rice, on the other hand, contains starch that leaves the stomach quickly and is then digested in a flash.)

Rice Krispies (GI 82) and some types of bread (e.g., white Turkish bread, GI 87) have very high GI values, meaning their effect on blood glucose levels is almost as high as that of an equal amount of pure glucose. See Figure 2.

Foods with a low GI value (such as lentils, GI 26–48) show a flatter blood glucose response when eaten, as shown in Figure 3. That means that the resulting peak blood glucose level is lower, and the return to baseline levels may be slower than with a high GI food.

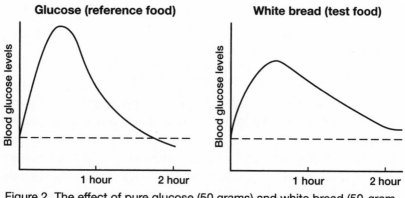

Figure 2. The effect of pure glucose (50 grams) and white bread (50-gram carbohydrate portion) on blood glucose levels

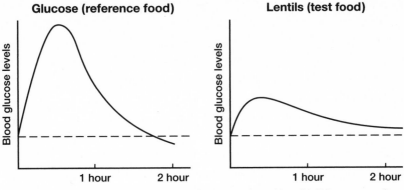

Figure 3. The effect of pure glucose (50 grams) and lentils (50-gram carbohydrate portion) on blood glucose levels

Why do we use the "area under the curve" in GI calculations? The area under the curve is the best way to take into account *all* the data available to us. It is preferable to taking just one or two points (e.g., the peak). It is reassuring to know, however, that the GI value is a good predictor of the actual peak level, as well as the absolute level of blood glucose at thirty minutes, sixty minutes, and ninety minutes. We also know that the higher the GI, the bigger the fall (i.e., from the peak to the trough).

The only way to know a food's GI value . . .

. . . is to test it. The GI cannot be predicted from the food's appearance, composition, carb content, or even the GI values of related foods.

Why Low GI Foods Are a Smart Choice

For most people, low GI foods have advantages over high GI foods. The slow digestion and gradual increase and decrease in blood glucose responses after eating a low GI food help control blood glucose levels in people with diabetes or glucose intolerance. This effect benefits healthy people as well, because it reduces the secretion of the hormone insulin over the course of the whole day. (We discuss this in greater detail in Chapters 4 and 12.)

Lower glucose levels over the course of the day also improve heart health. Abnormally high insulin levels resulting from a regular diet of high GI carbs promote high blood fats and high blood pressure, thus increasing the risk of heart attack. Keeping your blood glucose levels stable helps ensure that blood vessels remain elastic and supple, reducing the formation of fatty streaks and plaques that cause atherosclerosis, known more widely as hardening of the arteries. And good blood glucose management means your body is less likely to form blood clots in the arteries, which can precipitate a heart attack. Spikes in blood glucose levels also increase inflammation: a high glucose concentration stresses cells and triggers inflammatory responses.

You don't have to eat only low GI foods to benefit. Studies show that when a low and a high GI food are combined in one meal (e.g., lentils and rice), the overall blood glucose response is intermediate. You can keep both your glucose and insulin levels lower over the course of the whole day if you choose at least one low GI food at each meal.

For most people, low GI foods have advantages over high GI foods. The slow digestion and gradual increase and decrease in blood glucose responses after eating a low GI food help control blood glucose levels. Plus, slower digestion helps to delay hunger pangs, meaning you're less likely to overeat or make poor food choices as the result of hunger, which can promote weight loss if you're overweight.

Can the GI Be Applied to Everyday Meals?

Criticism of the GI has focused on unpredictable outcomes of blood glucose values in meals because of variations in fat, protein, and fiber levels. Most of our meals consist of a variety of foods, not just a single food. Even though GI values are derived from testing single foods in isolation, we and other scientists have found that it is possible to predict the blood glucose response for a meal that consists of several foods with different GI values.

Concerned about the methodology of recent studies showing unpredictable responses, we and our coresearchers at the University of Toronto's Department of Nutritional Sciences conducted studies with mixed meals on two groups of healthy subjects in Toronto and Sydney. We had previously done smaller studies, but we wanted to revisit the question, using more meals and variety in two different centers with judiciously selected foods. This time, fourteen different test meals were used in Sydney and Toronto, and the food combinations reflected a range of typical breakfast choices.

Despite the variations in food factors, blood glucose responses remained consistent with GI measures. In fact, we were startled by the degree of predictability. The carbohydrate, fat, and protein composition of the meals varied over a wide spectrum. The glucose responses varied over a fivefold range, and yet 90 percent of that variation was explained by the amount of carbohydrate in the meal and the GI values of the foods, as given in published GI tables. We found that the GI works just as predictably whether subjects consume a single portion of one item or a normal meal; we reported these findings in the June 2006 issue of the *American Journal of Clinical Nutrition*.

How Do You Estimate the Overall GI of a Meal?

Over the years, many readers—researchers and dietitians in the nutrition field, as well as laypeople—have asked us to explain how to estimate the total GI of a meal. So for their benefit, and for the more curious among you, we take a moment to walk you through two brief examples.

First of all, the GI value of a meal or recipe is not the sum of the GI values of each food in the meal, nor is it simply an average of their GI values. The GI of a meal, menu, or recipe consisting of a variety of carbohydrate foods is a weighted average of the GI values of each food. The weighting is based on the proportion of the total carbohydrate contributed by each food.

To estimate the GI of a mixed meal, you need to know the GI of the carbohydrate foods in the meal (information we provide in the tables in Part 5), plus the total carbohydrate content of the meal and the contribution of each food to the total carbohydrate. You will find this information in food-composition tables or nutrient-analysis computer programs. The following calculations may look complicated. In practice, you don't need to make these sorts of calculations to adopt the low GI way of eating, but dietitians and nutrition researchers sometimes have to.

Let's look at a snack of peaches (GI 42) and ice cream (GI 37–49). Depending on the amounts of each food, we could calculate the total content of these carbohydrates from food-composition tables. Let's say the meal contains sixty grams of carbohydrate, with twenty grams provided by the peaches (i.e., 33 percent) and forty grams by the ice cream (i.e., 67 percent). For the purposes of this calculation, we're using low-fat vanilla ice cream (GI 46).

To estimate the GI value of this dish, we multiply the GI value of peaches by their proportion of the total carbohydrate:

$$42 \times 33\% = 14$$

and multiply the GI value of ice cream by its proportion of the total carbohydrate:

$$46 \times 67\% = 31$$

We then add these two figures to give a GI value for this dish of 45.

Here's another scenario, for the classic combination of beans and rice. If half the carbohydrate in the mixed meal comes from a food with a GI value of 30 (e.g., black beans) and the other half from rice with a GI value of 80, then the mixed meal will have a GI of 55, determined as follows:

$$(50\% \text{ of } 30) + (50\% \text{ of } 80) = 55.$$

Our rice-and-beans example demonstrates that it's not necessary to avoid all high GI foods in order to eat a low GI diet. Nor is it necessary to calculate the GI value for every meal you eat. Rather, simply choose a low GI food in place of a higher GI food. Simply including one low GI food per meal is enough.

We'll share many more helpful dietary suggestions with you throughout the rest of the book, and in Part 4 you will find our guide to low GI eating.

Glycemic Index or Glycemic Load?

Your blood glucose rises and falls when you eat a meal containing carbohydrate. How high and how long it rises on any one occasion depends on two things: how much carbohydrate you eat and the GI of the carbohydrate you eat. The more carbohydrate you eat, the higher your blood glucose goes. The higher the GI of the food you eat, the higher your blood glucose goes. A small amount of a high GI food may raise your blood glucose as much as a large amount of a low GI food.

The glycemic load (GL), initially developed by researchers at Harvard University, takes in the amount of carbohydrate you eat *and* its GI to help predict how much a serving of food will raise blood glucose. If a serving of food has a GL of 10, it will raise blood glucose by as much as ten grams of glucose.

The GL of a food is a mathematical calculation—determined by multiplying the GI of a particular food by the available carbohydrate content (meaning the carbohydrate content minus fiber) in a particular serving size (expressed in grams), divided by 100. The formula is:

GL = (GI × the amount of carbohydrate) divided by 100.

Let's take a single apple as an example. It has a GI of 38 and it contains fifteen grams of carbohydrate.

$$GL = 38 × 15 ÷ 100 = 6$$

What about a small serving of French fries? Its GI is 75 and it contains twenty-nine grams of carbohydrate.

$$GL = 75 × 29 ÷ 100 = 22$$

So we can predict that our fries (GL 22) will pack nearly four times the glycemic punch of an apple (GL 6).

You can think of GL . . .
_____

. . . as the amount of carbohydrate in a food "adjusted" for its glycemic impact.

Proponents of the GL—both within the scientific nutrition community and beyond it—think that this concept should be used instead of the GI when comparing foods because it more fully reflects a food's glycemic potential. But a word of caution: we don't want people actively avoiding carbs and striving for a diet with the lowest GL possible. That's why we advocate sticking with the GI.

The problem with GL is that it doesn't distinguish between foods that are low carb (and thus higher in fat and/or protein) or slow carb (that is, low GI carbs). Some people whose diets have an overall lower GL are consuming more fat or protein and fewer carbohydrates of any kind, including healthy, low GI carbs.

Following a low GL path could mean that you're unnecessarily restricting foods, missing out on nutrients and the other proven benefits of a higher carbohydrate diet, and thus eating a less healthful diet—one that's too low in carbohydrates and full of the wrong types of fats and proteins.

Research also shows that by choosing carbs by their GI value—and opting primarily for those that are low GI—you'll get a healthy, safe diet with an appropriate quantity and quality of carbohydrate. In fact, you'll be increasing your intake of nutritional powerhouse foods, including fruits and vegetables, legumes (including beans, chickpeas, and lentils) and *whole* grains (see page 199). And by choosing moderate servings of low GI foods, you'll automatically be eating lower GL foods, too, so a low GI diet is a win–win situation, while a low GL diet is a "mixed bag."

Yes, a handful of high GI foods, such as watermelon, have a low GL, but we recommend that you don't limit any fruits or vegetables, other than some potatoes (see "This for That" on page 193).

A word here about portion sizes: some carb-rich foods such as pasta have a low GI but *could* have a high GL if the serving size is large. Portion sizes do count.

The bottom line . . .

. . . about glycemic index vs. glycemic load:

- Use the GI to identify your best carbohydrate choices.
- Keep your portion size in check to limit the overall GL.

3

What Determines Whether a Food Is High or Low GI?

FOR MANY YEARS, scientists have been studying what gives one food a high GI and another one a low GI. That research has generated a huge amount of information, which can be confusing. The table on page 22 summarizes the factors that influence the GI value of a food.

The physical state of the starch in a food is by far the most important factor influencing its GI value. This is why advances in food processing over the past two hundred years have had such a profound effect on the overall GI values of the carbohydrates we eat.

The Effect of Starch Gelatinization on the GI

The starch in raw food is stored in hard, compact granules that make it difficult to digest. This is why potatoes would probably give you abdominal pain if you ate them raw and why most starchy foods need to be cooked. During cooking, water and heat expand the starch granules to different degrees; some granules actually burst and free the individual starch molecules. (That's what happens when you make gravy by heating flour and water until the starch granules burst and the gravy thickens.)

If most of the starch granules have swollen and burst during cooking, the starch is said to be fully gelatinized. Figure 4 on page 23 shows the difference between raw and cooked starch in potatoes.

Factors That Influence the GI Value of a Food

FACTOR	MECHANISM	EXAMPLES OF FOOD WHERE THE EFFECT IS SEEN
Starch gelatinization	The less gelatinized (swollen) the starch, the slower the rate of digestion.	Al dente spaghetti, oatmeal, and cookies have less gelatinized starch.
Physical entrapment	The fibrous coat around beans and seeds and plant cell walls acts as a physical barrier, slowing down access of enzymes to the starch inside.	Pumpernickel and grainy breads, legumes, and barley.
High amylose to amylopectin ratio*	The more amylose a food contains, the less water the starch will absorb and the slower its rate of digestion.	Basmati rice and legumes contain more amylose and less amylopectin.
Particle size	The smaller the particle size, the easier it is for water and enzymes to penetrate.	Finely milled flours have high GI values. Stoneground flours have larger particles and lower GIs.
Viscosity of fiber	Viscous, soluble fibers increase the viscosity of the intestinal contents, and this slows down the interaction between the starch and the enzymes. Finely milled whole-wheat and rye flours have fast rates of digestion and absorption because the fiber is not viscous.	Rolled oats, beans, lentils, apples, psyllium husks, and Metamucil.
Sugar	The digestion of sugar produces only half as many glucose molecules as the same amount of starch (the other half is fructose). The presence of sugar also restricts gelatinization of the starch by binding water and reducing the amount of "available" water.	Social tea biscuits, oatmeal cookies, and some breakfast cereals (such as Kellogg's Frosted Flakes or Smacks) that are high in sugar have relatively low GI values.
Acidity	Acids in foods slow down stomach emptying, thereby slowing the rate at which the starch can be digested.	Vinegar, lemon juice, lime juice, some salad dressings, pickled vegetables, and classic sourdough bread.
Fat	Fat slows down the rate of stomach emptying, thereby slowing the digestion of the starch.	Potato chips have a lower GI value than boiled white potatoes.

* Amylose and amylopectin are two different types of starch. Both are found in foods, but the ratio varies (see page 24).

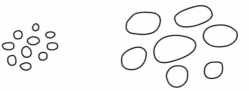

Figure 4. The difference between raw (compact granules, left) and cooked (swollen granules, right) starch in potatoes

The swollen granules and free starch molecules are very easy to digest, because the starch-digesting enzymes in the small intestine have a greater surface area to attack. The quick action of the enzymes results in a rapid blood glucose increase after consumption of the food (remember that starch is nothing more than a string of glucose molecules). As a result, food containing starch that is fully gelatinized will have a very high GI value.

In foods such as cookies, the presence of sugar and fat and very little water makes starch gelatinization more difficult, and only about half of the granules will be fully gelatinized. For this reason, cookies tend to have medium GI values.

The Effect of Particle Size on the GI

The particle size of a food is another factor that influences starch gelatinization and GI value. Grinding or milling grains reduces particle sizes and makes it easier for water to be absorbed and digestive enzymes to attack the food. This is why many foods made from fine flours tend to have a high GI value. The larger the particle size, the lower the GI value, as Figure 5 on page 24 illustrates.

One of the most significant alterations to our food supply came with the introduction, in the mid-nineteenth century, of steel-roller mills. Not only did they make it easier to remove the fiber from cereal grains, but also the particle size of the flour became smaller than ever before. Prior to the nineteenth century, stone grinding produced quite coarse flours that resulted in slower rates of digestion and absorption.

When starch is consumed in "nature's packaging"—whole intact grains that have been softened by soaking and cooking—the food will have a low GI. For example, cooked pearl barley's GI value is 25, and most cooked legumes have a GI of between 30 and 40 whether home cooked or canned.

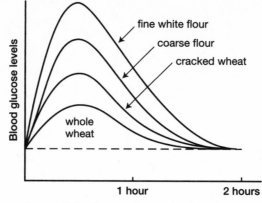

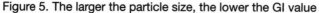

Figure 5. The larger the particle size, the lower the GI value

The Effect of Amylose and Amylopectin on the GI

There are two types of starch in food—amylose and amylopectin. Researchers have discovered that the ratio of one to the other has a powerful effect on a food's GI value.

Amylose is a straight-chain molecule, like a string of beads. These tend to line up in rows and form tight compact clumps that are harder to gelatinize (see page 21) and therefore harder to digest (see Figure 6 opposite).

Amylopectin, on the other hand, is a string of glucose molecules with lots of branching points, like you'd see in some types of seaweed or a piece of ginger root. Amylopectin molecules are therefore larger and more open, and the starch is easier to gelatinize and to digest. Foods that have little amylose and plenty of amylopectin in their starch have higher GI values—for example, jasmine rice and wheat flour. Foods with a higher ratio of amylose to amylopectin have lower GI values—for example, basmati rice and legumes.

The only whole (intact) grain food with a high GI is low-amylose rice, such as jasmine (GI 109). Low-amylose varieties of rice have starch that is very easily gelatinized during cooking and therefore easily broken down by digestive enzymes. This may help explain why we sometimes feel hungry not long after rice-based meals. However, some varieties of rice (basmati and long-grain white rice) have lower GI values, because they have a higher amylose content than normal rice. Their GI values are in the range of 50–59.

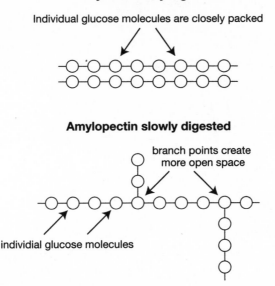

Figure 6. Amylose is a straight-chain molecule that is harder to digest than amylopectin, which has many branching points.

Why Does Pasta Have a Low GI Value?

Somewhat surprisingly, pasta in any shape or form has a relatively low GI value (30–60). Great news for pasta lovers! But portion size is important; keep it moderate to keep the GL (glycemic load) moderate. In the early days of GI research, we assumed that pasta has a low GI value because the main ingredient is semolina (durum or hard wheat flour) and not finely ground wheat flour.

Subsequent research has shown, however, that even pasta made entirely from plain wheat flour has a low GI value. The reason for the slow digestion rate and subsequent low GI value is the physical entrapment of the ungelatinized starch granules in a spongelike network of protein (gluten) molecules in the pasta dough. Pasta and noodles too are unique in this regard.

Overcooked pasta is very soft and swollen in size and will have a higher GI value than pasta cooked al dente. Adding egg to the dough lowers the GI further by increasing the protein content. Asian noodles such as hokkien, udon, and rice vermicelli also have low to medium GI values.

The Effect of Sugar on the GI

Table sugar or refined sugar (sucrose) has a GI of between 60 and 65. The reason: table sugar is a disaccharide (double sugar), composed of one glucose molecule coupled with one fructose molecule. (See Chapter 5 for a fuller explanation of the structure of sugars.) Fructose is absorbed and taken directly to the liver, where it is immediately oxidized (burned as the source of energy). The blood glucose response to pure fructose is very modest (GI 19). Consequently, when we consume sucrose, only half of what we've eaten is actually glucose; the other half is fructose. This explains why the blood glucose response to fifty grams of sucrose is approximately half that of fifty grams of corn syrup or maltodextrins—where the molecules are all glucose ones.

Many foods containing large amounts of refined sugar (sucrose) have a GI close to 60. This is the average of glucose (GI 100) and fructose (GI 19). It's lower than that of ordinary white bread, with a GI value averaging around 70. Kellogg's Cocoa Puffs, which contain 39 percent sugar, have a GI value of 77, lower than that of Rice Krispies (GI 82), which contain little sugar.

Most foods containing simple sugars do not raise blood glucose levels any more than most complex starchy foods like bread. This is one of the key findings of the GI, and it has "liberalized" the management of diabetes.

One of the spin-offs from research . . . .

. . . on the GI is the recognition that both sugary and starchy foods can raise your blood glucose.

The sugars that naturally occur in food include lactose, sucrose, glucose, and fructose in variable proportions, depending on the food. On theoretical grounds, it is difficult to predict the overall blood glucose response to a food, because stomach emptying is slowed by increasing the concentration of the sugars.

Some fruits, for example, have a low GI value (grapefruit's GI is 25), while others are relatively high (watermelon's is 76). The higher the acidity of the fruit, the lower the GI value. Consequently, it is not possible to lump all fruits together and say they will have a low GI value because they are high in fiber. They are not all equal. (For a comparison of all fruits, take a look at the fruit section of the table in Part 5, on pages 320–322.)

Many foods containing sugars are a mixture of refined and naturally occurring sugars—sweetened yogurt, for example. Their overall effect on blood glucose response is difficult to predict. This is why we've tested individual foods to determine their GI values rather than guessing or making generalizations about entire food groups.

The Effect of Fiber on the GI

The effect of fiber on a food's GI value depends on the type of fiber and its viscosity or thickness.

Dietary fiber comes from plant foods; it is found in the outer bran layers of grains (corn, oats, wheat, and rice, and in foods containing these grains), fruits, vegetables, nuts, and legumes (dried beans, peas, and lentils). There are two types—soluble and insoluble—and there is a difference.

Soluble fibers are the gel, gum, and often jellylike components of apples, oats, and legumes. Psyllium, found in some breakfast cereals and dietary fiber supplements such as Metamucil, is soluble fiber. These viscous fibers thicken the mixture of food entering the digestive tract. By slowing down the time it takes for the fiber to pass through the stomach and small intestine, foods with high levels of soluble or viscous fiber lower the glycemic response to, or glycemic impact of, food, which is why legumes, oats, and psyllium have a low GI.

Insoluble fibers are dry, branlike, and commonly thought of as roughage. All cereal grains and products made from them that retain the outer layer of the grain are sources of insoluble fiber (e.g., *whole-grain* bread and All-Bran), but not all foods containing insoluble fiber are low GI.

Insoluble fibers will only lower the GI of a food when they exist in their original, intact form—for example, in whole grains of wheat. Here they act as a physical barrier, delaying access of digestive enzymes and water to the starch within the cereal grain. Finely ground wheat fiber, such as in whole-wheat bread, has no effect whatsoever on the rate of starch digestion and subsequent blood glucose response. Breakfast cereals made with wheat flakes will also tend to have high GI values, unless there are other ingredients in the food that will lower the GI.

The GI Was Never Meant to Be Used in Isolation

At first glance, you might assume that some high-fat foods, such as chocolate, seem a good choice simply because they have a low GI value. Fat chance! This is absolutely not the case.

A food's GI value was never meant to offer the only criterion by which it is judged. Large amounts of fat (and protein) in food tend to slow the rate of stomach emptying and therefore the rate at which foods are digested in the small intestine. High-fat foods will therefore tend to have lower GI values than their low-fat equivalents. For example, potato chips have a lower GI value (54) than potatoes baked without fat (77). Many cookies have a lower GI value (55–65) than bread (70).

But clearly, in these instances, a lower GI value doesn't translate into a better, healthier choice. Saturated fat in these foods will have adverse effects on coronary health that are far more significant than the benefit of lower blood glucose levels. These foods should be treated as indulgences for special occasions, rather than as part of a regular diet.

We are not recommending that you avoid all fats. Just as there are differences in the nature of carbohydrates in foods (what we refer to as the quality, conveyed as the GI value), there are differences in the quality of fats. You should be just as choosy about the fats you eat as you are about carbohydrates.

Healthy fats, such as the omega-3 polyunsaturated fats, not only are good for you, but also help to lower the blood glucose response to meals. On the other hand, saturated fats increase your risk of obesity, heart disease, and other serious health conditions.

The Effect of Acid on the GI

Several research findings over the last decade have indicated that a realistic amount of vinegar or lemon juice as a salad dressing eaten with a mixed meal has significant blood glucose-lowering effects.

As little as one tablespoon of vinegar in a vinaigrette dressing (with two teaspoons of oil) taken with an average meal lowered blood glucose by as much as 30 percent. Our research shows that lemon juice is just as powerful. Vinegar or lemon juice may also be used in marinades or sauces.

These findings have important implications for people with diabetes or who are at risk for diabetes, coronary heart disease, or the metabolic syndrome (see Part 2).

The effect appears to be related to the acidity, because some other organic acids (like lactic acid and propionic acid) also have a blood glucose-lowering effect, but the degree of reduction varies with the type of acid.

Blood Glucose and the GI at a Glance

Blood glucose is the amount of glucose, or sugar, in your blood. It changes throughout the day depending on what you eat, and it can have a profound effect on your health—your mood, how hungry you are, and whether you develop conditions such as diabetes.

- Your body's blood glucose response to a meal is primarily determined by the meal's carbohydrate content. Both the quantity and the quality of carbohydrates in food influence the rise in blood glucose that you experience.

- Carbohydrates that break down quickly during digestion have high GI values. Their blood glucose response is fast and high.

- Carbohydrates that break down slowly, releasing glucose gradually into the bloodstream, have low GI values. In comparison to foods with high GI values, these are more desirable for optimal health.

- Avoiding carbohydrate foods is counterproductive. You will end up eating harmful foods and fats, and you'll miss favorite foods such as fruit, bread, and pasta.

Real sourdough breads made the traditional way, in which lactic acid and propionic acid are produced by the natural fermentation of starch and sugars by the bacterial starter culture, also can reduce levels of blood glucose and insulin by up to 25 percent compared to normal bread.

In addition, studies show that there's higher satiety—that is, people feel fuller and more satisfied—associated with breads that have decreased rates of digestion and absorption, like sourdough. There's significant potential to lower your blood glucose and insulin and increase satiety with sourdough breads, so incorporating them into your diet is a smart choice. (We discuss the concept of satiety more fully in Chapter 7.)

Real Sourdough

Sourdough bread is made without added yeast. By making a "starter" in which wild yeast can grow, the sourdough baker can get the bread to rise naturally, just as people did for thousands of years before they could run down to the local supermarket for a packet of yeast.

The tangy "sour" taste of sourdough bread comes from the lactic acid and acetic acid produced in the fermentation process.

When buying sourdough bread, make sure you are getting the real thing.

4
What's Wrong with Today's Diet?

YOU MAY BE WONDERING, *"What's wrong with the way I eat now?"* It's possible that you already follow a balanced, nutrient-dense diet that emphasizes whole foods and low GI carbs. But the simple truth is that the majority of North Americans do not; our lifestyle makes it all too easy to stray from a healthful regime. That's why it's so important to have a concrete, working knowledge of how to eat for optimum well-being.

We didn't always eat the way we do today. During the Paleolithic period, humans were hunter-gatherers, consuming the animals and plants found in their natural environment. Our ancestors were fussy about which parts of animals they ate. They preferred the hind legs of the largest animals and the females over the males because they contained more fat and were therefore juicier and more flavorful. They also enjoyed organ meats—liver, kidneys, brains—foods that are extremely rich sources of nutrients.

As humans evolved over time, they became more and more carnivorous. From the latest studies of modern hunter-gatherer diets, it appears that our ancestors obtained about two-thirds of their energy intake from animal foods (including fish and seafood) and only one-third from plant foods. Although they ate more protein and less carbohydrate than we do now, their fat intake, interestingly, was roughly the same as now, but the type of fat was primarily healthy unsaturated fat rather than unhealthy saturated fat (which we'll discuss shortly). This is because the fat of wild animals, including their organs, has much higher proportions of unsaturated fat than typically found in the farmed animals we consume today.

Our predecessors' carbohydrate intakes were lower, because the main plant foods they had available were fruits and vegetables rather than cereals. Wheat, rice, and other cereal grains were largely absent until after the introduction of agriculture and the domestication of crops and animals (sometimes called the Neolithic revolution), which began some 10,000 years ago.

So why does this matter to you? Because these findings have strong implications for current dietary recommendations. Although our ancestors ate plenty of animal foods, they also ate large amounts of micronutrient-rich plant foods (leaves, berries, nuts), which would have been gathered every day, ensuring that their overall diet was both naturally low GI and low GL. It doesn't mean that we all need to be meat eaters to be healthy, but it does imply that we need to consider carefully the types and amount of protein, carbohydrate, and fat we eat.

Beginning about 10,000 years ago, when we became farmers growing crops rather than hunter-gatherers, our diet changed in many ways. For the first time, starch entered the human diet, in a big way; large quantities of harvested cereal grains tipped the human diet ratio from being more animal to more plant. Those plants were what we would now call whole-grain cereals (wheat, rye, barley, oats, corn, and rice). The cultivation of legumes (beans), starchy roots, tubers, fruits, and berries also contributed to the now higher carbohydrate intake of our farmer ancestors.

But food preparation was simple: grinding food between stones and cooking it over the heat of an open fire. The result was that although we were eating a high-carbohydrate diet, all the carbohydrates in our food were digested and absorbed slowly; thus, the effects of these carbohydrate foods on our blood glucose were minimal.

This diet was ideal because it provided slow-release energy that helped to delay hunger pangs and provided fuel for working muscles long after a meal had been eaten. It was also easy on the insulin-producing cells in the pancreas. As far as we can tell, diabetes was rare.

Over time, our ancestors developed the technology to grind flours more and more finely, and to separate bran completely from white flour. Finally, with the advent of high-speed roller mills in the nineteenth century, it was possible to produce white flour so fine that it resembled talcum powder in appearance and texture. These fine white flours were—and are—highly prized because they make soft bread and delicious, airy cakes and pastries.

As incomes grew, the foods commonly eaten by our ancestors—barley, oats, and legumes—were cast aside; consumption of fatty meat increased. The composition of the average diet changed again. We began to eat more saturated fat, less fiber, and more easily digested carbohydrates.

Then something we didn't expect happened, too—blood glucose rises after a meal became higher and more prolonged, stimulating the pancreas to produce more insulin.

As a result of these developments, we not only experienced higher blood glucose spikes after a meal, but also experienced greater insulin secretion. As we've mentioned, our bodies require insulin to metabolize carbohydrate, but too much or too little spells trouble. Researchers believe that excessively high glucose and insulin levels are among the key factors responsible for heart disease and hypertension. And because insulin also influences the way we metabolize foods, it ultimately determines fat storage around the body.

Among the consequences of these major dietary changes, one is crucial for our discussion here: traditional diets all around the world contained slowly digested and absorbed carbohydrate—foods that we now know are low GI. On the other hand, our modern diet, with its rapidly digested carbohydrates, is based on high GI foods.

One of the most important ways . . .

. . . in which our diet differs from that of our ancestors is the speed of carbohydrate digestion and the resulting effect on our blood glucose and hence every cell of the body.

Insulin Plays Critical Roles in Our Health and Well-being

One important function of the pancreas, a vital organ near the stomach, is to produce the hormone insulin. Insulin plays several critical roles in our health and well-being.

First, it **regulates our blood glucose levels**. When you eat a meal containing carbohydrate, your blood glucose level rises. This causes the pancreas to secrete insulin (unless you have type 1 diabetes), which pushes the glucose out of the bloodstream and into the muscles and tissues, where it provides energy for you to carry out your regular activities. The movement of glucose out of the blood and into the body's cells (particularly the muscles and liver) is finely controlled. Just the right amount of insulin takes the glucose level back to normal.

Second, insulin **plays a key part in determining the fuel mix that we burn** from minute to minute—and whether we burn fat or carbohydrates to meet our energy needs. It does this by switching muscle cells from fat-burning to carb-burning. The relative proportions of fat to carbohydrate in your body's fuel mix are dictated by the prevailing levels of insulin in your blood. If insulin levels are low, as they are when you wake up in the morning, then the fuel you burn is mainly fat. If insulin levels are high, as they are after you consume a high-carbohydrate meal, then the fuel you burn is mainly carbohydrate.

Carbohydrates stimulate the secretion of insulin more than any other component of food. When carbohydrates are slowly absorbed by our bodies—which is the case with low GI foods—the pancreas doesn't have to work as hard and secretes less insulin. If it is overstimulated over a long period of time, which often occurs as a result of a diet rich in high GI foods, it may become "exhausted." Type 2 diabetes may develop in someone who is genetically susceptible and whose pancreas has been overworked. Even without diabetes, excessively high insulin levels increase the risk of heart disease in everyone.

What We Eat Now

Today's Western diet is the product of industrialization and many amazing inventions—pasteurization, sterilization, refrigeration, freezing, roller drying, and spray drying, to name just a few. In the cereal-foods world, there's also high-speed roller milling, flaking, toasting, high-temperature and high-pressure extrusion, puffing guns, short-time bread fermentation—you name it, it's been invented.

The benefits are many: we have a plentiful, affordable, palatable (some would say too palatable), and safe food supply. Gone are the days of monotonous meals, food shortages, and weevil-infested and otherwise spoiled food. Also long gone are such widespread vitamin deficiencies as scurvy and pellagra. Today's food manufacturers develop and sell delicious and safe products that satisfy just about everyone: foodies, the most health conscious, and everyday supermarket shoppers alike.

Many of today's low-cost foods are still based on our cereal staples—wheat, corn, and oats—but the original grain has been drastically altered to produce more palatable breads, cakes, cookies, crackers, pastries, breakfast cereals, and snack foods that bear no resemblance to the starting product. Cereal chemists and bakers know that fine, white flours produce the most prized and shelf-stable end product.

Our busy lives have also driven up the need for convenience—quick-cooking express and instant products—that take little time to prepare. Precooked oats, rice, and wheat products are now a common sight on supermarket shelves.

Unfortunately, these market forces have resulted in an unforeseen problem. Our bodies quickly digest and absorb many of the carbohydrate foods we consume the most—think corn flakes, white bread, instant rice. The resulting effect on blood glucose levels has created a problem of epidemic proportions.

With a Wave of the Fat Wand

We've placed quite a bit of emphasis on carbohydrates, but our health is also affected by another key component in food, which often goes hand in hand with carbohydrates: fat.

Food manufacturers, bakers, and chefs know we love to eat fat. We love its creaminess and feel in the mouth and find it easy to consume in excess. Fat makes meat more tender, vegetables and salads more palatable, and sweet foods even more desirable. And fat makes numerous carbohydrates even tastier: with a wave of the fat wand, bland high-carbohydrate foods such as rice, potatoes, and oats are magically transformed into highly palatable, energy-dense foods such as fried rice, French fries, and high-fat granola. In fact, when you analyze it, much of our diet today is an undesirable but delicious combination of fat and high GI carbohydrates.

One problem with fat is the amount we eat, sometimes without knowing it. Fat provides a lot of calories—more than any other nutrient per gram—and it is the least satiating nutrient. This is great for someone who's starving, but it's a real disadvantage for those of us who constantly verge on eating too much. Fat provides nine calories per gram—more than twice the energy of protein or carbohydrate. And the main form in which our bodies store those extra calories is, you guessed it, fat.

Whatever the fat content of your diet, the type of fat you eat matters; monounsaturated fats, found in nuts, seeds, olive oil, avocadoes, etc., should dominate. Eating more fat from these sources gives you a nutritional profile more like a Mediterranean diet, which will also help you lower your triglyceride levels and increase your HDL (good) cholesterol. However, you need to remember that the Mediterranean diet carries a risk of weight gain (if it's not calorie controlled) and in the long run may not benefit your glycemic control.

For the past twenty-five years, health authorities have wanted people to reduce the amount of saturated fat they eat. Unfortunately, *all* fats have been lumped together as bad—the message "reduce fat" was easier to give than "reduce saturated fat." Today, we know that this simplified message was counterproductive. People have avoided even the most essential of fats, the highly polyunsaturated, long-chain fats such as *omega-3*s that are fundamental to human health. Dietitians restricted fat because of its high energy content and tendency to be overeaten—only to replace it with large quantities of high GI carbs that have adverse effects of their own. We fooled ourselves into thinking that any low-fat diet—especially one formulated with the help of a sophisticated food industry—was automatically a healthy diet. But it's not.

It's Not Just the Calories We Take in . . .

We need to balance our food intake with the rate our bodies use it, that is, to eat the amount of calories from food that our bodies need. Consuming more calories than we use is a recipe for gaining weight and experiencing health problems. That balance, as many of us know, is difficult to achieve.

Why? It's extremely easy to overeat in our modern world. Refined foods, convenience foods, and fast foods are often delicious (well, to many of us!) and tend to lack fiber and chewiness; as a result, we often overdose on calories long before we realize we're full.

It's even easier not to exercise: it takes longer to walk somewhere than it does to drive, and our schedules are often so full that making time for physical activity seems impossible. That means we burn even fewer calories than we should, even as we're eating more. Our appetite meter no longer works properly and the more we ignore hunger, the more we end up overstuffed. The result: our calorie intake exceeds our energy needs on a regular basis, and we gain weight.

Despite what many would have you believe, the answer to weight maintenance is not dieting most of the time, that is, reducing your food intake to a low level that matches a low level of energy expenditure. That's a recipe for failure. It's a sad fact but true that nineteen of twenty people who lose weight by dieting will regain the lost weight. Nutritionists and public health experts are beginning to appreciate that a healthy diet comes in many different forms that may differ greatly in terms of proportions of fat, protein, and carbohydrate. As a result, finding a solution that works for you has never been easier or more viable. We encourage you to choose nutritious foods that suit your lifestyle and cultural and ethnic origins, as these are the ones you are most likely to stick with for life.

We need to balance . . .

. . . our food intake with the rate our bodies use it.

Eat Well, Move More

One of the golden rules is to accumulate sixty minutes of physical activity every day, including incidental activity and planned exercise. This will help you control your weight for a whole host of reasons. To make a real difference to your health and energy levels, exercise has to be regular and some of it needs to be aerobic. But every little bit counts, and, best of all, any extra exercise you do is a step in the right direction.

Though some people can make a serious commitment to thirty-plus minutes of planned exercise three or four times a week, most of us have a long list of excuses. We're too busy, too tired, too rushed, too stressed, too hot, too cold to go to the gym or take a walk or do a regular exercise routine. But there's good news. Research tells us that the calories we burn in our everyday activities are important too, and that any amount of movement is better than none at all.

Coupling a healthy, flexible diet you can live with in the long term with an active lifestyle is the best way to stay healthy and fit. That doesn't mean spending an hour at the gym six days a week. Instead, it means grabbing the opportunity for physical activity wherever you can: using the stairs instead of escalators, using a treadmill while you watch the news, working in the garden, parking a little distance from the office, or taking the dog for a walk. We know you have heard all this before. But, be creative with whatever works for you; just *do it*. Even housework burns calories. Small bursts of activity accumulate to increase fat burning. You don't have to exercise too strenuously—just do it regularly in a way you enjoy.

There are two fundamental principles to eating well: the carbo-hydrates are slow release and the fat is relatively unsaturated (even when the intake is high). But no diet plan will work in the long term if it eliminates your favorite foods, whether these are bread or potatoes, ice cream or chocolate. The next chapter begins to tell you how you can eat a balanced and healthy diet, one tailored to *your* tastes and *your* needs, without your feeling deprived. Part 4, Your Guide to Low GI Eating, shows how easy it is to make the switch to low GI eating for lifelong health and well-being. You might be pleasantly surprised at just how simple and enjoyable your meals can be.

5

Carbohydrate—The Big Picture: What It Is, Why We Need It, How We Digest It

BESIDES WATER, carbohydrate is the most widely consumed substance in the world. One of three main macronutrients (protein and fat are the other two), carbohydrate is the most important source of energy found in plants, including fruit, vegetables, cereals, and grains. There is virtually no carbohydrate in animal foods, apart from dairy foods. The simplest form of carbohydrate is glucose, which is:

- a universal fuel for most organs and tissues in our bodies,
- the only fuel source for our brain, red blood cells, and a growing fetus, and
- the main source of energy for our muscles during strenuous exercise.

Some plant foods contain large amounts of carbohydrate (rice, corn, and potatoes, for instance), while others, such as beans, broccoli, and carrots, have much smaller amounts of carbohydrate.

Breast milk, cow's milk, and milk products (but not cheese) contain carbohydrate in the form of milk sugar or lactose.

As we explained at the beginning of this book, not all carbohydrates are created equal; in fact, they can behave quite differently in our bodies, and the GI is how we describe this difference. When you switch to eating low GI carbs that have less "glycemic punch," you help to keep your blood glucose on an even keel and your energy levels perfectly balanced, and you'll feel fuller for longer periods between meals.

What Exactly Is Carbohydrate?

Carbohydrate is a part of food. Starch is a carbohydrate; so, too, are sugars and nearly all dietary fiber. Starches and sugar are nature's reserves created by energy from the sun, carbon dioxide, and water.

The simplest form of carbohydrate is a single-sugar molecule called a **monosaccharide** (*mono* meaning one, *saccharide* meaning sweet). **Glucose** is a monosaccharide that occurs in food (as glucose itself and as the building block of starch) and is the most common source of fuel for the cells of the human body. **Fructose** and **galactose** are also monosaccharides.

If two monosaccharides are joined together, the result is a **disaccharide** (*di* meaning two). **Sucrose**, or common table sugar, is a disaccharide, as is **lactose**, the sugar in milk, and **maltose**. As the number of monosaccharides in the chain increases, the carbohydrate becomes less sweet. Maltodextrins are **oligosaccharides** (*oligo* meaning a few). They taste only a little sweet and are commonly used as a food ingredient.

Starches are long chains of sugar molecules joined together like the beads in a string of pearls. They are called **polysaccharides** (*poly* meaning many). Starches are not sweet tasting at all.

Dietary fibers are large carbohydrate molecules containing many sorts of monosaccharides. They are different from starches and sugars because they are not broken down by human digestive enzymes. Dietary fiber is not digested in the small intestine; it reaches the large intestine without changing its form. Once there, bacteria begin to ferment and break it down. As we noted in Chapter 3, different fibers have different physical and chemical properties. **Soluble fibers** are those that can be dissolved in water; some soluble fibers, such as cellulose, are not soluble in water and do not directly affect the speed of digestion.

Just as a car runs on fuel, your body uses fuel (the food you eat). The fuel your body burns is derived from a mixture of the macro-nutrients—protein, fat, carbohydrates, and alcohol—that you consume. If you want to function well, be healthy, and feel your best, you need to fill your fuel tank—your body—with the right amount and the right kind of fuel every day.

Sugars Found in Food	
Monosaccharides (single-sugar molecules)	Disaccharides (two single-sugar molecules)
Glucose	Maltose = glucose + glucose
Fructose	Sucrose = glucose + fructose
Galactose	Lactose = glucose + galactose

Your body burns the macronutrients in a specific order—its fuel hierarchy. Because your body has no place to store unused alcohol, it tops the list. Excess protein comes second, followed by carbohydrate; fat comes in last. In practice, your body's fuel is usually a mix—a combination of carbohydrate and fat, in varying proportions. After meals, it's predominantly carbohydrate, and between meals, it's mainly fat.

Your body's ability to burn all the fat you eat is the key to weight control. If fat burning is inhibited, fat stores gradually accumulate. Because of this, the relative proportions of fat to carbohydrate in your body's fuel mix are critical (as we discussed on pages 35–36).

The Sources of Carbohydrate

The carbohydrate in our diet comes primarily from plant foods—cereal grains, fruits, vegetables, and legumes (dried beans, chickpeas, and lentils). Milk and foods made from milk (yogurt and ice cream, for example) also contain carbohydrate in the form of milk sugar, or lactose. Lactose is the first carbohydrate we encounter as infants; human milk contains more lactose than the milk of any other mammal, and it accounts for nearly half the energy that an infant will use.

Foods that are high in carbohydrate include:

- **Cereal grains:** rice, wheat, corn, oats, barley, rye, and anything made from them—bread, pasta, noodles, flour, breakfast cereal
- **Fruits:** apples, bananas, grapes, apricots, peaches, plums, cherries, pears, mango, kiwi
- **Starchy vegetables:** potatoes, sweet potatoes, sweet corn, yams
- **Legumes:** all dried beans (kidney, black, cannellini), lentils, chickpeas, split peas
- **Dairy products:** milk, yogurt, ice cream

Turning Food into Fuel

To be able to use the carbohydrate in foods, your body has to break it down into a form that it can absorb and that the cells can use; that process is digestion. To illuminate exactly what happens when your body digests food, here's how you digest a piece of bread:

1. When you chew the bread, it combines with saliva. Amylase, an enzyme in saliva, starts the process of chopping up the long-chain starch molecules into smaller-chain ones, such as maltose and maltodextrins (see page 40 for the definitions of these molecules).

2. When you swallow the bread, it lands in your stomach; there it gets pummeled and churned, much like clothes in a washing machine. The stomach's job is to deliver its load, bit by bit, to the small intestine. If the bread has viscous fibers in it (such as oats and flax) or is acidic (like sourdough), mixing takes longer and the stomach empties more slowly.

3. Once the bread is in your small intestine, an avalanche of digestive juices does the majority of the work involved in digestion. Starch is broken down into smaller and smaller chains of glucose. Many starches are rapidly digested, while others are more resistant, and thus the process is slower. The starch inside any whole kernels in the bread will be protected from attack and take longer to be broken down to glucose.

    If the mixture of food and enzymes is highly viscous or sticky, owing to the presence of viscous fiber, mixing slows down, and the enzymes and starch take longer to make contact. The products of starch digestion will also take longer to move toward the wall of the intestine, where the last steps in digestion take place.

4. At the intestinal wall, the short-chain starch products together with the sugars in foods are broken down by specific enzymes. The monosaccharides that finally result from starch and sugar digestion include glucose, fructose, and galactose. These are absorbed from the small intestine into the bloodstream, where they are available to the cells as a source of energy.

5. Within minutes of eating, glucose appears in the bloodstream. The rate at which it appears (i.e., in a big gush, or as just a little trickle)

is determined by the rate of digestion, as well as the rate at which food is emptied from the stomach. Together, these factors influence the GI of the food.

Sources of Carbohydrate

APPROXIMATE PERCENTAGE OF CARBOHYDRATE (grams per 100 grams of food)

apple	12%	peas	8%
baked beans	11%	pear	12%
banana	21%	plum	6%
barley	61%	potato	15%
bread	47%	raisins	75%
corn flakes	85%	rice (raw)	79%
flour	73%	split peas	45%
grapes	15%	sugar	100%
ice cream	22%	sweet corn	16%
milk	5%	sweet potato	17%
oats	61%	tapioca	85%
orange	8%	water cracker	71%
pasta (raw)	70%	wheat biscuit	62%

Carbohydrate Is Brain Food

Carbohydrate (glucose) is your brain's primary fuel source. If you are starving or deliberately avoiding carbs, under some circumstances the brain will make up the shortfall by burning compounds called "ketones."

Your brain is the most energy-demanding organ in your body, responsible for about one-quarter of your obligatory energy requirements that keep your body functioning. Unlike muscle cells, which can burn either fat or carbohydrate, the brain does not have the metabolic machinery to burn fat. If you fast for twenty-four hours or decide not to eat carbohydrates, your brain will initially rely on small stores of carbohydrate in your liver; but within hours, these are depleted, and the liver begins synthesizing glucose from noncarbohydrate sources, including your muscle tissue. It has only a limited ability to do this, however, and any shortfall in glucose availability has consequences for brain function.

The benefits of carbohydrate on mental performance are well documented. Medical research shows us that people's intellectual performance dramatically improves after they eat carbohydrate-rich foods (or a glucose load). In recent studies, subjects were tested on various measures of cognitive function, including word recall, maze learning, arithmetic, short-term memory, rapid information processing, and reasoning. All types of people—young people, college students, people with diabetes, healthy elderly people, and those with Alzheimer's disease—showed an improvement in mental ability after they ate glucose or a carbohydrate meal. Interestingly, research shows that low GI carbohydrates enhance learning and memory more than high GI carbs, probably because there is no rebound fall in blood glucose.

Too little glucose can have serious physical consequences, as well; for a complete discussion, see Chapter 11, where we discuss hypoglycemia, which results from low blood glucose.

What's Wrong with a Low-Carbohydrate Diet?

Low-carbohydrate diets are nothing new: a low-carb diet to lose weight was first published in 1864. Low-carb diets are either high in protein or high in fat or both. They cannot be anything else, because we have to get our energy from something (and alcohol, the only other macronutrient, won't keep you alive for long).

There are several variations of a low-carbohydrate diet; we'll confine our discussion to those where the reduction of carbohydrate is significant. This includes those that are low in carbohydrate, containing less than a hundred grams of carbohydrate per day and others that are *very low*, with reductions to as little as twenty to thirty grams of carbohydrate per day (ketogenic diets). The latter is the case with the first phase or "kick start" of various popular diet books and is not recommended by us or most health authorities.

Without enough carbohydrate in your diet, you may experience in the short term:

- muscle fatigue, causing even moderate exercise to be an exceptional effort,
- insufficient fiber intake and therefore constipation,
- headaches and tiredness due to low blood glucose levels,
- bad breath due to the breakdown products of fat (ketones), and
- bad moods and even clinical depression.

A recent review of low-carb diets has concluded that they are relatively safe and effective for weight loss in the short term, but there were potential risks in the long term (longer than six months).

One major concern is its high saturated fat intake and the repercussions. Even a single meal high in saturated fat can have an adverse effect on blood vessels by inhibiting vasodilation, the normal increase in the diameter of blood vessels that occurs after a meal. A short-term and long-term effect of a low-carb diet includes an increase in LDL cholesterol. Compounding this, there may be a low intake of micronutrients that are protective against disease. For this reason, a vitamin and mineral supplement is an essential accompaniment to a low-carb diet.

Low-carb diets are often high in protein (although not all high-protein diets are low in carbohydrate). In people with diabetes, higher long-term protein loads (over six months) may accelerate decline in kidney function and increase calcium loss in urine, potentially increasing the risk of osteoporosis and kidney stones.

To ensure that blood glucose levels can be maintained between meals, your body draws on the glucose stored in the liver; that form of glucose is called glycogen. Supplies of glycogen are strictly limited and must be replenished from meal to meal. If your diet is low in carbohydrate, your glycogen stores will be low and easily depleted.

Once your body has used up its glycogen stores, which occurs twelve to twenty-four hours after you begin a fast, it will start breaking down muscle protein to create glucose for your brain and nervous system to use. However, this process can't supply all of the brain's needs. As mentioned earlier, under these circumstances, the brain will make use of ketones, which are a by-product of the breakdown of fat. The level of ketones in the blood rises as the fast continues. You can even smell the ketones on the breath.

In people who are losing weight on a low-carb diet, the level of ketones in the blood rises markedly, and this state, called ketosis, is taken as a sign of success. But the brain may not be at its best, and one result is that mental judgment is impaired. In low-carb diet studies, volunteers complained of headaches and physical and mental lethargy. Researchers from Tufts University found that low-carb dieters had slower reaction times in tests performed two days and one week after starting the diet and a gradual decline in memory recall. In Australia, scientists found poorer mood and even depression one year after the start, even though the dieters had achieved significant weight loss. Finally, since your muscle stores of glycogen will have been depleted, you'll also find strenuous exercise almost impossible, and you may tire easily. See Chapter 7 for more information on low-carb diets.

Ketosis and Pregnancy

Ketosis is a serious concern for pregnant women. The fetus can be harmed and its brain development impaired by high levels of ketones crossing from the mother's blood via the placenta. Because being overweight is often a cause of infertility, women who are losing weight may get pregnant unexpectedly. One of the primary reasons we advocate a healthy, low GI diet for pregnant women is that there are absolutely no safety concerns for mother and baby. Indeed, there is some evidence that a low GI diet will help the mother control excessive weight gain during pregnancy.

6
How Much Carbohydrate Do You Need?

MOST OF THE WORLD'S POPULATION eats a high-carb diet based on staples such as rice, corn, millet, and wheat-based foods, including bread or noodles. In some African and Asian countries, carbohydrates may form as much as 70 percent to 80 percent of a person's energy intake, though this is probably too high for optimum health. In contrast, most people in industrialized countries eat less than half their energy as carbs. Our diets typically contain about 45 percent of energy in carbohydrate form.

Is this too low, too high, or just right?

How Much Carbohydrate Should You Be Eating?
Doctors and public health nutritionists now agree that your carbohydrate intake can vary over quite a wide range. They specify that the *type* and *source* of the carbohydrate and fat are more important than the proportions. The actual range shouldn't be lower than 40 percent or higher than 65 percent of energy as carbohydrate, i.e., moderate to high. This is a long way from a low- or very low-carbohydrate diet, which may contain as little as 10 percent to 25 percent of energy in the form of carbs.

If you look carefully at diets all around the world, it's clear that both high and moderate intakes of carbohydrate are commensurate with good health; the choice is ultimately up to you. Both types of diets, however, need to emphasize low GI carbs and healthy fats. The way of eating that you'll enjoy and tend to follow over the long term is the one that is closest to your usual diet. Our low GI approach has built-in flexibility when it comes to the amount of carbohydrate you eat.

In 2002, the National Institutes of Health (NIH) published new nutritional guidelines suggesting a range of carbohydrate intakes that could adequately meet the body's needs while minimizing your disease risk. We like the NIH's figures in part because they allow for individual tailoring. Specifically, they advised the following ranges:

- **Carbohydrate:** 45 percent to 65 percent of energy
- **Fat:** 20 percent to 35 percent of energy
- **Protein:** 10 percent to 35 percent of energy

Source: www.health.gov/dietaryguidelines

If you have diabetes, carbohydrate can be as low as 40 percent, according to the newest guidelines of the prestigious Joslin Diabetes Center in Boston. Chances are your diet already falls within these flexible ranges; if so, we encourage you to stick with what you have. If your preference is for more protein or more fat and fewer carbs, then go ahead. Just be choosy about the quality. (For more about protein, see pages 50 and 51.) We believe that you are the best judge of what you can live with.

However, we do recommend that you consume at least 125 grams of carbohydrate a day, even if you are on a weight-loss program. Whatever the amount, the type of carbohydrate is important, and that's where the GI, whole grains (see page 199), and fiber come into the story.

How to Find a Dietician

For specific information about your own energy and exact carbohydrate needs, you should consult a registered dietitian (RD). Your primary care physician or a medical specialist you see for a specific condition may have one or more dietitians in his or her practice. Alternatively, look in the *Yellow Pages* under Dietitians or contact the American Dietetic Association: www.eatright.org; 1-800-877-1600. Make sure that the person you choose has the letters RD after his or her name.

Is a High-Carbohydrate–Low-Fat Diet for You?

Is consuming 50 percent or more of your calories from carbohydrates and less than 30 percent from fats (the remaining 15 percent or more should come from protein) realistic for you? That depends. If you have always been health conscious and avoided high-fat foods, or if you follow an Asian or Middle Eastern diet, then chances are you're already eating a high-carbohydrate diet, and it's a good choice for you.

Of course, the number of calories and the amount of carbohydrate vary with your weight and activity levels. If you're an active person—as we hope you are!—with average energy requirements who is not trying to lose weight (i.e., with an average intake of 2,000 calories per day), you'll be eating 275 grams of carbohydrate. If you are trying to lose weight and are consuming a low-calorie diet (in other words, you're a small eater on 1,200 calories per day), that means you would be eating about 150 grams of carbohydrate a day.

Is a Moderate Carbohydrate Diet for You?

While many Australians and New Zealanders prefer more moderate carbohydrate intakes, North Americans tend to eat too many calories from all food sources. The reason: typical American portions of carbohydrate and protein are oversized (and should be reduced). A Mediterranean-type diet is higher in fat and provides only 45 percent of energy as carbohydrate. In the past, most nutritionists would have frowned upon this, but that's no longer the case, as research has shown that this type of diet can have important health benefits. As long as you carefully consider the types of fat and the types of carbohydrate you're eating, then this level of carbohydrate intake is perfectly commensurate with good health. At this level, you'll consume at least 125 grams of carbohydrate a day if you are a small eater and 225 grams if you are an average eater. See page 139 for an idea of how many servings of bread, cereal, pasta, or rice will provide these amounts of carbohydrate.

To determine the percentage of calories you get from carbohydrate in a food, multiply the grams of carbohydrate by four (the number of calories supplied per gram of carbohydrate) and then divide by the total number of calories.

The Real Deal on Protein and Health

Adding more protein to your diet makes good sense for weight control. In comparison with carbohydrate and fat, protein makes us feel more satisfied immediately after eating it and reduces hunger between meals. In addition, protein increases our metabolic rate for one to three hours after eating. This means we burn more energy by the minute compared with the increase that occurs after eating carbs or fats. Protein foods are also excellent sources of micronutrients, such as iron, zinc, vitamin B12, and omega-3 fats.

Which Foods Are High in Protein?

The best sources of protein are meats (beef, pork, lamb, chicken), fish, and shellfish. As long as these are trimmed of fat and not served with creamy sauces, you can basically eat sensibly to suit your appetite, though you'll find your appetite for lean protein will have a natural limit. When buying protein foods, choose the leanest cuts, remove all the visible fat, and grill, bake, braise, stir-fry, or pan-fry.

Another excellent source of protein is any type of legume (beans, chickpeas, or lentils)—a low GI food that is easy on the budget, versatile, filling, nutritious, and low in calories. Legumes are high in fiber, too—both soluble and insoluble—and are packed with nutrients, providing a valuable source (in addition to protein) of carbohydrate, B vitamins, iron, zinc, magnesium, and phytochemicals (natural plant chemicals that possess antiviral, antifungal, antibacterial, and anticancer properties). Whether you buy dried beans, lentils, and chickpeas and cook them yourself at home, or opt for the very convenient, time-saving canned varieties, you are choosing one of nature's lowest GI foods.

Dairy products are also good sources of protein, and the combination of protein and calcium that is unique to dairy foods can aid weight management. Research has shown that the more calcium or dairy foods (it's hard to separate the two) people eat, the lower their weight and fat mass. Calcium is intimately involved in burning fat—a process we want to encourage. Choose low-fat dairy products, including milk, yogurt, and cottage cheese. Go easy on high-fat cheeses such as cheddar, feta, Camembert, and Brie, though you don't have to cut them out entirely. It's better to have a small serving of one of these cheeses than a giant serving of a reduced-fat version that doesn't taste anywhere near as good.

Nuts are excellent sources of protein, dietary fiber, and micro-nutrients—and they contain very little saturated fat (the fats are predominantly mono- or polyunsaturated). Take care not to overeat nuts, because they're energy dense—meaning they pack a lot of calories into a small weight. Any nut will do, but research shows that eating one ounce of walnuts every day can help lower cholesterol and reduce heart attack risk. If you eat them as a snack, put a small handful in a bowl; don't eat them straight from the package. (See pages 205–206 for more recommendations about eating nuts.)

Eggs have been shedding their undeservedly bad reputation brought on because of their cholesterol content; in fact, they are a great source of protein and several essential vitamins and minerals. We now know that high blood cholesterol results from eating large amounts of saturated fat (rather than cholesterol) in foods. And if you select omega-3–enriched eggs, you will increase your intake of this valuable fat as well as your protein intake.

Can You Eat Too Much Protein?

The American Institute of Medicine recommends that no more than 35 percent of energy in our diets come from protein. That is 175 grams of pure protein for a person consuming 2,000 calories a day. In practice, most people will have no desire to eat beyond 20 percent to 25 percent of energy as protein.

A high protein intake has been criticized because it might also mean a high intake of saturated fat, which shouldn't happen if you stick to lean meat and low-fat dairy products.

Concerns about the effect of high protein intake on kidney function are limited to people who have compromised kidney function—some people with diabetes, the very elderly, and infants.

For example, take a container of yogurt with twenty-five grams of carbohydrate:

$$25 \times 4 \div 180 = 55\% \text{ of calories from carbohydrate}$$

The Best Ways to Eat Carbs

To ensure that you are eating enough carbohydrates and the right kind of carbohydrate, eat:

■ at least one low GI food at each meal,
■ lots of vegetables at least twice a day, and
■ fruit at least twice a day.

If you are looking for ways to improve your own diet, here are two important things for you to remember:

■ Identify the sources of carbohydrate in your diet and reduce the high GI foods. Don't go to extremes; there is room for your favorite high GI foods.
■ Identify the sources of fat and look at ways you can reduce saturated fat. Choose monounsaturated and polyunsaturated fats, such as olive oil and sunflower oil, instead of saturated fats like butter. Again, don't go overboard.

How to Switch to a Lower GI Diet Today

Here's a list of the foods our readers and clients choose to achieve a low GI diet:

■ grainy breads,
■ low GI breakfast cereals,
■ more fruit,
■ yogurt,
■ pasta,
■ legumes (baked beans make a good start), and
■ vegetables.

In Part 4, Your Guide to Low GI Eating, we give you many ways to make the change to a low GI diet (see Chapter 18), along with the low GI food finder, pantry planner, cooking tips, and fifty fast, delicious recipes making the most of low GI ingredients.

If you look carefully at diets . . .

. . . all around the world, it's clear that both high and moderate intakes of carbohydrates are commensurate with good health; the choice is ultimately up to you.

PART 2

The GI
and Your Health

■

How the GI Can Help You with Weight Control

The GI and Diabetes

The GI and Prediabetes

Pregnancy and Having a Healthy Weight Baby

Hypoglycemia

Heart Health and the Metabolic Syndrome

Polycystic Ovarian Syndrome (PCOS)

How Children, Athletes, and People Who Exercise
Can Use the GI

Plus the Latest Research Findings on the GI

7
The GI and Weight Control

IT IS SAD BUT TRUE that nineteen of twenty people who lose weight by dieting will regain the lost weight. Those who succeed are those who adopt a lifestyle solution to weight concerns, not another temporary fix. A low GI diet is about changing the way you eat for good.

Being slim or normal weight is no longer the norm. Between half and two-thirds of adults in the United States and Canada are classified as overweight or obese. Men are worse off than women, and our children are affected, too. Approximately one in four weighs much more than he or she should for age and height.

First, One of the Loudest Messages in This Chapter Is Don't "Diet"

Don't severely restrict food intake, *don't* skip breakfast, *don't* skip meals, *don't* follow fad diets; you are just asking for trouble. Instead, we want you to adopt simple lifestyle "maneuvers," only some of which are specific to food. Our focus is on eating *well* and moving *more*. The aim is to maximize your muscle mass (increase your engine size), minimize your body fat (decrease the cushioning), and keep you burning the optimal fuel mix for lifelong weight control (high-octane energy with built-in engine "protectants").

Why People Become Overweight: You and Your Genes

Let's take a look at the role our genes play in weight control. There are many overweight people who tell us resignedly, "Well, my mother's the same," "I've always been overweight," or "It must be in my genes." In fact, these comments have some truth behind them.

There is plenty of evidence to back up the idea that our body weight and shape are at least partially determined by our genes. A child born to overweight parents is much more likely to be overweight than one whose parents are not overweight. Most of this knowledge comes from studies of twins. Identical twins tend to be similar in body weight even if they are raised apart. Twins adopted as infants show the body-fat profile of their biological parents rather than that of their adoptive parents.

We also know that when naturally lean people are fed 10 percent more energy than they need, they increase their metabolic rate and their body *resists* the opportunity to gain weight, while overweight people, fed the same excess energy, pile on the pounds. The information stored in our genes governs our tendency to burn off or store excess calories.

The Importance of Resting Metabolic Rate

Our genetic makeup underlies our metabolic rate—how many calories we burn per minute. Bodies, like cars, differ in this regard. An eight-cylinder car consumes more fuel than a small four-cylinder one. A bigger body requires more calories than a smaller one. When a car is stationary, the engine idles, using just enough fuel to keep the motor running. When we are asleep, the "revs" are even lower and we use a minimum number of calories. Our resting metabolic rate (RMR)—the calories we burn by just lying completely at rest—is fueling our large brain, heart, and other important organs. When we start exercising or even just moving around, the number of calories (the amount of fuel we use) increases. But the greatest proportion of the calories used in a twenty-four-hour period are those used to maintain our RMR.

Since our RMR is where most calories are used, it is a significant determinant of body weight. The lower your RMR, the greater your risk of gaining weight, and vice versa. Whether you have a high or low RMR is genetically determined and runs in families. We all know someone who appears to eat like a horse but is positively thin. Almost in awe, we comment on the person's fast metabolism, and we may not be far off the mark.

Men have a higher RMR than women because their bodies contain more muscle mass and are more expensive to run; body fat, on the other hand, gets a free ride. These days, too many men and women have undersized muscles that hardly ever get a workout. Increasing muscle mass with weight-bearing (resistance) exercise will raise your RMR and is one of the secrets to lifelong weight control.

Interestingly, we know that our genes dictate the fuel mix we burn in the fasting state (overnight). Some of us burn more carbohydrate and less fat, even though the total energy used is the same. Scientists believe that subtle deficiencies in the ability to burn fat (as opposed to carbs) lie behind most states of being overweight and obese.

Indeed, according to the latest research, if you have one copy of a high-risk gene called FTO, geneticists have found you are 30 percent more likely to become overweight. If you have two copies, then you are 67 percent more likely! That is the strongest association yet of a common gene with obesity. Unfortunately, one in six people of European descent carry two copies and are therefore more prone to gain weight in the current environment.

This doesn't mean that if your genes are to blame you should resign yourself to being overweight too. But it may help you understand why you have to watch what you eat while other people don't. Furthermore, the current epidemic of obesity can't be blamed on our genes. Our genes haven't mutated in twenty-five years, but our environment has. So while genetics writes the code, environment presses the buttons. Our current sedentary lifestyles and food choices press all the wrong buttons.

If you were born with a tendency to be overweight, what you eat matters more. Genes can be switched on or off. By being choosy about carbohydrates and fats, you will maximize your insulin sensitivity, *up*-regulate the genes involved in burning fat, and *down*-regulate those involved in burning carbs. By moving your fuel "currency exchange" from a "carbohydrate economy" to a "fat economy," you increase the opportunity of depleting fat stores over carbohydrate stores. This is exactly what will happen when you begin to eat a nutritious, low GI diet.

If your genes are to blame, . . .

. . . you shouldn't resign yourself to being overweight. But it may help you understand why you
have to watch what you eat while other people
don't.

Food Choices Affect Your Appetite

Foods affect your appetite; they dictate when and how much you eat.
If digestion takes time and involves lower parts of your intestine, you
stimulate natural appetite suppressants. Consequently, both quality
and quantity of food are important for weight control.

Among all four major sources of calories in food (protein, fat,
carbohydrate, and alcohol), fat has the highest energy content per unit
of weight, twice that of carbohydrate and protein. A high-fat food is
therefore said to be "energy dense," meaning there are a lot of calories
in a standard weight of food. A typical croissant made with wafer-thin
layers of buttery pastry contains about five hundred calories—a whop-
ping 20 percent to 25 percent of total energy needs for most people
for twenty-four hours! To eat the same amount of energy in the form
of apples, you have to eat about six large apples. So, getting more
energy—calories—than your body needs is relatively easy when eating
a high-fat food. That's why there has been so much emphasis on low-
fat diets for weight control.

However, what really matters is not the fat content per se but a
food's "energy density" (calories per gram). Some diets, such as traditional Mediterranean diets, contain quite a lot of fat (mainly from olive
oil), but are not so energy dense, because the oil comes with a large
volume of watery fruits and vegetables. On the other hand, many new
low-fat foods on the market are energy dense. Indeed, some have much
the same energy density as the original high-fat food because two
grams of carbohydrate have replaced every gram of fat. If a low-fat food
has the same calories per serving as a high-fat food, then it's just as
easy to overeat. Nutritionists have therefore had to fine-tune the message about fat and weight control:

- Higher fat intake is compatible with healthy weight loss.
- The type of fat is more critical than the amount.

- Only saturated fat and trans fat need to be limited.
- Think energy density per serving, not high fat or low fat.

Why Insulin Resistance Is a Big Deal

Many overweight people, but not all, are insulin resistant (see page 74). This condition has genetic underpinnings and results in high insulin secretion after every meal. In time, even fasting insulin levels tend to rise. Having persistently high insulin levels is likely to make you fatter and fatter, undermining all your efforts at weight control. It is the very reason why people with diabetes and polycystic ovarian syndrome (PCOS) find it so hard to lose weight.

The higher your insulin levels, the more carbohydrate you burn at the expense of fat. This is because insulin has two powerful actions: one is to "open the gates" so that glucose can move into the muscle cells and be used as the source of energy. The second role of insulin is to *inhibit* the release of fat from fat stores. Unfortunately, the burning of glucose inhibits the burning of fat (and vice versa).

These actions persist even in the presence of insulin resistance because the body overcomes the hurdle by just pumping out more insulin into the blood. Unfortunately, the level that finally drives glucose into the cells is many times more than is needed to switch off the use of fat as a source of fuel. If insulin is high all day long, as it is in insulin-resistant and many overweight people, then the cells are being forced to use glucose as their fuel source, drawing it from either the blood or stored glycogen. Blood glucose therefore swings from low to high and back again, playing havoc with our appetite and triggering the release of stress hormones. Our limited stores of carbohydrate in the liver and muscles also undergo major fluctuations over the course of the day. When you don't get much chance to use fat as a source of fuel, it is not surprising that fat stores accumulate around different parts of the body.

A healthy low GI diet plus physical activity . . .

. . . is the most powerful way of optimizing insulin sensitivity and decreasing insulin levels over the course of the whole day.

Low GI Smart Carbs Help You Lose Weight

In previous editions of this book, we discussed the benefits of low GI diets mainly in terms of appetite and blood glucose control. Now we can argue confidently, on the basis of good scientific evidence, that the GI helps people lose weight, specifically that dangerous fat around the belly we mentioned earlier. There is concrete evidence that a low GI diet increases the rate of weight loss compared to a conventional low-fat diet. The confirmation comes from our own weight-loss studies at the University of Sydney, as well as research from the Children's Hospital in Boston and Hotel Dieu Hospital in Paris.

What's more, well-designed studies published in major medical journals have confirmed that the fat loss is maintained over the long term. This was especially evident in those overweight volunteers who secreted more insulin during meals. That is a critically important point because it is where the other diets have failed. Let's take a close look at all the facts supporting a healthy low GI diet.

The Filling Power of Low GI Carbs

One of the biggest challenges to losing weight is ignoring that gnawing feeling in your gut: hunger. Indeed, it is impossible to deny extreme hunger. Food-seeking behavior is wired into our brains to ensure we survive when energy intake is too low. Extreme hunger followed by binge eating can develop into a vicious cycle, and that is one reason we discourage rapid weight loss.

The low GI diet is based on an important scientifically proven fact—that foods with low GI values are more filling than their high GI counterparts. They not only give you a greater feeling of fullness instantly, but delay hunger pangs for longer and reduce food intake during the remainder of the day. In contrast, foods with a high GI can actually stimulate appetite sooner, increasing consumption at the next meal.

When it comes to filling power, foods are not created equal. Some foods and nutrients are simply more satiating than others, calorie for calorie. In general, protein packs the greatest punch, followed by carbohydrate and fat. Most of us can relate to the fact that a good steak has greater filling power than a croissant, despite the fact that they provide an equal number of calories.

There are also foods that are "addictive"—corn chips and potato chips, for example. We can't stop at one, just as the advertisement says. Fatty foods, in particular, have only a weak effect on satisfying appetite relative to the number of calories they provide. This has been demonstrated clearly in experiments where volunteers were asked to eat until their appetite was satisfied. They ate far more calories if the foods were high in fat than when they were starchy or sugary foods. Even when the fat and carbohydrate were disguised in yogurts and puddings, people consumed more energy from the high-fat option. This may surprise you, but remember that a gram of fat contains twice as many calories as a gram of protein, starch, or sugar.

In our laboratory at the University of Sydney, we developed the world's first satiety index of foods. Volunteers were given a range of individual foods that contained equal numbers of calories, and then their satiety responses and subsequent food intake were compared. We found that the most important determinant of satiety was the actual weight or volume of the food—the higher the weight per 240 calories, the higher the filling power. So foods that were high in water (and therefore the least energy dense), such as oatmeal, apples, and potatoes, were the most satiating. When water contents were equal, however, protein and carbohydrate were the best predictors of satiating power.

Then, if carbohydrate contents were similar, the GI became the most important determinant. Low GI foods were more satiating than high GI foods. (It is true that potatoes, despite their high GI, are high on the satiety index scale, but in theory, a low GI potato would be even more satiating.)

Eating to lose weight . . .

. . . with low GI smart carbs gives you freedom, flexibility, and security. What's more, it's sustainable.

Invariably, foods that provided a lot of calories per gram (energy-dense foods such as croissants, chocolate, and peanuts) were the least satisfying. These foods are more likely to leave us wanting more and to lead to what scientists call "passive overeating" without us realizing it. In developing our low GI diet, we made good use of these findings, encouraging food choices that will keep you feeling fuller for longer.

In addition to our own research, at least twenty other studies worldwide have confirmed that low GI foods, in comparison to their nutrient-matched high GI counterparts, are more filling, delay hunger pangs longer, and/or reduce energy intake during the remainder of the day. There are several explanations: low GI foods can take longer to chew, remain longer in the stomach, and reach much lower parts of the small intestine, triggering receptors and hormones that produce natural appetite suppressants. Many of these receptors are present only in the lower gut. It doesn't take a genius to appreciate that a food that dissolves and disappears from the gut quickly won't satisfy for hours on end.

We now know that low GI meals are associated with higher levels of two helpful hormones, known by their abbreviations CCK and GLP-1. Both produce feelings of pleasant fullness after eating and reduce food intake over the course of the day. GLP-1 has a further beneficial effect: it improves insulin sensitivity, a factor that helps facilitate weight control over the long term.

Here's the deal on GI and appetite:

- Low GI foods are more filling because they remain longer in the gut.
- High GI foods may stimulate hunger because the precipitous fall in blood glucose levels stimulates counterregulatory responses.
- Stress hormones such as adrenalin and cortisol are released when glucose levels rebound after a high GI food. Both stimulate appetite.
- Low GI foods may be more satiating simply because they are often less energy dense than their high GI counterparts. The naturally high water and fiber content of many low GI foods increases their bulk without increasing their energy content.

Fat Loss Is Faster with Low GI Foods

There are now a dozen or more studies showing that people who eat low GI foods lose more body fat than those eating high GI foods. In one study conducted by Harvard scientists, overweight adults were instructed to follow either a conventional high-fiber low-fat diet or a low GI diet containing more good fats and and low GI carbs. The low GI group's diet emphasized foods such as oatmeal, eggs, low-fat dairy products, and pasta. In contrast, the low-fat diet emphasized high-fiber cereal products, potatoes, and rice. Both diets contained the same number of calories and were followed for eighteen months (six months of intense intervention and twelve months of follow-up). At the end, changes in weight were similar in both groups. But, among the subjects who had high insulin levels (half of them), those on the low GI diet lost nearly six kilograms (over thirteen pounds) of weight compared to only one kilogram (two pounds) on the conventional low-fat diet. Moreover, they lost three times more body fat and had greater improvements in cardiovascular risk factors. In our own research unit at the University of Sydney, we have made similar findings in a group of young overweight adults who followed one of the four popular diets. To ensure dietary compliance, we gave them most of the food they needed for the whole twelve-week period. At the end, we found that weight and body fat loss were over 50 percent greater in those following our low GI diet than those following the conventional low-fat approach. Those instructed to follow a high-protein diet also lost more body fat but showed adverse blood lipid effects. Fortunately, the cholesterol-raising effect of the high-protein diet could be prevented by simultaneous consumption of low GI carbs.

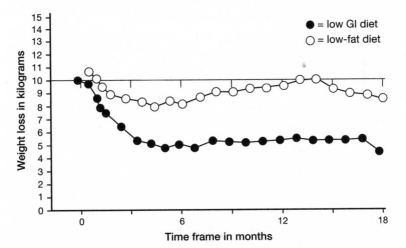

Figure 7: In a study of overweight adults with relatively high insulin levels, those on a low GI diet lost more weight and sustained that weight loss over time better than those on a conventional low-fat diet.

Why do low GI diets work so well for weight loss? The most important reason is likely to be the effect on daylong insulin levels; low GI foods result in lower levels of insulin over the course of the whole day.

The hormone insulin not only is involved in regulating blood glucose levels, but also plays a key part in fat storage. High levels of insulin mean the body is forced to burn carbohydrate rather than fat. Thus, over the course of a day, even if the total energy burned is the same, the proportions of fat to carbohydrate are different. Oxidizing carbohydrate won't really help you lose weight, but burning fat will.

These are not idle claims. Dr. Emma Stevenson's research with Loughborough University in the U.K. demonstrated over and over that, compared with healthy conventional meals, low GI meals were associated with greater fat oxidation during episodes of moderate exercise in overweight volunteers.

People who are overweight have been shown to have high glycogen (carbohydrate) stores that undergo major fluctuations during the day. This suggests that glycogen is a more important source of fuel for them. If glycogen is being depleted and replenished on a regular basis (before and after each meal, for example), it is displacing fat from the engine. Each meal restores glycogen (especially if the food has a high GI value) and the cycle repeats itself. Carbohydrate "balance," as it's called, is turning out to be one of the best predictors of future weight gain.

The benefits of a low GI diet for weight control go beyond appetite and fat burning. When you first begin a diet, your metabolic rate drops in response to the reduction in food intake, which makes weight loss slower and slower. Research shows your metabolic rate drops much less, however, on a low GI diet than on a conventional diet. If your engine revs higher, you'll not only lose weight faster, you'll also be much less likely to regain it.

The fall in metabolic rate that occurs whenever we restrict our energy intake is part of our body's natural response to food scarcity. This brings us to two new and profound concepts in the obesity research field, described in lay terms as the "famine reaction" and the "fat brake."

The "Famine Reaction"

The invisible enemy of any dieting effort is a natural physiological phenomenon that makes it progressively more difficult for dieters to keep losing weight, and even more difficult for them to keep it off. Dr. Amanda Sainsbury-Salis, obesity researcher at the Garvan Institute in Sydney, calls this the "famine reaction": it's a survival mechanism that's been helping the human race to survive famines and food shortages for millions of years. The famine reaction is the reason that, after each dieting effort, you end up doing battle with ravenous hunger, cravings for fattening foods, guilt-ridden binge eating, lethargy, weight plateauing, and rapid rebound weight gain. These are all classic signs of the famine reaction in full swing. It has nothing to do with lack of commitment or willpower. It's why conventional dieting advice fails.

In her book *The Don't Go Hungry Diet*, Dr. Sainsbury-Salis explains the origin of these telltale symptoms—a naturally occurring hormone called neuropeptide Y. Its secretion causes irrepressible increases in hunger, the hallmark feature of the famine reaction, but also acts to prevent further weight loss and promote fat accumulation, regardless of whether or not the person continues to follow a program of diet and physical activity. Neuropeptide Y is just one of a whole army of hormones and brain chemicals that bring on the famine reaction. All conspire to make sure you hit the wall of resistance to further weight loss. Drinking water, moving, and eating more fiber only serve to make the famine reaction stronger: more hunger, more cravings, more lethargy, and an even slower metabolic rate and longer plateau.

How do you switch off the famine reaction? Simple. It can be switched off by *eating freely*, eating sensibly to appetite. In other words, eating enough to satisfy your physical hunger, including your favorite foods. Nothing more complicated than that. The science behind this concept is new but rock solid. And it provides another explanation for the long-term success of our low GI diet, i.e., a diet underpinned by sensible *eating to appetite*, enjoying foods that make you feel fuller for longer because they take many more hours to be digested and absorbed.

The "Fat Brake"

Here is another crucial piece of scientific research with the potential to change your life for the better. According to Dr. Sainsbury-Salis, not only does your body have the potential to mount a famine reaction to stop your weight loss, it also possesses a remarkable system that protects you from gaining weight. She calls it the "fat brake." If you can pick up the fat-brake signals, it will actually be difficult for you to get fat. Just as there are brain chemicals and hormones that control the famine reaction, there is an opposing army of brain chemicals controlling the fat brake. The commander is a hormone called leptin that has the opposite effects to neuropeptide Y. It acts to blunt the appetite, increase the tendency to be active, and boost the metabolic rate. So you should heed not only the signals that say "eat more" but also those that say "eat less" and "don't eat yet."

Low GI and Weight Regain

Many people who successfully lose weight find themselves gradually putting the weight back on. Scientists are now focusing on this critical period, trying to determine the optimal dietary strategy for maintaining weight loss and preventing weight regain. The findings of the largest study of its kind, the Diogenes Study, led by Professor Arne Astrup at the University of Copenhagen, are just beginning to emerge. This collaborative project from eight countries in the European Union included over eight hundred overweight or obese individuals, all of them parents of young children. One or two parents in each family underwent an eight-week weight-loss diet using a low-calorie diet formula, which was designed to achieve a weight loss of 8 percent of their original starting weight (about twenty-four pounds). If the parents were successful in meeting this target, they were offered the opportunity to participate in the next stage of the study, which investigated the problem of weight regain. In this part of the study, volunteers were assigned to one of five different dietary regimes, designed to test the relative effectiveness of the GI as well as protein content in weight control.

The diets were:

Group 1: Low protein, low glycemic index
Group 2: Low protein, high glycemic index

Group 3: High protein, low glycemic index
Group 4: High protein, high glycemic index
Group 5: Control diet, medium protein and medium glycemic index

Over the course of twelve months, the investigators found that both low GI diets *and* high-protein diets were equally effective in preventing weight regain (see Figure 8). But they also found something that took them by complete surprise. The third diet group that combined both low GI *and* high-protein strategies continued to lose weight throughout the one-year follow-up. This was something never, ever seen before in any study of weight maintenance after weight loss. Furthermore, this group had the lowest dropout rate of any of the groups, a testament to the fact that not only was this diet effective, but it was acceptable to the volunteers and their families—not too difficult, complex, or hard to sustain. Interestingly, the Diogenes Study achieved only a moderately small reduction in GI (from about 58 to 50), yet it was sufficient to produce these outstanding results.

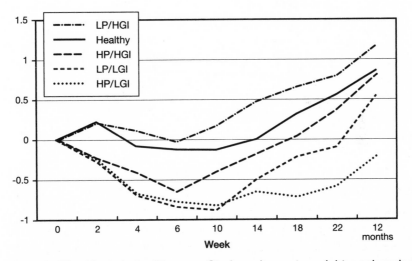

Figure 8: All subjects in the Diogenes Study underwent an eight-week period of fast weight loss before starting on one of five dietary strategies to prevent weight regain. (Week 0 in the figure represents the end of the eight-week period.) The two low-GI diet groups continued to lose weight in the first six months, but the best outcome after twelve months was the combination of a low GI and high-protein diet (HP/LGI in the figure).

Low GI Carbs and Lifelong Weight Control

One of the best reasons to adopt a low GI diet is the value-added benefits you get for long-term weight control. People who *naturally* eat a diet with a low GI have been found to be at much lower risk of being overweight and gaining weight in the future. Studies in the United States, Denmark, and Japan tell us that low GI diets *are* sustainable and have distinct advantages over other types of diets. There is no evidence that high protein intake, for example, benefits weight in the long term.

These types of studies (called epidemiological or observational) control or adjust for all the known confounding factors associated with weight gain: age, family history, physical activity, alcohol intake, fiber intake, etc. Hence, it is highly unlikely that a low GI diet is just a coincidental marker of a group of people at low risk of weight gain. The remarkable fact is scientists are finding that the higher the GI and/or GL, the higher the risk of developing disease like type 2 diabetes, stroke, and heart disease. In most cases, scientists find that the total carbohydrate, sugar, protein, and fat content of the diet are NOT predictive of future risk.

Epidemiological studies also prove to us that many people are already eating a diet that has a low GI. In other words, it is practical and feasible to select low GI foods from the vast array of foods currently on supermarket shelves. You don't have to jump through a hoop or turn yourself inside out to adopt a diet that gives you the benefits of lifelong health and weight control.

Make Healthy Eating a Habit

Make healthy eating a habit. Motivation is what gets you started. Habit is what helps to keep you going. Here are some key tips:

- Make breakfast a priority.
- If it's healthy, keep it handy.
- Don't buy food you want to avoid.
- Eat small portions regularly. Eat when you are hungry and stop when you are full (you don't have to leave a clean plate).

In Part 4, Your Guide to Low GI Eating, we give you all the information you need to make it happen for you and your family: how you can make the change to a low GI diet, along with the low GI food finder, pantry planner, cooking tips, and fifty delicious recipes making the most of low GI ingredients.

For our twelve-week, low GI weight-loss program, we encourage you to consult *The Low GI Diet Revolution*, which covers topics such as why restrictive diets fail, how much weight you should aim to lose, the optimal diet for weight loss, and how a low GI diet helps prevent weight regain. *The Low GI Diet Cookbook* also provides delicious, easy, smart-carb recipes.

Quite simply, . . .

. . . the low GI diet is not a fad, but a blueprint for healthy eating for the rest of your life.

Veronica's Story

I lost almost forty-five pounds on the low GI diet. I had tried various diets before—low fat, detox, etc., but they never made any difference to my weight and they were often quite restrictive in what they allowed me to eat. So I could never keep them up for long. With the low GI diet, it took one year to lose the weight with once-a-week exercise, and now, two years later, I still have not regained the weight. My diet is varied, enjoyable, and helps me keep the weight off. The great thing about the low GI diet is that it is not restrictive—you only need to modify your diet slightly, like eating grainy bread instead of white bread. I find that low GI foods taste better, too. I am eating foods I would never have eaten before because I thought they were too fattening. This diet has given me more freedom in what I eat and more energy.

8

The GI and Diabetes

DIABETES IS ON ITS WAY TO BECOMING one of the most serious and most common health problems in the world. A type 2 diabetes epidemic is gaining momentum in many developed and newly industrialized nations. Worldwide, the total number of people with diabetes is 246 million, and the International Diabetes Federation predicts it will affect 380 million people by 2025. In some developing countries, half of the adult population already has type 2 diabetes. Even in developed countries, the rate of type 2 diabetes is increasing at an alarming rate. An estimated 23.6 million people in the United States and 1.3 million Canadians have diabetes. Additionally, 57 million Americans have prediabetes.

The prediction is that one of every three people in the United States born in the year 2000 will develop type 2 diabetes. Australia and New Zealand are not lagging too far behind in statistics like these. In the absence of any sort of preventive intervention, a high proportion of people with prediabetes will eventually develop diabetes. The GI has far-reaching implications for diabetes and prediabetes (see Chapter 9). Not only is it important in treating people with diabetes, but it may also help prevent people from developing type 2 diabetes in the first place and possibly even prevent some of the complications of diabetes.

What Is Diabetes?

Diabetes is a chronic condition in which there is too much glucose in the blood. Keeping your blood glucose levels normal requires the right amount of a hormone called insulin. Insulin gets the glucose out of the blood and into your body's muscles, where it is used to provide energy for the body. If there is no insulin, not enough insulin, or if the insulin does not do its job properly, diabetes develops.

Type 1 diabetes (formerly referred to as insulin-dependent diabetes, or juvenile onset diabetes) is an autoimmune disease triggered by as yet unknown environmental factors (possibly a virus) that usually develops in childhood or early adulthood. In type 1 diabetes, the pancreas cannot produce any insulin, because the body's immune system has attacked and destroyed its insulin-producing beta cells. About 10 percent of people with diabetes have type 1 diabetes. To survive, everyone with type 1 diabetes requires insulin, delivered through injections or an insulin pump.

Type 2 diabetes (formerly known as noninsulin-dependent diabetes or maturity onset diabetes) has a large genetic component, but overeating, being overweight, and not exercising enough are important lifestyle factors that can contribute to its development, particularly in people who have a family history of diabetes. Eighty-five to 90 percent of people with diabetes have type 2.

Typically, type 2 diabetes develops after the age of forty. However, our society's increasing physical inactivity and obesity have led to the diagnosis in younger and younger people. Even children under ten years of age are developing type 2 diabetes.

People develop type 2 diabetes because they have developed insulin resistance (see box on page 74). As type 2 diabetes progresses, the body may struggle to make the extra insulin needed and then may ultimately develop a shortage of insulin. Treatments for type 2 diabetes aim to help people make the best use of the insulin their bodies produce and to try to make it last as long as possible. In some cases, oral medications and insulin injections may be necessary to treat this type of diabetes.

What Is Insulin Resistance?

Insulin resistance means that your body is insensitive, or "partially deaf," to insulin. The organs and tissues that ought to respond to even a small increase in insulin remain unresponsive. So your body tries harder by secreting more insulin to achieve the same effect. This is why high insulin levels are found in people with type 2 diabetes who are insulin resistant.

Why Do People Get Type 2 Diabetes?

As our ancestors settled down to become farmers and began to grow food crops 10,000 years ago, their diet was no longer protein-based. It was more carbohydrate-based, in the form of whole cereal grains, vegetables, and beans. Such a dietary change would also have changed the glucose levels in their blood. While they ate a high-protein diet, the glucose levels in their blood would not have risen significantly after a meal.

When they started eating carbohydrate regularly, their blood glucose levels would have increased after meals. The amount by which the glucose levels in the blood increased after a meal would have depended on the GI of the carbohydrate. Crops such as spelt wheat grain, which our ancestors grew, had a low GI value. These foods would have had a minimal effect on glucose levels in the blood, and the demand for insulin would have been similarly low.

As we discussed in Chapter 4, the second major change in our diet came with industrialization and the advent of high-speed steel-roller mills in the nineteenth century. Instead of whole-grain products, the new milling procedures produced highly refined carbohydrate, which we now know increases the GI value of a food and transforms a low GI food into one with a high GI value. When this highly refined food is eaten, it causes a greater increase in blood glucose levels. To keep blood glucose levels normal, the body has to make large amounts of insulin. The vast majority of the commercially packaged foods and drinks that most people eat today have a high GI value. All of this strains the body's insulin-making capabilities.

Our bodies adapted to such major changes in diet over long periods of time. Because our European ancestors had thousands of years to adapt to a diet with a lot of carbohydrate, they were in a better position to cope with the changes in the GI values of foods. We believe that's why people of European descent have a lower prevalence of type 2 diabetes than people whose diets have recently changed to include lots of high GI foods. There is, however, only so much that our bodies can take. As we continue to consume increasing quantities of foods with high GI values, plus excessive amounts of fatty foods, our bodies are coping less well. The result can be seen in the significant increase of people developing diabetes.

Large-scale studies at Harvard University, in which thousands of men and women have been studied over many years (see page 110 for information on one major study), have shown that people who ate large amounts of refined, high GI foods were two to three times more likely to develop type 2 diabetes or heart disease. The most dramatic increases in diabetes, however, have occurred in populations that have been exposed to these lifestyle changes over a much shorter period of time. In some groups of Native Americans and populations within the Pacific region, up to one adult in two has diabetes because of the rapid dietary and lifestyle changes they have undergone in the twentieth and twenty-first centuries.

Treating Diabetes

Watching what you eat is essential if you have diabetes. For some people with type 2 diabetes, diet, along with exercise, is *the* most critical way to keep their blood glucose levels in the normal range (70–130 mg/dL; 4–6 mmol/L). Others also need to take tablets or insulin. Everyone with type 1 diabetes must receive insulin, no matter what their diet. Regardless of the type or degree of their diabetes and their doctor-approved treatment, everyone with diabetes must carefully consider what they eat in order to keep their blood glucose levels under control. There's no question about it, research shows that good (also called "tight") blood glucose control helps to prevent the dire complications that can arise: heart attacks, strokes, blindness, kidney failure, and leg amputations.

It wasn't until the 1970s that carbohydrate was considered to be a valuable part of the diabetic diet. Researchers found that a higher carbohydrate intake brought both improved nutritional status and insulin sensitivity. In the early 1980s, with Dr. David Jenkins's development of the glycemic index, described in Chapter 1, the foundations were established for our present-day understanding of the real effect of those carbohydrates on blood glucose levels.

Some people think that because carbohydrate raises blood glucose levels, people who have diabetes shouldn't eat it at all. We cannot stress enough that this is simply not correct. Carbohydrate is a useful component of a healthy diet, helps maintain insulin sensitivity, and provides physical endurance. Mental performance is also better when meals contain carbohydrate rather than just protein and fat. (See "Carbohydrate Is Brain Food" on pages 43–44).

Fundamentally, the GI shows that the way for people with diabetes to incorporate more carbohydrates into their diet—while keeping tight control on their blood glucose levels—is to choose low GI carbs.

Lowering the GI of your diet is not as hard as it seems, because nearly every carbohydrate food that we typically consume has an equivalent food with a low or lower GI value. Our research has shown that blood glucose levels in people with diabetes are greatly improved if foods with a low GI value are substituted for high GI foods—the "This for That" approach we talk about in Chapter 18 (see pages 193–209).

We showed a group of people with type 2 diabetes how to replace the high GI foods they normally ate with low GI foods. After three months, we found a significant drop in their average blood glucose levels. They did not find the diet at all difficult; rather, they commented on how easy it had been to make the change and how much more variety had been introduced into their diet.

Similar results have been reported by other researchers studying both type 1 and type 2 diabetes. For example, large studies in Australia, Europe, and Canada of people with type 1 diabetes have shown that the lower the GI of the diet, the better the diabetes control.

The improvement in diabetes management seen after changing to a low GI diet is often better than that achieved with some of the newer, expensive diabetes medications and insulins. Making this type of change in your everyday diet does not mean that your diet has to be restrictive or unpalatable. Many people with type 2 diabetes end up taking oral medication and/or insulin to control blood glucose levels. An increased intake of low GI carbs can sometimes make these drugs unnecessary. Sometimes, however, despite your best efforts with diet, medication will be necessary to obtain good blood glucose control. This is eventually the case for most people with type 2 diabetes as they grow older and their insulin-secreting capacity declines further.

What Should People with Diabetes Be Eating?

- A low GI diet containing whole-grain breads (made with intact kernels), cereals like oats, pearl barley, couscous, cracked wheat, legumes like kidney beans and lentils, and all types of fruit and vegetables.

- Only small amounts of saturated fat. Limit cookies, cakes, butter, potato chips, take-out fried foods, full-fat dairy products, and fatty meats and sausages, which are all high in saturated fat. The poly- and monounsaturated olive, canola, and peanut oils are healthier types of fats that can be eaten in moderation.

- A moderate amount of sugar and sugar-containing foods. It's okay to include your favorite sweetener or sweet food—small quantities of sugar, honey, maple syrup, jam—to make meals more palatable and pleasurable.

- Only a small quantity of alcohol (see Step 10, page 209 for guidelines)

- Only a small amount of salt and salted foods. Try lemon juice, freshly ground black pepper, garlic, chili, herbs, and other flavors instead of relying on salt.

For more recipes and ideas about eating the low GI way to manage your diabetes, see Part 4, Your Guide to Low GI Eating. You also may find it helpful to consult *The New Glucose Revolution for Diabetes* or other books in our series that include many recipes, including *The Low GI Diet Revolution, The Low GI Cookbook, The New Glucose Revolution Low GI Family Cookbook*, and *The New Glucose Revolution Low GI Vegetarian Cookbook*.

Lowering the GI of your diet . . .

. . . is not as hard as it might seem, because nearly every carbohydrate food has an equivalent food with a low or lower GI.

John's Story

I was diagnosed with type 2 diabetes a little over a year ago. The diet that my local diabetes association recommended wasn't working, and my symptoms—including blurry vision, weight gain, and high blood pressure—weren't getting better. Then I began following a low GI diet. Since then, I gradually reduced my insulin requirements until I no longer needed it. Today, my blood pressure and weight are back to normal, and my liver, kidney, and urine tests yielded healthy results. Following a GI diet approach has truly helped me manage my diabetes, and I plan on eating this way for the rest of my life!

The Dreaded Diabetes Complications

As we mentioned earlier, heart attacks, leg amputations, strokes, blindness, and kidney failure are more common in people with diabetes. The reason: poor blood glucose control can damage the blood vessels in the heart, legs, brain, eyes, and kidneys—all parts of the body that are susceptible to vascular damage. Poor blood glucose control can also damage the nerves in the feet, leading to pain and irritation, numbness, and loss of sensation.

In addition to high blood glucose levels, many researchers believe that high levels of insulin also contribute to the damage of the blood vessels of the heart, legs, and brain. High insulin levels are thought to be one of the factors that might stimulate muscle in the wall of blood vessels to thicken. Thickening of this muscle wall causes the blood vessels to narrow and can slow the flow of blood to the point that a clot can form and stop blood flow altogether. This is what happens to cause a heart attack or stroke.

We know that high GI foods cause the body to produce larger amounts of insulin, which results in higher levels of insulin in the blood. Eating low GI foods not only helps to control blood glucose levels, but also does so with lower levels of insulin. Lower levels of both blood glucose and insulin may have the added benefit of reducing large-vessel damage, which accounts for many of the problems that people with diabetes tend to experience.

The GI and Snacks

The GI is especially important when you eat carbohydrate by itself and not as part of a mixed meal. Carbohydrate tends to have a stronger effect on blood glucose levels when it is eaten alone rather than as part of a meal with protein foods, for example. This is the case with between-meal snacks, which most people with diabetes eat.

Many people taking insulin or oral medications may need to eat some form of carbohydrate between meals to prevent their blood glucose from dropping too low.

Snacks, when chosen wisely, can make a significant nutrient contribution even if you're not taking any diabetes medication. We recommend them especially for small children, to ensure a sufficient energy intake. Even for adults, regular snacks can prevent extreme hunger and help to reduce the amount of food eaten at a single sitting, which can help manage blood glucose levels.

Studies that have looked at the effects of small, frequent meals (rather like grazing) versus two or three large meals each day have found that in people with type 2 diabetes, blood glucose and blood fat levels improve when meal frequency increases. There's also evidence that you will reap metabolic benefits by eating at regular set times rather than haphazardly.

Snacking isn't a license to eat more food. Rather, it is a way to spread the same amount of food over more frequent and smaller meals. Research indicates that if you spread your nutrient load more evenly over the course of a day, you may reduce the need for insulin in the disposal and uptake of carbohydrates. Researchers have seen this effect in people without diabetes, too. Although it has not been proven by controlled trials, it may also be that small, frequent meals could reduce your risk of developing diabetes by reducing the periodic surges in insulin that follow large meals.

Choose Low GI Foods for a Between-Meal Snack

An apple, with a GI of 38, is better than a slice of white toast, with a GI of around 70, and will result in a smaller jump in the blood glucose level. Other low-fat, low GI snack ideas include:

- A fruit smoothie
- A low-fat milkshake

- An apple
- Low-fat fruit yogurt
- 5 or 6 dried apricot halves
- A small banana
- 1 or 2 oatmeal cookies
- An orange
- A scoop of low-fat ice cream in a cone
- A glass of low-fat milk

Hypoglycemia—the Exception to the Low GI Rule

We discuss hypoglycemia in greater detail in Chapter 11, but we want to mention it here briefly because people with diabetes who use insulin or oral medication may sometimes experience hypoglycemia, which occur when blood glucose levels drop below 70 mg/dL (4 mmol/L), the lower end of the normal range. Symptoms of hypoglycemia differ from person to person, but can include feeling hungry (even ravenous), feeling shaky, sweating, having a rapid heart beat, and being unable to think clearly.

To Treat Hypoglycemia . . .

Raise your blood glucose levels quickly with rapid-acting carbohydrate such as:

- Glucose tablets or gels (ten to twenty grams)
- ½ cup of regular (not diet) soft drink, fruit juice, or sweetened fruit beverage
- 4 large jelly beans or 7 small jelly beans
- 2–3 teaspoons of sugar

Follow within fifteen to twenty minutes with carbohydrate foods that will maintain blood glucose levels:

- 1 slice of low-GI bread
- 1 banana or apple
- A container of unsweetened yogurt (6–8 ounces) or ½ a container (3–4 ounces) of sweetened yogurt
- 1 glass of low-fat milk

Hypoglycemia (also known as low blood sugar) is a potentially dangerous situation that must be treated immediately by eating approximately fifteen grams (one-half ounce) of an easily absorbed source of carbohydrate. If you aren't about to eat your next meal or snack, follow up with another fifteen grams of lower GI carbohydrates, like an apple, to keep your blood glucose from falling again until you next eat.

Symptoms of hypoglycemia . . .

. . . differ from person to person, but can include feeling hungry (even ravenous), feeling shaky, sweating, having a rapid heart beat, and being unable to think clearly.

Frank's Story

The managers of my workplace insisted that people were their best asset, and to prove their point, they provided a health assessment for their staff. I took one, and my health was perfect, except my urine sample turned out sugary. I was advised to consult my physician as soon as possible. When I came home and told my wife and daughters the news, my wife took my medical condition very seriously—her father had died at fifty-nine due to diabetes. I went to see my physician, and after the blood tests, I was formally diagnosed with diabetes. I was advised to shed eleven pounds. I lost eight pounds over two years through a strict diet and exercise regime. Soon after the diagnosis, during a routine eye inspection, my left retina was found to have developed a cataract due to my diabetes. On my wife's insistence, I finally underwent an operation where a plastic lens was implanted.

Ever since I became diabetic, my food tastes have revolved around the glycemic index. My latest results indicate very good self-control, but I have to monitor it regularly. Exercise is also an important factor in tackling diabetes. I walk four to five miles a day. I competed in my first competitive run—Sydney's City to Surf—at the prime age of sixty, although it was more fun than run. I clocked 152 minutes. I am aiming to do it in under 120 minutes in the future.

If You're Having Trouble Controlling Your Blood Glucose Levels . . .

Many factors can affect your blood glucose levels—what you eat and drink, your weight, your stress levels, how much exercise you're getting, and the medications you're taking. So if you have diabetes and you're finding it hard to achieve "tight control" of your blood glucose levels, we cannot stress strongly enough how important it is to seek help. Treating diabetes really is a team effort. Ideally, on your team, there will be a doctor (and possibly an endocrinologist or specialist physician), a diabetes educator, a dietitian, a podiatrist, an exercise specialist, an eye doctor, and a dentist. There may also be a counselor (psychologist or psychiatrist) to help you cope with living with a chronic disease. Working with a healthcare team like this is the best way you can avoid the serious complications that diabetes can cause. That's the clear message from numerous studies of people with diabetes in recent years.

The most important member of your team . . .

. . . is you, and knowledge is your best defense. Only you can make sure you know as much as possible about your diabetes and only you can act on the advice you are given.

Jane's Story

Low blood glucose in the night was a real problem for me. My evening insulin doses had been adjusted to try to stop my blood glucose from going too low at night, but I thought that experimenting with my supper carbohydrate could also help. After trying all sorts of different foods and many 3 a.m. blood tests, I found the answer that the GI predicted would work—milk! Before going to bed, a large glass of milk rather than my usual plain crackers was easy and maintained my blood glucose at a good level through the night.

9

The GI and Prediabetes

IF YOU HAVE PREDIABETES (the term used to describe impaired glucose tolerance and/or impaired fasting glucose), it means that you have blood glucose levels somewhere between normal and diabetes. It's diagnosed by either a fasting blood glucose test or an oral glucose tolerance test.

- Impaired fasting glucose (IFG) is diagnosed if the fasting glucose is 100–125 mg/dL (5.6–6.9 mmol/L).
- Impaired glucose tolerance (IGT) is diagnosed after a glucose tolerance test if the two-hour glucose level is 140–199 mg/dL (7.8–11.0 mmol/L). Studies around the world show that there are twice as many people with prediabetes as with diabetes. In fact, it is currently estimated that there are about 300 million people worldwide with prediabetes (with 57 million in the United States). So it is a major public health problem that's only going to get worse unless something is done.

Left untreated, prediabetes can develop into type 2 diabetes. It also puts you at risk of some of the complications associated with diabetes, such as heart attacks and stroke. That's why, in addition to making lifestyle changes to deal with prediabetes, you could also benefit from advice on how to prevent heart disease and stroke.

The good news is that there is very strong evidence that you can prevent, or at the very least delay, getting type 2 diabetes—and all of its complications. In fact, several large studies have shown that three of five people with prediabetes can prevent the development of type 2 diabetes—very good odds indeed.

Be Well, Know Your BGL (blood glucose level)

Normal ranges for:

Fasting glucose	63–99 mg/dL (3.5–6.0 mmol/L)
Nonfasting glucose	<200 mg/dL (less than 11.1 mmol/L)
Glycated hemoglobin	<7.0 percent (4.0–6.0 percent)

Risk Factors for Developing Prediabetes

If there's type 2 diabetes in your family, you probably already know that you have an increased chance of getting it too. But genes alone don't account for the current diabetes/prediabetes epidemic. Instead, it's what's being called our "diabetogenic environment"—the food we eat and our sedentary lifestyle. The most obvious trigger is that we're all getting heavier, and carrying extra body fat goes hand in hand with prediabetes and type 2 diabetes. People who are overweight, particularly around their middle, have up to three times more chance of developing type 2 diabetes than people who are in the healthy weight range.

Risk Factors You Cannot Change
- A family history of diabetes
- Your ethnic background (people of Native American, Puerto Rican, Mexican American, African American, Cuban, and Pacific Island backgrounds have a greater risk)
- Having polycystic ovarian syndrome (PCOS)
- Having diabetes in pregnancy or giving birth to a big baby (more than eight pounds)
- Having heart disease, angina, or having had a heart attack

Risk Factors You Can Do Something About
- Being overweight, especially if that weight is around your middle
- Being sedentary

- Smoking
- Having high blood pressure
- Having high triglycerides
- Having low HDL (good) cholesterol
- Having high total LDL cholesterol
- Unhealthy eating

Of course not every overweight person is going to develop prediabetes or type 2 diabetes (many don't), but the underlying metabolic problem in prediabetes and type 2 diabetes—that is, insulin resistance—is exacerbated by being overweight.

As we explain in Chapter 8, insulin resistance means your body cells are resistant to the action of insulin (plenty of keys but the locks are malfunctioning). They don't let glucose in as easily as normal, so the blood glucose level tends to rise. To compensate, the pancreas makes more and more insulin. This eventually moves the glucose into the cells, but the blood insulin levels stay high. Having high insulin levels all the time spells trouble.

Being overweight makes this situation worse because the excess fat "blocks" the action of the insulin, putting added pressure on the body's ability to maintain optimal blood glucose levels.

What's the Best Way of Preventing It?

A healthy lifestyle, of course. There's nothing you can do about the inherited risk factors or family history. But you can do something about your weight, the food you eat, and a sedentary lifestyle. And if you smoke, you can quit.

Several studies around the world (in China, Finland, the United States, Japan, and India, for example) have shown conclusively that people with prediabetes can delay or prevent the development of diabetes. All of these studies were based on people who made lifestyle changes. People increased their level of activity, ate a healthier diet, and achieved modest weight loss (about ten to twenty pounds). All these changes are achievable with a little effort, and the long-term benefit is enormous—not having to live with diabetes and reducing your risk of heart attack and stroke.

Living with Prediabetes

What can you do about prediabetes? Plenty. Lifestyle changes—moderate weight loss, healthy eating, and regular physical activity—will go a long way.

Aim for Moderate Weight Loss

For most people with prediabetes, the first priority has to be reducing body weight. You don't have to lose a lot of weight for it to help. Research has shown that people with prediabetes who lose 5 percent to 10 percent of their body weight at diagnosis can prevent or delay the onset of type 2 diabetes.

Lower Your Saturated Fat Intake

We know that people who develop type 2 diabetes are more likely to have a high saturated fat intake. Saturated fat promotes insulin resistance, making it harder for insulin to do its job of regulating your blood glucose levels. To eat less saturated fat:

> **Use low-fat dairy products.** Routinely purchase low-fat milk, cheese, ice cream, and yogurt rather than their regular forms.
>
> **Choose your snack foods wisely.** Don't buy chocolates, cookies, potato chips, cereal bars, snack bars, etc. See Chapter 18 for healthy snack options.
>
> **Cook with the good oils.** The healthier oils to use are olive, canola, and mustard seed oils.
>
> **Take care when you are eating away from home.** Give up the French fries and potato wedges with sour cream, along with other deep-fried foods, pizza, and pies.
>
> **Eat lean meats.**

Boost Your Omega-3 Intake

While high fat intakes are associated with diabetes, there is one type of fat that's the exception—the very long chain omega-3 fatty acids. Dietary trials in animals and people have shown that increased omega-3 intake can improve insulin sensitivity and therefore could reduce diabetes risk.

Our bodies make only small amounts of these unique fatty acids, so we rely on dietary sources, especially fish and seafood, for them. Aim to include fish in your diet at least twice a week, such as a main meal of fresh fish *not* cooked in saturated fat, plus at least one sandwich-sized serving of, say, canned salmon or tuna. See Chapter 18.

In addition to eating these great sources of long-chain omega-3s, you can also increase your total omega-3 intake by eating short-chain omega-3s, which are found in canola oil and margarine, nuts and seeds (particularly walnuts and flaxseeds), and legumes such as baked beans and soybeans.

Lower the GI of Your Diet

Studies show that people who base their diet on carbohydrates with a low GI are the least likely to develop type 2 diabetes. The findings of some studies suggest that simply changing the bread you eat can make a difference. See Part 4 for some key ways to lower the GI of your diet.

Increase Your Fiber Intake

Higher fiber intakes are also associated with a lower incidence of type 2 diabetes. Specifically, higher intakes of whole-grain cereals (see page 199), fruits, and vegetables are recommended.

Get the benefit of whole grains (grains that are eaten in nature's packaging or close to it) with foods such as:

- Barley. Try pearl barley in soup or in recipes such as barley risotto or a barley salad.
- Whole wheat or cracked wheat such as bulgur in tabbouleh
- Rolled oats for breakfast in oatmeal or muesli
- Whole-grain breads—the ones with chewy grains and seeds (low GI versions are best)

If you don't eat many fruits or vegetables at the moment, aim for at least one piece of fruit and two servings of vegetables each day; then build up gradually by eating one extra piece of fruit and one extra serving of vegetables each week. If you are already eating a lot of fruits and vegetables, increase your intake until you reach two servings of fruit and five servings of vegetables every day.

Get Regular Physical Activity

All the studies that have proven that a healthy lifestyle can prevent the development of type 2 diabetes have included a comprehensive exercise program in their definition of a healthy lifestyle. You need 150–210 minutes of moderate-level physical activity each week, which is of course around thirty minutes of activity each day. The kinds of activities that proved most useful to people with prediabetes included walking, jogging, cycling, swimming, dancing, and ball games.

Encourage Your Children to Exercise

Type 2 diabetes is increasing in young people, so encouraging your children to be more active is a very important part of reducing their risk of later developing prediabetes or diabetes. Turning off the TV and computer and getting kids outside to play may be one of the most health-promoting things you can do as a parent.

Physical activity has many benefits, including increasing your lean body mass (giving you more muscles) and decreasing your body fat stores, which lead to lower insulin resistance and better insulin sensitivity. You get these benefits with regular exercise even if you don't lose weight. And being physically active is not just about playing sports. Be more active in as many ways as you can. Think of movement as an opportunity, not an inconvenience, and make it part of your day.

The good news . . .

. . . is that there is very strong evidence that you can prevent, or at the very least delay, getting type 2 diabetes—and all of its complications.

Karen's Story

I have been a yo-yo dieter for twenty years and have gradually gained more and more weight. I began to do a "no no," that is, not eat, thinking it would help me lose weight. This only led to prediabetes and gaining much more weight. I tried every diet and exercise regime but kept putting on weight. It wasn't until I began to get low blood glucose levels and often felt like I was going to pass out that I saw my doctor. But he didn't help; he just said, "Keep dieting." So I persisted for the sake of my hubby and children—forty-two is too young to be on the road to diabetes and heart disease. My family needs their wife and mom. When I had had enough, I went to a different doctor, who told me about the low GI diet. I was amazed to discover that within a week of beginning the diet (plus some moderate exercise), I began shedding the pounds. Moreover, my blood glucose levels were finally normalizing after ten years.

I lost twenty-three pounds in seven months with "eating." This is simply amazing! With the continual support from the Website (www.glycemicindex.com) and the wonderful recipes in the newsletter (http://ginews.blogspot.com), it makes the process so much easier. I no longer think I am on a "diet," but eating the "low GI way." I have gone from possibly eating only one meal a day if I was lucky to eating three meals and three snacks a day, and from being so unhealthy and on the road to diabetes and other associated heart and circulatory diseases to being healthy with normal blood glucose levels and so much energy.

10
The GI and Pregnancy

DURING PREGNANCY, a woman's need for almost all nutrients increases and, while her ability to absorb them increases appreciably, the key is the food she eats. Most people are aware of the importance of nutrients such as iron, calcium, folate, and iodine, but what might not be so clear is that the quality of carbohydrate in the diet can also have a significant impact on the growth and development of the baby. There's even evidence that the type of carbohydrate a woman eats can play a role in increasing her fertility.

To understand the connection between the GI of carbohydrate and pregnancy, we need to have a closer look at the importance of glucose to babies.

Babies and Blood Glucose

A woman's body changes during pregnancy to ensure a steady supply of glucose to her baby. Glucose is the main fuel the baby uses to grow, and it crosses freely from mother to baby through the placenta. How much glucose the baby receives depends directly on the mother's blood glucose level and the rate of placental blood flow. The higher the glucose concentration in the mother's blood, the more glucose is transferred to the baby.

In any pregnancy, insulin resistance and increased insulin secretion are normal, as insulin requirements increase by two to three times the mother's normal needs. But for women with a predisposition to diabetes, problems can arise. For example, if the degree of insulin resistance in the mother is too great or if she is unable to make enough extra insulin to meet the demand, her glucose levels will remain elevated. What's more, they will become more elevated as her pregnancy progresses, with insulin demand increasing markedly from twenty-eight weeks' gestation—the stage when gestational diabetes is most commonly diagnosed.

Gestational Diabetes

Gestational diabetes is the name given to the diagnosis of elevated blood glucose levels during pregnancy. It is more likely if a woman has risk factors such as: a family history of diabetes; overweight; older in age; of certain ethnic origin (particularly Native American, Hispanic, African American, Asian American, Pacific Islander, Southern European, Middle Eastern or Southeast Asian descent).

Currently, an estimated 5 to 8 percent of all pregnant women are diagnosed with gestational diabetes. A new study led by the Northwestern University Feinberg School of Medicine in Chicago tracked 23,000 pregnant women in nine countries to determine if the measurements currently used to diagnose gestational diabetes fail to take into account additional risks to mothers and babies. The researchers determined that blood glucose levels previously considered safe or normal in pregnant women actually pose a threat to both the women and their babies. The Northwestern researchers estimate that under the more stringent new measurements, more than 16 percent of pregnant women would be diagnosed with the condition—a doubling or tripling of the current percentage.

The Problem with High Blood Glucose During Pregnancy

Although gestational diabetes doesn't usually develop until twenty-eight weeks' gestation, higher than normal blood glucose levels are a concern whenever they occur in pregnancy. Increased glucose is associated with an increased rate of high blood pressure, preeclampsia, and infection of the placenta (chorioamnionitis).

Furthermore, if a woman's blood glucose level is high, then higher levels of glucose will also be transferred to her baby. From about fifteen weeks, babies make their own insulin to handle glucose. So, extra glucose stimulates the baby's pancreas to make extra insulin. The extra glucose is metabolized and stored, making the baby grow bigger and fatter than normal.

An overly fat baby can present problems for labor and delivery, and the newborn infant is also at risk of low blood glucose (hypoglycemia), low blood calcium (hypocalcemia), jaundice (hyperbilirubinemia), respiratory distress, and a high red-blood-cell count (polycythemia). Any of these conditions may necessitate special medical intervention.

A baby's exposure to high blood glucose also has serious longer term consequences. Children of women who have had gestational diabetes are at greatly increased risk of obesity and glucose intolerance as they grow up. The risk of children becoming overweight adults rises in step with the levels of blood glucose they were exposed to during pregnancy. Untreated gestational diabetes, for example, doubles a child's risk of being overweight or obese by five to seven years of age.

The good news for pregnant women is that by treating elevated glucose levels during pregnancy, the risk of any problems drops considerably. And this is where the GI comes to the fore. Foods with a low GI typically evoke a lower rise in blood glucose levels, making maintenance of normal glucose levels easier. Lower blood glucose elevations after meals mean a lower demand for insulin too, which can lessen the load when the mother's pancreas is struggling.

A recent study in just over 1,000 pregnant women confirmed a relationship between the GI of the women's diets and their glucose levels. The researchers found that the lower the GI of the mom-to-be's diet, the lower her average blood glucose (HbA1c) and the lower her response to a glucose load. So the good news is that following a low GI diet means lower blood glucose levels during pregnancy.

The benefit of a low GI diet in pregnancy has been further demonstrated by an Australian study. The researchers, led by endocrinologist Dr. Robert Moses, compared the outcomes of pregnant women eating either low or high GI diets. Both types of diet were equally nutritious. The babies of mothers eating a low GI diet were of normal size, but were smaller and had less body fat than the babies of mothers eating the moderate to high GI high-fiber, low-sugar diet. This study showed that the GI appears to have a more important effect on birthweight than any single dietary factor, including the amount of protein, fat, or carbohydrate.

The Future Impact of Gestational Diabetes

If you've had gestational diabetes in one pregnancy, you are likely to get it in subsequent pregnancies. You also have a high risk of developing type 2 diabetes at some point later in life. Depending on your risk factors, such as your age, ethnic background, weight, and your glucose levels during pregnancy, that point could be closer than you think. A recent study found one-third of women had developed type 2 diabetes within five years of having gestational diabetes.

If you have had gestational diabetes, . . .

. . . see your doctor every year to be screened for diabetes.

Diabetes Before Pregnancy

When diabetes exists before pregnancy, it greatly increases the risk of birth defects. However, this risk depends almost entirely on a mother's glycemic control before and during her pregnancy. One of the most critical times for good glucose control is during the first seven to eight weeks' gestation, because this is when the baby's major organs are formed.

One of the major events at this time is the formation of the neural tube (the baby's future brain and spinal cord). At this early stage, the baby's pancreas hasn't started working, so its concentration of glucose is a direct reflection of the mom-to-be's blood glucose. When the mother's blood glucose levels are high, the baby is flooded with extra glucose at a rate much greater than normal. Breaking down this glucose requires oxygen, but so much glucose means the baby uses oxygen faster than it can be delivered. The resulting shortage of oxygen is one of the reasons that cells die and malformations occur.

With careful management of blood glucose levels, a woman with diabetes can have a perfectly healthy pregnancy. But, as you might imagine, an unplanned pregnancy along with poor glycemic control could have serious consequences for the unborn child. If the pregnancy is unexpected, a woman can be eight weeks or more pregnant before she knows about it, and if her blood glucose levels are high, damage may already have been done.

The message should be clear:

... if you have diabetes and could get pregnant, make sure you have good blood glucose control first!

If you have diabetes, prediabetes, or even a risk of diabetes, plan pregnancy with good blood glucose levels in mind. Following a low GI diet could help you achieve this. Neural tube defects are linked to poor glycemic control, and a U.S. research study has suggested a link between the GI of a woman's diet during early pregnancy and the risk of her baby developing a neural tube defect.

Reducing Your Risk of Gestational Diabetes

Although pregnancy can unmask a predisposition to diabetes, developing gestational diabetes may not be inevitable, even if you are at risk. Gestational diabetes is the result of a combination of factors—your genetic susceptibility plus risk factors such as a high-fat diet and sedentary lifestyle. So living a healthy lifestyle could reduce your risk.

We know, for example, that being overweight increases your risk of gestational diabetes, but research suggests that eating a diet with a high glycemic load is just as risky. In a U.S. study of more than 10,000 predominantly Caucasian women, those who had a high-glycemic-load diet with low fiber content were twice as likely to develop gestational diabetes as other, similar women, independent of their body mass index.

Eating Well During Pregnancy

In Part 4, we include our ten steps to low GI eating, but here are some extra tips for eating well during pregnancy. We set out clearly the types of foods you need to eat and what a typical day on a healthy low GI diet looks like.

- Eat small, frequent meals.
- Choose low GI breads, breakfast cereals, and rice, and include pasta, fruit, legumes, and low-fat milk and milk products as low GI sources of carbohydrate.
- Include good sources of protein in meals, such as lean meat, poultry, fish, and seafood, eggs, nuts, low-fat cheese, and cottage cheese.

- Eat plenty of vegetables and salads.
- Limit foods high in saturated fat such as cakes, cookies, pastries, sausage, salami, fries, take-out foods, butter, and cream. High saturated fat diets are linked with the development of insulin resistance.
- Limit food and drinks containing large amounts of refined or added sugar or starch with low nutritive value, such as soft drink, sweets, chips, and other packaged snacks.
- Avoid alcohol. Drink plenty of water.
- Use iodized salt—sparingly—in cooking to help prevent iodine deficiency.

Getting Pregnant

If you're having difficulty getting pregnant due to problems with ovulation, a low GI diet could help. Glucose control and insulin sensitivity are important determinants of ovulation and fertility. A study published in *Obstetrics & Gynecology* in 2007 suggested that modifications to diet and lifestyle could prevent most cases of ovulatory infertility. Key dietary aspects favoring fertility were higher consumption of monounsaturated fats rather than trans fats, vegetables rather than animal protein sources, and low GI carbohydrates.

Rachel's Story

About halfway through my second pregnancy, I found out that I had gestational diabetes. I was putting on weight fast and was told that if I didn't change my eating habits, I would be putting the baby—and myself—at risk. I had to see a nutritionist and learn what foods had a low GI. I learned how to eat so my blood glucose stayed level and so my baby continued to gain weight at a healthier pace. The health of my baby was a huge motivator, so I was able to stick to my diet and lose weight everywhere else on my body as my belly expanded a little more slowly. My baby was born a bit large (over nine pounds), but had no blood glucose problems after birth. (Whew!) And I was so pleased with what the low GI diet had done to the rest of my body (my thighs and backside had literally shrunk) that I stayed the course and lost more weight. Within a year of giving birth, I had dropped four sizes from my pre-pregnancy weight. My husband recently joined me in eating more low GI foods, and he's looking and feeling healthier than he has in years.

Your Daily Food Guide for Healthy Eating During Pregnancy

A healthy, low GI diet during pregnancy includes:

- 6–10 servings of low GI breads, cereals, and other starchy carbs
- 2–3 servings of fruit
- 2–3 servings of low-fat milk products or alternatives
- 3 servings of lean meat or alternatives
- 3 servings of healthy fats
- 5–6 servings or more of vegetables

A menu for the day might look something like this:

Breakfast

	Example
1 serving of fruit	4 oz fruit juice
2 servings of low GI bread	2 slices of low GI toast,
1 serving of healthy fats	each spread with 1 teaspoon of canola margarine
1 serving of vegetables	1 large grilled tomato
½ serving of meat or alternative	1 poached egg

Snack

	Example
1 serving of fruit	3 fresh apricots
1 serving of healthy fats	10 almonds

Lunch

	Example
2 servings of low GI carbs	1 cup of steamed basmati rice
1 serving of meat or alternative	4 oz canned tuna or salmon
1 serving of vegetables	1 cup of salad vegetables, such as
1 serving of fat	strips of red pepper, shallots, cucumber, and carrots dressed with 1 tablespoon of oil/vinegar dressing
1 serving of milk or milk product	1 glass of low-fat milk

Snack

	Example
1 serving of milk or milk product	A cup of low-fat fruit yogurt

Dinner	Example
1½ servings of protein	5 oz lean beef steak or chicken
3 servings of vegetables	1½ cups of steamed broccoli, snow peas, carrots, and baby squash dressed with lemon juice
3 servings of low GI carbs	3 baby new potatoes and 1 ear of fresh sweet corn

Snack	Example
1 serving milk product or fruit	A cup of low-fat chocolate milk or a cup of fresh fruit salad

11
The GI and Hypoglycemia

YOUR BODY NEEDS to maintain a minimum threshold level of glucose in the blood at all times to keep the brain and central nervous system functioning. If for some reason blood glucose levels fall below this threshold (specifically, below 70 mg/dL [4 mmol/L], the low end of the normal range), you experience hypoglycemia. It derives from the Greek words *hypo* (meaning under) and *glycemia* (meaning blood glucose)—hence *blood glucose level below normal*.

If you already have diabetes and are treating it with medication, you probably already know all about hypoglycemia. If you don't have diabetes but you have vague health problems, including fatigue and depression, and you think you may have hypoglycemia or someone tells you that you probably have "low blood sugar," you need to see your doctor and get a proper diagnosis.

Hypoglycemia has a variety of unpleasant consequences. Many of these are stresslike symptoms such as anxiety, trembling, sweating, palpitations, dizziness, and nausea. Poor concentration, drowsiness, and lack of coordination may also be experienced. For people with type 1 diabetes, treatment with readily absorbed carbohydrate is essential. Without this, coma and even death may ensue.

This is not the case, however, for people without diabetes who experience "reactive" hypoglycemia, which occurs after eating and is the most common form of hypoglycemia. When blood glucose levels rise too quickly after eating, they cause an excessive amount of insulin to be released. This draws too much glucose out of the blood and causes the blood glucose level to fall below normal. The result is hypoglycemia.

The diagnosis of reactive hypoglycemia *cannot* be made simply on the basis of symptoms. Instead, it requires the detection of low blood glucose levels while the symptoms are actually being experienced. A blood test is required to do this; a home blood glucose meter is not considered precise enough for the diagnosis of hypoglycemia in people without diabetes. Because it may be difficult—or almost impossible— for someone to be in the right place at the right time to have a blood sample taken while experiencing the symptoms, a glucose tolerance test (GTT) is sometimes used to try to make the diagnosis. This involves drinking pure glucose, which causes the blood glucose levels to rise. If too much insulin is produced in response, a person with reactive hypoglycemia will experience an excessive fall in his or her blood glucose level. Sounds simple enough, but there are pitfalls.

Testing must be done under strictly controlled conditions; low blood glucose is best demonstrated by measuring properly collected blood samples. If your doctor uses an oral glucose tolerance test to diagnose hypoglycemia, you have to continue it for at least three to four hours (the normal time is two hours). Your insulin levels would be measured at the same time.

- Hypoglycemia is far less common than once was thought (unless you have diabetes).
- Hypoglycemia due to a serious medical problem is rare.

Treating Hypoglycemia

The aim of treating reactive hypoglycemia is to prevent sudden, large increases in blood glucose levels. If the blood glucose level can be prevented from rising quickly, then excessive, unnecessary amounts of insulin will not be produced and the blood glucose levels will not plunge to abnormally low levels.

Smooth, steady blood glucose levels can readily be achieved by switching from high GI foods to low GI foods. This is particularly important when you eat foods that contain carbohydrates by themselves.

Low GI foods such as whole-grain bread (see page 199), low-fat yogurt, and low GI fruits are best for snacks.

If you can stop the big swings in blood glucose levels, then you will not get the symptoms of reactive hypoglycemia, and chances are you will feel a lot better.

Notably, hypoglycemia due to a serious medical problem is rare. Such conditions require in-depth investigation and treatment of the underlying medical problem causing hypoglycemia. But having an irregular eating pattern is the most common dietary habit seen in people who have hypoglycemia.

How to Help Prevent Hypoglycemia

- Eat regular meals and snacks; plan to eat every three hours.
- Include low GI carbohydrate foods at every meal and for snacks.
- Mix high GI foods with low GI foods in your meals; the combination will give an overall intermediate or medium GI.
- Avoid eating high GI foods on their own for snacks. This can trigger reactive hypoglycemia.

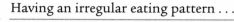 Having an irregular eating pattern . . .

. . . is the most common dietary habit seen in people who have hypoglycemia.

Anne's Story

My life has always been controlled by my hypoglycemia attacks, which almost always occurred in the late afternoon. They were so bad that I couldn't go anywhere without a blood glucose "fix" in my pocket, be it an apple, a package of chocolate-covered nuts and raisins, or a carton of juice. The attacks were awful—I'd lose the ability to concentrate and often even to function because I was so shaky and fatigued—yet my doctors claimed nothing was wrong with me. Finally, I started following a diet that incorporated low GI snacks or meals every two hours. Somewhat to my surprise, my hypoglycemia drastically improved. I still experience minor fluctuations in blood glucose from time to time, but I'll have a little yogurt or an apricot and feel better within minutes. A low GI eating approach has truly changed my life.

12
The GI, Heart Health, and the Metabolic Syndrome

HEART DISEASE is the single biggest killer of people in North America. According to the American Heart Association, every twenty-nine seconds an American has a heart attack or goes into cardiac arrest.

Most heart disease is caused by atherosclerosis, also referred to as "hardening of the arteries." Most people develop atherosclerosis gradually during their lifetime. If it occurs slowly, it may not cause any problems at all, even into old age. But if its development is accelerated by one or more of many processes (such as high cholesterol or high blood glucose levels), it can develop faster and cause trouble sooner.

Knowing your blood glucose level . . .

. . . is just as important as knowing your cholesterol level in helping to prevent heart disease.

Atherosclerosis leads to reduced blood flow through the affected arteries. In the heart, this can mean that the heart muscle does not receive enough oxygen to provide the power for pumping blood, and it changes in such a way that it causes pain (in particular, central chest pain, or angina pectoris). Elsewhere in the body, atherosclerosis has a similar blood-flow–reducing effect: in the legs, it can cause muscle pains during exercise; in the brain, it can cause a variety of problems, from irregular gait to strokes.

An even more serious consequence of atherosclerosis occurs when a blood clot forms over the surface of a patch of atherosclerosis in an artery. This process, called thrombosis, can result in a complete blockage of the artery, with consequences ranging from sudden death to a small heart attack from which the patient recovers quickly.

Thrombosis can happen elsewhere in the body, and the extent of it determines how serious it is. The probability of developing thrombosis depends on the tendency of the blood to clot versus the natural ability of the blood to break down clots (fibrinolysis). These two counteracting tendencies are influenced by a number of factors, including the level of glucose in the blood.

People who have gradually developed atherosclerosis of the arteries to the heart (which are called the coronary arteries) may gradually develop reduced heart function. For a while, the heart may be able to compensate for the problem, so there are no symptoms, but eventually the heart begins to fail. It might start with shortness of breath, initially on exercise, and there may sometimes be swelling of the ankles.

Modern medicine has many effective drug treatments for heart failure, so this consequence of atherosclerosis does not now have quite the same serious implications it had in the past.

Why Do People Get Heart Disease?

Atherosclerotic heart disease develops early in life when the many factors that cause it have a strong influence. Over many decades, doctors and scientists have identified the risk factors (what we call red flags) in healthy people as well as in those with established heart disease. Your risk of developing heart disease is determined by things you cannot change, such as genetic (inherited) factors, and things you can do something about.

Risk Factor: Smoking

Smokers have more than twice the risk of heart attack as nonsmokers and are much more likely to die if they suffer a heart attack. Smoking is also the most preventable risk factor for heart disease. Smokers tend to eat fewer fruits and vegetables compared with nonsmokers (and thus miss out on vital protective antioxidant plant compounds). Smokers also tend to eat more fat and more salt than nonsmokers. While these dietary differences may put the smoker at greater risk of heart disease, there is only one piece of advice for anyone who smokes: quit.

Risk Factor: High Blood Pressure

High blood pressure is the most common heart disease risk factor. High blood pressure (hypertension) is harmful because it demands that your heart work harder and it damages your arteries.

An artery is a muscular tube. Healthy arteries can change their size to control the flow of blood. High blood pressure causes changes in the walls of arteries, which makes atherosclerosis more likely to develop. Blood clots can then form, and the weakened blood vessels can easily develop a thrombosis (clot) or rupture and bleed.

Risk Factors for Heart Disease

Risk factors you cannot change:
- Being male
- Being older
- Your ethnic background
- A family history of heart disease
- Being postmenopausal

Risk factors you can do something about:
- Smoking
- High blood pressure
- Diabetes or prediabetes
- High blood cholesterol, high triglycerides, and low levels of the "good" (HDL) cholesterol
- Elevated CRP (C-reactive protein) levels (a marker of low-grade chronic inflammation somewhere in the body)
- Being overweight or obese, or having extra fat around your abdomen
- Being sedentary

Risk Factor: Diabetes and Prediabetes

Diabetes and prediabetes cause inflammation and hardening of the arteries. High levels of glucose in the blood, even short-term spikes after a meal, can have many undesirable effects and are a predictor of future heart disease. A high level of glucose in the blood means:

- The cells lining the arteries absorb excessive amounts of glucose.
- Highly reactive charged particles called "free radicals" are formed, which gradually destroy the machinery inside the cell, eventually causing the cell's death.
- Glucose adheres to cholesterol in the blood, which promotes the formation of fatty plaque and prevents the body from breaking down cholesterol.
- Higher levels of insulin develop, which in turn raise blood pressure and blood fats, while suppressing "good" (HDL) cholesterol levels. High insulin levels also increase the tendency for blood clots to form. This is why so much effort is put into helping people with diabetes achieve normal control of blood glucose levels. Even when cholesterol levels appear to be normal, other risk factors, such as triglycerides, can be highly abnormal.

Even moderately raised blood glucose levels before or after a meal have been associated with increased risk of heart disease in normal "healthy" people.

Risk Factor: High Blood Cholesterol

Cholesterol is vital for healthy cells. It is so important that our bodies can make most of the cholesterol we need—about 1,000 mg per day. But in certain circumstances, we make more than necessary. This causes the level of cholesterol in our blood to build up, and that's when we have a problem. When the body accumulates too much cholesterol, it can be deposited on the walls of the arteries, which become bloated, damaged, and may become blocked.

Having high blood cholesterol is partly determined by our genes, which can "set" the cholesterol level slightly high and which we cannot change, and partly by lifestyle or dietary factors, which push it up further—which we can do something about.

A diet high in saturated fat is the biggest contributor. Diets recommended for lowering blood cholesterol are low in saturated fat, high in good carbohydrate (particularly whole grains; see page 199), and high in fiber.

There are some relatively rare genetic conditions in which particularly high blood cholesterol levels occur. People who have inherited these conditions need a thorough examination by a specialist doctor followed by a rigorous cholesterol-lowering eating plan combined with drug treatment to reduce and control the risk of heart disease.

Even moderately raised blood glucose levels . . .

. . . before or after a meal have been associated with increased risk of heart disease in normal "healthy" people.

What about the Good HDL Cholesterol?

HDL (high-density lipoprotein) cholesterol seems to protect us against heart disease because it clears cholesterol from our arteries and helps its removal from our bodies. Having low levels of HDL in the blood is one of the most important markers of heart disease.

What about LDL Cholesterol—the Bad Cholesterol?
LDL (low-density lipoprotein) cholesterol does the most damage to the blood vessels. It's a red flag for heart disease.

What about Triglycerides?
The blood also contains triglycerides, another type of fat linked to increased risk of heart disease. Having too much triglyceride is often linked with having too little HDL cholesterol. Although people can inherit the tendency to have excess levels of triglycerides, it's most often associated with being overweight or obese.

Risk Factor: CRP (C-Reactive Protein)
Scientists have recently established that CRP in the blood is a powerful risk factor for heart disease. A measure of chronic low-grade inflammation anywhere in the body, it shows the damaging effect of high glucose levels and other factors on the blood vessel walls.

Studies at Harvard University have shown that CRP levels are higher in women consuming high GI/high GL diets. That's one more good reason to choose low GI!

Risk Factor: Being Overweight or Obese,
or Having Extra Fat around Your Abdomen

Overweight and obese people are more likely to have high blood pressure and diabetes. They are also at increased risk of developing heart disease. Some of that increased risk is due to high blood pressure and the tendency to diabetes, but there is a separate, "independent" effect of the obesity.

When increased fatness develops, it can be distributed evenly all over the body or it may occur centrally—in and around the abdomen. The latter is strongly associated with heart disease. In fact, you can have "middle-age spread"—a potbelly or a "muffin top"—and still be within a normal weight range. But that extra fat around the middle is playing havoc with your metabolism. Abdominal fat increases your risk of heart disease, high blood pressure, and diabetes. In contrast, fat on the lower part of the body, such as hips and thighs, doesn't carry the same health risk.

A Healthy Waist

The International Diabetes Foundation has established new criteria for defining metabolic syndrome that reduce waist circumference thresholds, making it easier for doctors to identify people who have the condition. (A person with metabolic syndrome will have abdominal obesity plus at least two of the following other risk factors: high triglycerides, low HDL cholesterol, elevated blood pressure, and/or increased blood glucose.) The recommended limits of waist measurement are:

For people of European origin:
Men   37 inches (94 cm)
Women   31.5 inches (80 cm)

For people from South Asia, China, and Japan:
Men   35.5 inches (90 cm)
Women   31.5 inches (80 cm)

More information is available at www.idf.org/home.

Risk Factor: Being Sedentary

People who aren't active or don't exercise have higher rates of death and heart disease compared with people who perform even mild to moderate amounts of physical activity. Even gardening or going for a walk can lower your risk of heart disease.

Exercise and activity speed up your metabolic rate (increasing the amount of energy you use), which helps to balance your food intake and control your weight. Exercise and activity also make your muscles more sensitive to insulin (you'll need less to get the job done) and increase the amount of fat you burn.

Treating Heart Disease

When heart disease is detected, two types of treatment are typically given. First, the effects of the disease are treated (for example, medical treatment with drugs and surgical treatment to bypass blocked arteries); and, second, the risk factors are treated in order to slow down further progression of the disease.

Treatment of risk factors after the disease has already developed is secondary prevention. In people who have not yet developed the disease, treatment of risk factors is primary prevention.

Preventing Heart Disease

Thankfully, more and more people have their blood pressure tested and are checked for diabetes regularly. Increasingly, blood-fat tests are done to check people's risk factors for heart disease as well. If you haven't been checked recently, ask your doctor for these tests.

A good health professional will offer lifestyle advice that can reduce your risk of heart disease, including stopping smoking, regular exercise, and eating a healthy diet. But often, people find it difficult to follow this advice for long. This is especially true if heart disease isn't an immediate and life-threatening problem. But remember that it's better to take steps to be healthy today than to wait until heart disease has dramatically impaired your health.

The effect of exercise doesn't end when you stop moving. People who exercise have higher metabolic rates, and their bodies burn more calories per minute even when they are asleep.

Understanding the Metabolic Syndrome and Insulin Resistance

Surveys show that one in two adults over the age of twenty-five has at least two features of what is seen to be a silent disease: the metabolic syndrome, or insulin resistance syndrome. This syndrome (sometimes called syndrome X) is a collection of metabolic abnormalities that can "silently" increase your risk of heart attack. The list of features is getting longer and longer, and the number of diseases linked to insulin resistance is growing.

People with metabolic syndrome are three times as likely to have a heart attack or stroke compared with people without the syndrome, and they have a fivefold greater risk of developing type 2 diabetes (if it's not already present).

The metabolic syndrome is a cluster of risk factors for a serious heart attack, recognized as a "cardiovascular time bomb." In 2005, the International Diabetes Federation agreed on a definition of metabolic syndrome to make it easier for doctors to identify people who are at risk. A person with metabolic syndrome will have extra fat around the abdomen plus two of the following risk factors:

- High triglycerides
- Low HDL cholesterol
- Raised blood glucose
- Raised blood pressure

The key to understanding metabolic syndrome is insulin resistance, which we discussed in Chapter 8. Tests on people with the metabolic syndrome show that insulin resistance is very common. If your doctor has told you that you have high blood pressure and prediabetes (formerly, you might have been advised you have "a touch of sugar" or "impaired glucose tolerance"), then you probably have metabolic syndrome.

Carol's Story

I just came from a visit with my dietitian. I got a positive report. My A1c is at 6.7 and overall cholesterol is down from 195 to 61. Triglycerides 11—down from 161; LDL 117—down from 133. At two hundred pounds, it was a big adjustment for me to regulate my diet. I had lost seventeen pounds in the first ten days. I continued to stay away from coffee, sugar (refined), or any processed food.

It was difficult to prepare my own meals; I received pointers from my dietitian, but my daughter-in-law had done some low GI eating, and she pointed me in the right direction. Soon I was able to prepare and freeze low GI meals for myself on the weekends.

After recommending the New Glucose Revolution *books, my dietitian remarked how well I had done. She said I should be the poster child for the low GI diet because with my evening snack of plain yogurt, strawberries, and almonds, I have incorporated six small frequent meals into my day. In doing so, I have lost fifty-five pounds, and my body mass index (BMI) has gone from 35 to 25. I am no longer considered obese, and I am only 1 point away from a normal BMI. Only four more pounds!*

The GI and Heart Health

The GI is vitally important for coronary health and the prevention of heart disease. First, it has benefits for weight control (see Chapter 7), helping to satisfy appetite and preventing overeating. Second, it helps reduce post-meal blood glucose levels. This improves the elasticity of the walls of the arteries, making dilation easier and improving blood flow. Third, blood fats and clotting factors can also be improved by low GI diets. Studies have shown that HDL levels are correlated with the GI and GL of the diet. People with the lowest GI diets have the highest and best levels of HDL—the good cholesterol.

 By working on several fronts at once, . . .

. . . a low GI diet has a distinct advantage over other types of diets or drugs that target only one risk factor at a time.

Furthermore, research studies in people with diabetes have shown that low GI diets reduce triglycerides in the blood, a factor strongly linked to heart disease. Last, low GI diets have been shown to improve insulin sensitivity in people at high risk of heart disease, thereby helping to reduce the increase in blood glucose and insulin levels after eating.

The Weight of Evidence

One major study provides the strongest evidence in support of the role of GI in heart disease. Conducted by Harvard University and commonly referred to as the Nurses' Health Study, this ongoing, long-term study follows over 100,000 nurses, who every few years provide their personal health and diet information to researchers at Harvard School of Public Health.

The Nurses' Health Study found that those who ate more high GI foods had nearly twice the risk of having a heart attack over a ten-year period of follow-up compared with those eating low GI diets. This association was independent of dietary fiber and other known risk factors, such as age and body mass index, or BMI (see page 351). In other words, even if fiber intake was high, there was still an adverse effect of high GI diets on risk. Importantly, neither sugar nor total carbohydrate intake showed any association with risk of heart attack. That means there was no evidence that lower carbohydrate or lower sugar intake was beneficial.

One of the most important findings of the Nurses' Health Study was that the increased risk associated with high GI diets was largely seen in those with a BMI over 23. There was no increased risk in those under 23. The great majority of adults, however, have a BMI greater than 23; indeed, a BMI of 23 to 25 is considered normal weight. The implication then is that the insulin resistance that comes with increasing weight is an integral part of the disease process.

If you are very lean and insulin sensitive, high GI diets won't make you more prone to heart attack. This might explain why traditional Asian populations, such as the Chinese, who eat high GI rice as a staple food, do not show increased risk of heart disease. Their low BMI and their high level of physical activity work together to keep them insulin sensitive and extremely carbohydrate tolerant.

Research shows that low GI diets not only improve blood glucose in people with diabetes, but they also improve the sensitivity of the body to insulin.

In a recent study, patients with serious disease of the coronary arteries were given either low or high GI diets before surgery for coronary bypass grafts. They were given blood tests before their diets and just before surgery. During surgery, small pieces of fat tissue were removed for testing. The tests on the fat showed that the low GI diets made the tissues of these "insulin insensitive" patients more sensitive. In fact, they were back in the same range as normal control patients after just a few weeks on the low GI diet.

In another study, young women in their thirties were divided into those who did and those who did not have a family history of heart disease and had not yet developed the condition. They had blood tests, followed by low or high GI diets for four weeks, after which they had more blood tests. When they had surgery (for conditions unrelated to heart disease), pieces of fat were removed and tested for insulin sensitivity. The young women with a family history of heart disease were insensitive to insulin originally (those without the family history of heart disease were normal), but after four weeks on the low GI diet, their insulin sensitivity was back within the normal range.

In both studies, the diets were designed to try to ensure that all the other variables (total energy, total carbohydrates) were not different, so that the change in insulin sensitivity was likely to have been due to the low GI diet rather than any other factor.

Recent research reported . . .

. . . in the *British Journal of Nutrition* found that eating just one extra low GI item per meal can lower blood glucose levels and reduce the risk of metabolic syndrome.

Work on these exciting findings continues, but what is known so far strongly suggests that a low GI diet not only improves body weight and blood glucose in people with diabetes, but also improves the body's sensitivity to insulin.

It will take many years of further research to show that this simple dietary change to a low GI diet will definitely slow the progress of atherosclerotic heart disease. In the meantime, it is already clear that risk factors for heart disease are reduced by a low GI diet.

Low GI diets are consistent with the other required dietary changes needed for prevention of heart disease. For an even more in-depth discussion of the metabolic syndrome, heart health, and the GI, you may want to consult *The New Glucose Revolution Low GI Guide to Metabolic Syndrome and Your Heart.*

And as we've already stressed, you'll find much dietary guidance about how to adopt and eat the heart-healthy, low GI way in Part 4, Your Guide to Low GI Eating.

A low GI diet . . .

. . . not only improves body weight and blood glucose in people with diabetes, but it also improves the body's sensitivity to insulin.

13

The GI and Polycystic Ovarian Syndrome (PCOS)

POLYCYSTIC OVARIAN SYNDROME, or PCOS, often goes unrecognized, yet it is very common. Elements of the disease are believed to affect one in four women in developed nations; the severe form affects one in twenty. It is a health condition linked with hormone imbalance and insulin resistance.

The signs range from subtle symptoms, such as faint facial hair, to a "full house" of symptoms—lack of periods, heavy body-hair growth, obstinate central body fat, and infertility. They can occur at any age and can even be seen in girls as young as ten or women as old as seventy. (Contrary to popular belief, PCOS does not suddenly disappear at menopause.)

Not only are the symptoms distressing, but PCOS has also been tied to an increased risk of heart disease and type 2 diabetes. You may also see it referred to as polycystic ovarian disease, Stein-Leventhal syndrome, or functional ovarian hyperandrogenism.

Only a doctor can diagnose PCOS. If you have any of the following symptoms, you should see your general practitioner and ask him or her to refer you to an endocrinologist for proper diagnosis and treatment:

- Delayed (or early) puberty
- Irregular or no periods
- Acne

- Excess body or facial hair
- Unexplained fatigue
- Excess weight around the waistline
- Infertility
- Mood swings
- Hot flashes in young women
- Sleep disorders such as sleep apnea or insomnia
- Recurrent spontaneous miscarriages
- Inappropriate lactation
- Drop in blood pressure when standing up or with exercise
- Rough, dark skin in the neck folds and armpits, a mark of severe insulin resistance from any cause
- Hypoglycemia (low blood glucose) after meals. (The most common symptoms are light-headedness, sweating, sudden fatigue, and a "butterflies in the stomach" feeling.)

It is vital to diagnose and treat PCOS as early as possible to prevent it from developing to the "full house" stage. Keep in mind that some women do not show the classic signs at all, which is why consulting a doctor who knows the many facets of PCOS is so important.

Insulin Resistance and PCOS

Most women with PCOS have severe insulin resistance (see Chapter 8) and, as a result, high insulin levels. The problem is that insulin stimulates the growth and multiplication of cells in the ovary—in particular, those that make up the bulk of the ovary in which the eggs are embedded, causing them to become cystic. This flood of insulin leads to a vicious cycle of hormonal imbalance that creates the symptoms of PCOS.

The receptors for insulin in the ovaries are different from those in other tissues; when blood insulin levels are high, the ovary fails to adjust insulin receptor numbers accordingly or reduce their activity. The action of insulin continues unabated, and ovarian cells grow, multiply, and increase their metabolic activity. The result is excessive production of both male sex hormone (testosterone) and female sex hormone (estrogen).

High testosterone levels in women bring about male characteristics in women, such as weight gain and excessive hair on the face and in other areas. Excess insulin and sex hormones also stimulate an area in the brain called the hypothalamus, making it more sensitive and causing it to secrete more luteinizing hormone. This stimulates the ovaries' hormone production even more, causing a vicious cycle. Breaking that cycle is the key to managing PCOS successfully.

Insulin resistance . . .

. . . leads to a vicious cycle of hormonal imbalance that creates the symptoms of PCOS.

Insulin resistance is more common in some people than others; for example, people of Asian descent have been found to be more resistant than Caucasians. Native American, Australian Aboriginals, and Pacific Islanders are more insulin resistant than others. Not surprisingly, PCOS also runs in families and may have a genetic link.

Environmental factors such as diet and a lack of physical exercise may also play a role. We also know that weight gain can trigger insulin resistance and PCOS, as can certain steroid medications. While being overweight or obese increases the degree of insulin resistance, you can be lean and still have PCOS.

Managing PCOS

Although there's no cure as such for PCOS, keeping the symptoms under control is well within your grasp by making some diet and lifestyle changes that will encourage hormonal stabilization.

When you see your doctor, you'll find that any medical management is usually tailored to your symptoms and to some extent your priorities—regular periods, a much-wanted pregnancy, or simply a reduction in facial hair. It usually involves lifestyle changes such as eating well and moving more, along with insulin-sensitizing medication, such as metformin, to:

- Improve your PCOS symptoms—regulating menstrual cycles and reducing acne and excess hair growth.
- Achieve and maintain a healthy weight.
- Control your blood glucose and insulin levels.
- Stabilize your hormone levels.

- Boost fertility.
- Give you more control and improve your quality of life.

The one thing women with PCOS say again and again is that they feel "out of control"—gaining weight, being unable to get pregnant, growing an excessive amount of body hair in areas where it shouldn't be, and so on. The good news is that by making some basic lifestyle changes—like choosing the right kinds of foods and exercising more—you'll find yourself back in the driver's seat again. An additional benefit of making these changes is that you will reduce your future risk of developing diabetes and heart disease. Here are some steps toward taking charge.

Step 1: Manage Your Weight

Managing your weight is essential if you have PCOS. That's because being overweight increases insulin resistance and worsens the symptoms of PCOS. You don't need to lose a lot of weight—or body fat—to improve your symptoms. Studies show that losing as little as 5 percent of body weight can help improve menstrual function, reduce testosterone levels, reduce excess hair growth, and lessen acne. How much weight does this actually mean? Well, if you weigh 200 pounds, this means losing about 10 pounds of body fat can make a difference; if you're 154 pounds, losing just 8 pounds would bring about a change.

So what's the healthiest way to lose weight? First of all, aim to lose body *fat* rather than simply *weight*. Put the scales away and get out the tape measure, or even go by how your clothes fit. Remember, muscle weighs more than fat, so as you begin to exercise more, you may be shedding fat but adding muscle, meaning the scale might not reflect just how much you're changing.

Second, don't think about going on a restrictive diet, as it will only make you feel deprived and lead to a binge. Instead, incorporate low GI foods into a healthy diet.

Third, be patient; it takes time to lose weight.

And last, get moving. Regular physical activity every day not only will help you get fit and trim, but will also improve your heart and bone health, reduce your risk of diabetes, and help you manage stress.

Step 2: Eat the Healthy, Low GI Way

The GI plays a key role in helping you beat PCOS symptoms because it focuses on carbohydrates—their quantity and quality, and their overall effect on your blood glucose. Controlling your blood glucose levels is the first step to increasing your insulin sensitivity. If you base your diet on eating balanced low GI meals, you will make it easier for your body to burn fat and less likely for the fat to be stored in places where you don't want it.

A healthy, low GI eating plan should include the following foods every day:

- Fresh vegetables and salads
- Fresh fruit
- Low GI whole-grain breads (with lots of grainy bits and/or made with intact kernels) and cereals
- Low-fat dairy products or nondairy alternatives like soy
- Fish, lean meat, chicken, eggs, legumes, and soy products
- Small amounts of healthy fats such as nuts, seeds, avocados, olives, olive oil, canola oil, or peanut oil

If you find it hard to get started, get help from a registered dietitian (see "How to Find a Dietitian," on page 48).

Step 3: Move More

Activity and exercise are crucial if you want to manage PCOS, as they help you control your weight, manage your insulin, and make a real difference in your health and energy levels. Exercise improves insulin sensitivity so that your body needs to secrete less insulin each time you eat. Ideally, you should try to fit in activity on most days.

Research shows that just thirty minutes of moderate intensity exercise each day can help improve your health, lowering your risk of heart disease and diabetes, among many other health problems. Busy schedule? Break the thirty minutes down into two sessions of fifteen minutes or even three sessions of ten minutes, and you'll still enjoy the same benefits. That said, if you're trying to lose weight, the more you can exercise, the better!

A balanced exercise program, including aerobic, resistance or "strength" training, and flexibility/stretching exercises will give you the best results. And don't forget to vary your activities; the body becomes efficient at anything it does repeatedly, so after a while, you won't see results unless you vary the type of activity or intensity.

Step 4: Take Care of Yourself

Eating well and being active are the cornerstones of managing PCOS, but there are a few other things you can do to help yourself. Stress reduction is at the top of the list.

Stress is a part of life for most of us and can't be avoided. The key is to be able to manage it effectively, which is absolutely crucial for women with PCOS, because too much stress can affect hormonal balance, increase blood glucose levels, and lead to overeating. You can get a handle on the stress in your life by starting a stress-reduction program, getting regular exercise, taking time out for activities you enjoy, and finding someone to talk to about your feelings. If need be, talk to a counselor or therapist.

Enough good-quality sleep is also important. A lack of sleep—that means less than eight hours for the average person—can reduce immunity, increase stress hormones, and worsen insulin resistance. If you've cut down on stress, started exercising regularly, and don't drink alcohol or caffeinated beverages before bed but still have difficulty sleeping, see your doctor to find out if you may have a sleep disorder, or if medication and/or cognitive behavioral therapy may help.

For more information, see *The Low GI Guide to Living Well with PCOS*.

Karen's Story

About eighteen months ago, at age twenty-eight, I was diagnosed with PCOS. I'd been overweight for most of my twenties and had a history of irregular periods. It had been six months since my last period and I knew I wasn't pregnant, so my doctor ran some tests. Then she broke the news—it was PCOS in combination with insulin resistance. It was a real wake-up call. The doctor suggested the drug metformin to help with my weight and regulate my periods. The concept of being on a daily medication for the rest of my life just to combat my symptoms was unacceptable. So I began to educate myself on my condition and alternatives to medication. I learned about the GI and the importance of regular exercise. Then I set about changing my life by incorporating both, and, surprisingly, it wasn't that hard to do. Now, three weeks away from my thirtieth birthday, I can honestly say I am the happiest I've ever been. I exercise most days; eat a healthy, low GI diet; and have a normal menstrual cycle. Not to mention I've lost over twenty-eight pounds!

14
The GI and Children

IF CHILDREN LEARN to combine regular physical activity with healthy, low GI eating, they will be in top condition throughout their lives. It's never too late to start. The importance of teaching children about good nutrition by providing healthy nutritious foods and by setting a good example cannot be overemphasized. It's a win-win situation, too: if you set a good example by eating well and being active, you will also feel fitter and healthier.

Children need our guidance . . .

. . . to learn how to respect their health and look after their bodies. Helping them develop good eating habits and be active every day is part of this.

Children growing up in the United States and Canada today face very different challenges and health concerns from those of any previous generation. About 30 percent of children and teenagers in the United States are overweight—a statistic that reflects a more than threefold increase in the percentage of overweight children and adolescents since the mid-1960s. But today's diet and lifestyle aren't just creating obesity:

■ School children are showing signs of risk factors for heart disease.

- Type 2 diabetes, once known as "maturity onset diabetes," is appearing in children as young as eight.
- A U.S. study found that one in five teenagers (fifteen- to sixteen-year-olds) has raised insulin levels, putting him or her at risk of type 2 diabetes; 9 percent of boys in this age group have signs of liver damage, and 10 percent have raised blood fats.

The increasing proportion of calories children consume from high GI carbs like doughnuts, white bread, burger buns, corn flakes, cookies, pastries, potato chips, snacks, corn chips, and French fries is a key aspect of today's diet linked to increasing their risk of diabetes, heart disease, and obesity. Managing these lifestyle diseases requires a holistic approach.

Many young people, . . .

. . . toddlers to teens, eat fast food up to four times a week.

In this chapter, you will discover how healthy low GI eating has benefits for all children, just as it does for adults, and how it can make a difference to your family's long-term well-being.

Of course, most of us (parents and children) need to make sure we turn off the television and shut down the computers and move more, too. On page 125, we look at the active side of the equation, and in Chapter 15, we cover the fat-burning benefits of exercise.

How Can the GI Help?
Children Who Are Overweight or Obese
It's no fun being fat in a world that equates attractiveness with body shape. Maintaining high self-esteem can be very difficult for overweight or obese children. They need support, acceptance, and encouragement from their parents. They need to know that they are okay, whatever their weight. If you have a child who is overweight or obese, the best approach is to get the whole family living a healthier lifestyle.

There's no simple solution to this problem, but part of any management plan for school children and teenagers who are overweight or obese is altering the balance.

First of all, we can't stress enough the importance of physical activity, and we discuss this further on page 125, "The Active Side of the Healthy Kids Equation." Remember, your kids may not always hear what you tell them to do, but they sure notice what you do (or don't do) when it comes to activity and healthy eating.

Second, don't put your child on a diet unless under the guidance of a qualified health professional who has experience in managing childhood obesity. An overweight child may not need to lose a lot of weight, but her weight gain may need to slow down while she grows into her existing weight.

The proportion of overweight or obese children in the population has tripled in the last forty years. In the United States, on average, one in five children is overweight or obese, but in some areas, it is as high as one in three. And high GI diets could be making things worse. When we eat foods with a high GI, the peaking glucose and insulin levels can stimulate a sequence of hormonal changes that can trigger overeating.

Dr. David Ludwig, director of the Optimal Weight for Life Program at the Children's Hospital Boston in the United States, demonstrated this effect by asking obese teenage boys to eat high, medium, or low GI breakfasts and then observing their food intake for the rest of the day. As expected, after the high GI breakfast of instant oatmeal, the boys' blood glucose and insulin levels rose the highest, then crashed back down. When their first meal had been high GI, the boys then consumed almost twice as many calories in the food they chose in the later part of the day. (See diagram below.)

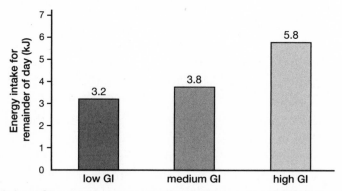

Figure 9: Low GI meals are more satiating. Voluntary food intake in twelve obese teenage boys following test breakfast and lunch of varying GI.

Falling blood glucose levels and other hormones send us in search of something else to eat. To make matters worse, the high insulin levels after a high GI meal temporarily switch off the release of fatty acids from fat tissue, making it even harder to burn off those extra calories.

In a study from the U.K., researchers confirmed that a low GI breakfast is more satiating for children than a high GI breakfast. On days when children ate a low GI breakfast, they ate a significantly smaller lunch and vice versa; when breakfast was high GI, they reported feeling significantly more hungry at lunchtime.

A Low GI Versus a High GI Breakfast

Giving children a low GI breakfast can reduce their food intake for the rest of the day; it's as simple as changing their cereal. The following examples are the actual breakfast choices offered to children in the U.K. study:

Low GI	High GI
All-Bran	Corn Flakes
Muesli	Cocoa Krispies
Traditional oatmeal	Rice Krispies
Soy-flaxseed bread	Regular white bread

In his outpatient obesity management program, Ludwig has confirmed that children eating a low GI diet lose significantly more weight than those on a standard reduced-fat diet. On a low GI diet, the children feel less hungry and decrease their food intake naturally without being told to restrict calories deliberately.

Children Who Have Fatty Liver

Another condition linked to obesity is the increasing prevalence of fatty liver in children. Nonalcoholic fatty liver disease (so named because it is liver disease in the absence of regular alcohol consumption), or NAFL, is estimated to affect one in three obese children.

The buildup of fat in the liver can progress to hepatitis, scarring of the liver, cirrhosis, and liver failure. Researchers have speculated that our high GI diet may be contributing to this condition. By boosting insulin levels, a high GI diet signals the liver to make fat from food energy and store it. Insulin levels are far higher in obese children than in nonobese, and there is evidence from animal studies that a high GI diet increases fat deposits throughout the body, including the liver.

Trials are currently underway in children to investigate whether a low GI diet can reverse fatty liver disease. By improving insulin sensitivity, a low GI diet could, at the very least, improve the metabolic conditions that contribute to this condition.

Children with Type 2 Diabetes

Along with obesity come escalating numbers of children with type 2 diabetes. The link between type 2 diabetes in children and obesity is very strong; around 80 percent of children with the condition are obese.

Because the development of type 2 diabetes lags several years behind that of obesity, we are just experiencing the beginning of the type 2 diabetes epidemic in children and adolescents. Given the current obesity rates, it is almost inevitable that there will be an epidemic of type 2 diabetes if we don't start doing something about it—right now!

What's so bad about developing type 2 diabetes at a young age? Children with type 2 diabetes are believed to face the same risk of heart attack, stroke, impotence, blindness, and kidney disease as adults. But don't these health problems only happen to old people? The shocking thing is, these people won't be old; children with type 2 diabetes will be developing these complications at the peak of their adult lives when their working and earning capacity is greatest. The implications for an individual are shocking, and the public health burden is overwhelming.

If you have type 2 diabetes, then your children are at risk, as there is a strong family link.

Children with Type 1 Diabetes

At present, half the people with type 1 diabetes are diagnosed before they are sixteen years old. For young people who are still growing and developing, it's vital to do everything possible to achieve and maintain optimal blood glucose levels. Poorly managed diabetes, particularly before puberty, can mean that children don't achieve their full growth potential. And they don't get a chance to go back and try again!

It's no mean feat keeping blood glucose levels within the recommended range without too many episodes of hypoglycemia or hyperglycemia. But studies in the United States and Australia show that the quality of the carbohydrate consumed can be particularly relevant to glycemic control in children with type 1 diabetes.

For example, in Heather Gilbertson's study of almost a hundred children with type 1 diabetes at the Royal Children's Hospital in Melbourne, the children and their parents reported that a low GI eating plan was more flexible and family-friendly than the traditional carbohydrate exchange regime, and the researchers found it achieved significantly lower HbA1c levels.

For children with type 1 diabetes, their blood glucose response to foods can vary dramatically, depending on the GI of the food (of course, it can vary depending on lots of other factors as well). For example, regular white bread will result in two and a half times the increase in blood glucose compared to eating the same amount of carbohydrate from barley or chickpeas.

In theory, lowering the GI of the diet in type 1 diabetes could be useful to:

- Reduce blood glucose levels after meals
- Decrease the chance of hypoglycemia (low blood glucose)
- Reduce insulin requirements
- Reduce the risk of diabetes complications

The Active Side of the Healthy Kids Equation

Of course, what children eat is only one-half of the equation to a healthy lifestyle. Regular physical activity is important for adults and no less so for children. Although they tend to run around and move a lot naturally, influences of modern society such as electronic games, computers, and DVDs can have an insidious effect by decreasing children's exercise. Reduced physical activity is a major contributor to obesity, and children who are less physically active are also more insulin resistant (increasing their risk of type 2 diabetes). When looking at your child's lifestyle, think about ways to decrease sedentary behavior and increase both planned and incidental activity.

Decreasing the sedentary side of the equation usually means limiting TV (and other small- or big-screen) time. There is very good evidence relating TV viewing to obesity. One study found that children who watched TV for more than two hours per day were more likely to consume high-energy snacks and drinks and less likely to participate in organized sports. The current viewing average for children ages eight to eighteen in the United States is about four hours per day, which doesn't paint a very good picture for the future of obesity in our children.

To successfully increase incidental and planned activity for your children, you need to exercise yourself. Parental activity is a strong predictor of a child's activity, so take a look at your own lifestyle and how you could be more active.

For incidental activity, get your children involved in helping with household tasks, including dressing themselves and doing laundry once they are old enough, and in active family activities such as shopping, maintaining the garden, and walking the dog.

Planned activity can mean participating in organized sports such as basketball, football, baseball, hockey, etc. But if your child is not interested, there are plenty of other things he can do, like riding a bike, going for a swim, or a walk, dancing, or practicing a martial art. Whatever your children choose, make sure they enjoy it; if they don't, try something else.

Like adults, children need to do at least thirty minutes of some kind of physical activity most days of the week just to maintain good health. To lose weight, they need to at least double that.

Helping Kids Keep Thinking

When you realize that our brains require a steady supply of glucose to function properly, it makes sense that the GI of a meal and the ensuing blood glucose levels can affect our ability to think. Studies in adults have suggested that low GI meals resulted in better mental performance. To investigate this in children, researchers gave six- to eleven-year-olds either a low GI breakfast (All-Bran, GI 42) or a high GI breakfast (Cocoa Krispies, GI 77). Following breakfast, the children were asked to complete a number of computerized tests of attention and memory for the next three hours. The results indicated, perhaps not surprisingly, that the children's thinking skills declined during the morning, but the rate of the decline was significantly slower following the low GI cereal breakfast, compared to the high GI cereal.

The message is clear: . . .

. . . to keep children thinking better for longer
during the school morning, make sure they eat
a low GI breakfast!

Putting the GI to Work in Children's Diets

A low GI diet is safe and adaptable for everyone, including children. It is adaptable to different cultural backgrounds and is, by nature, packed with nutrients essential to good health.

A healthy diet for children:

- allows for good health and growth,
- satisfies the appetite,
- establishes good eating habits,
- allows for varied and interesting meals and snacks,
- accommodates the child's usual routines and activities, and
- maintains a healthy body weight.

To put the GI to work in your family, all you really need to focus on are your children's carbohydrate choices; choose low GI breads, cereals, cookies, rice, potatoes, etc. The low GI options are listed in the tables at the back of this book. However, it's difficult, even for us, to talk about using low GI foods without looking at how they fit into the rest of the diet.

The foods children eat are very much a factor of their age and stage, their family and peer group, and what is available to them. In the following paragraphs, you'll see what you might need to remove as well as add to create a healthy low GI diet.

It's Never Too Soon to Start a Low GI Diet

A critical time for a mother to prevent problems such as obesity in her children may be before birth and possibly before conception. Studies suggest that, by starting pregnancy at a healthy body weight and eating a low GI diet during pregnancy, you are more likely to give birth to a baby with a healthier body weight and a lower risk of obesity and diabetes later in life.

Newborns

All you really need to know at this stage is that breast milk and infant formula are low GI. The World Health Organization recommends these as the sole source of nourishment for babies for the first six months of life, with continuation of breast-feeding for the first twelve months.

At This Stage, It May Be a Good Idea to Think about Your Role as a Parent in Feeding Children

On the whole, children can eat only what we make available to them. As adults, we know, or have the ability to learn, what foods are necessary for good health, and as parents, we have a responsibility to expose our children to a wide variety of nutritious foods. This happens naturally when a mother breast-feeds her baby, because the flavors of the foods she eats are transferred through her breast milk (so if you want baby to eat veggies in a few months' time, eat lots of them yourself). When we do begin introducing solid foods, it's important that we don't give the responsibility of food choice to our toddlers. Just because he or she relishes a cookie doesn't make it an appropriate food for him or her.

"As parents, . . .

. . . we have the responsibility of choosing when, where, and what is available to eat. Children have the responsibility of choosing how much and whether they eat it."

—Ellyn Satter, nutritionist

Infants and Toddlers

From six months of age, the world of food is just opening up, and it's time for your little one to explore. Take it slowly and keep it simple. A child's key need is for an increasing dietary source of iron, available from commercial fortified cereals and baby foods to which you can add single vegetables, fruits, and, later, meats. Keep the foods real—fruit, vegetables, milk, pasta, oatmeal, meat, etc., *not* commercial cookies, chips, deep-fried foods, candy, or other junk food.

- Give a slice of low GI bread rather than a cookie.

- Offer a range of chopped pieces of fruit every day.
- Include full-fat dairy products up to age two and reduced-fat products up to age five. Milk, yogurt, and pudding are calcium-rich, low GI snacks.
- Try oatmeal as a low GI cereal, but mix it with some iron-fortified cereal such as a rice cereal to help meet iron requirements.
- Plain cooked pasta is a low GI meal accompaniment or snack that is easily eaten, hot or cold, with fingers.

At This Stage, It May Be a Good Idea to Think about Avoiding Battles over Food

Children are naturally "neophobic," meaning it is normal for them to refuse new foods, vegetables included! This is believed to be a protective instinct, but it can be excruciatingly frustrating for parents.

The tendency to reject new foods can be overcome with frequent exposure so the new food is no longer unfamiliar. What this means is that you have to be persistent.

Offer a new food five to ten times in small amounts without pressuring the child to eat it; gradually you should see some acceptance. Praise any efforts at tasting new foods.

Make sure you are a good role model. Eat the same foods that you would like your children to eat. Avoid classifying foods as "good" or "bad" or forbidding certain foods. Instead, teach kids the concept that all foods can be eaten, some every day; others, sometimes.

Avoid using food, for example, dessert, as a reward. Withholding a child's favored food can make him feel powerless and is likely to increase his desire for it. Pushing children to eat everything on their plate with the temptation of a treat afterward can condition them—despite their excellent built-in ability to sense when they are full—to overeat.

Schoolchildren

Children, especially younger ones, eat mostly what's available at home. That's why it's important to control the supply lines—the foods that you serve for meals and have on hand for snacks. You can influence the GI of their diet with your choice of bread, breakfast cereal, noodles, dairy desserts, and the inclusion of fruit every day.

- Make your children's sandwiches with low GI white or grainy bread.
- Give fruit at least twice a day, washed, chopped, and looking attractive, without competition (like cookies).
- Make or buy some healthy granola bars (look for the GI symbol).
- Give fruit-filled, rather than cream-filled, cookies.
- Avoid packaged snacks such as chips, shaped crackers and cereal, and snack bars as much as possible. The low-fat varieties of these are not filling and are not a good alternative.
- Don't completely ban your children's favorite snacks; make them one of the "keep for a treat" foods.
- Limit fruit juice and soft drinks. Offer water and plain, low-fat milk instead.

At This Stage, It May Be a Good Idea to Think about Getting Your Children Involved with Food

Teach children how to cook and help them grow some of their own vegetables. Little cherry tomatoes, strawberries, or lettuce can easily be grown in pots, and they taste delicious. Take them to a farm or orchard when it's picking season. Let them select a new fruit or vegetable to try in the grocery store or market. Have them shop for food with you (sometimes). If you visit small local shops, get to know the shopkeepers at your butcher or market, bakery or deli. If you're a regular, many shopkeepers are only too pleased to give a little one a taste of something.

Teenagers

Teenagers are going to eat a lot, so if you can make even half their carbs low GI, you'll be doing really well.

- Expect teenagers to eat what you eat, so set a good example.
- Invite them into the kitchen and ask them to do something so that they learn how to cook.
- Keep a range of packaged low GI cereals available; a bowl of cereal is an excellent snack any time of day.

- Make sure there's always a loaf of low GI bread in the cupboard, plus plenty of tempting spreads, from jams and nut butters to honey.
- Buy low-fat milk and expect everyone over five years of age in the house to use it.
- Keep cartons of low-fat custard, flavored yogurt, and low-fat ice cream alongside a bowl of fruit salad or canned fruit in the fridge.
- Instant noodles or pasta topped with some grated cheese are filling low GI snacks that most teens can prepare for themselves.

At This Stage, It May Be a Good Idea to Think about Family Meals

Independent teenagers may turn up their noses at the prospect of a family meal, but studies have found that the predictability of family meals makes them a comforting ritual in the often tumultuous life of a teenager. They also offer parents a chance to catch up with their children. You might be able to tempt a reluctant teen by suggesting she invite a friend to dinner or involving her in planning the menu and cooking.

Kids who take part in regular family meals are:

- more likely to eat fruit, vegetables, and whole-grains (see page 199)
- less likely to snack on unhealthy foods, and
- less likely to smoke, use marijuana, or drink alcohol.

What counts as a family meal? Any time you and your family eat together, whether it's take-out food or a home-cooked meal. Maybe this means you have to eat a little later to wait until someone gets home from work or perhaps you set aside breakfast on the weekend as a leisurely family affair. Whenever it is, strive for nutritious food and a pleasant atmosphere (without the TV).

If you need individualized dietary guidance on managing any of the disorders in children discussed in this chapter, we suggest you seek the services of an accredited practicing dietitian (see page 48). There are no quick-fix pills or potions that are going to remedy these conditions; they are generally lifelong and require a holistic approach. And remember, the child is part of a family; if everyone eats the same way, it's better for the child, eases food preparation, and benefits the entire family's health.

If children learn . . .

. . . to combine regular physical activity with healthy low GI eating, they will be in top condition throughout their lives.

15
The GI and Exercise

WHETHER YOU ARE a professional athlete or exercising for health and fitness or to lose some weight, having a good nutrition program—the type, timing, and amount of food you eat before and after exercise—will help you achieve your goals whatever they are.

And that's where the GI comes in. It's a scientifically proven tool in sports and exercise nutrition that can help you to select the best carbs for your training or exercising program. (For this chapter, we worked closely with Dr. Emma Stevenson of the School of Psychology and Sports Sciences at Northumbria University to bring you the very latest research on the GI and exercise.) However, if the GI is to make any difference at all, your training diet needs to contain sufficient carbohydrate to start with.

Fueling Exercise

When you are exercising, your muscles rely on carbohydrate and fat as their main sources of fuel.

- Carbohydrate is stored in your muscles as glycogen, but the stores are limited and about ninety minutes of high-intensity exercise will deplete them.
- Fat, which provides the largest nutrient store in the body, can fuel one hundred to two hundred hours of exertion, but at a lower intensity.

In high-intensity sports, the availability of carbohydrate stores generally limits performance. The relative contribution of carbohydrate and fat as fuels while you are exercising depends on both the intensity and length of your exercise session. Generally, your body's use of carbohydrate as fuel increases as your exercise intensity increases and decreases the longer your exercise session lasts.

Aerobic training and fitness increase your body's ability to use fat as a fuel source. This is a plus, as it conserves your limited carbohydrate stores and allows you to exercise longer or at a higher intensity.

What you eat affects your muscle glycogen reserves and the amount of fat and carbohydrate you use up during exercise. If you are training on a regular basis, then every meal you eat becomes an important part of your cycle of recovery and preparing for the next exercise session. That's why you need to plan carefully to boost glycogen stores and promote fat burning during exercise. And this is where you can use GI to your advantage as a useful tool to plan your pre- and postworkout meals.

GI and Pre-exercise Carb Intake

The carbs you eat in the hours before exercise top off your muscle and liver glycogen stores so you can perform at your best during your exercise session. The findings of a number of studies show that eating low GI foods in the hours before exercise help extend endurance in athletes.

In one study, cyclists ate a pre-event meal of lentils (low GI) on one occasion and potatoes (high GI) on another, one hour before cycling at 65 percent of their maximum capacity. After the low GI meal, the athletes could cycle for twenty minutes longer than after the high GI meal. During exercise after the low GI meal, they also maintained their blood glucose concentrations at a higher level and used more fat.

Many other studies with male athletes support the findings of this study. Although not all studies have shown improvements in performance after a low GI pre-exercise meal or single food, they do consistently show differences in the ratio of carbohydrate and fat in the athletes' fuel mix. A high GI pre-exercise meal increases the carbohydrate used and thus reduces the amount of fat burned. It is also likely that the body's limited glycogen stores will be used up faster, leading to earlier fatigue.

A recent study by Dr. Emma Stevenson and Professor Clyde Williams at Loughborough University in the U.K. has come up with a couple of important findings about low GI foods and exercise. First, the benefits of low GI foods on exercise metabolism don't just apply to male endurance athletes like cyclists exercising at high intensity. Second, the effects of the GI aren't restricted to single foods; they also apply to having mixed meals in the hour before exercising.

In their study, Stevenson and Williams gave women recreational exercisers (for health and fitness) a high GI or low GI breakfast three hours before exercise. The meals were made up of a variety of foods in the typical combinations that people eat at breakfast:

- The high GI breakfast consisted of corn flakes and milk, toast and jam, and a carbohydrate-based sports drink (GI 78).
- The low GI breakfast included muesli and milk, apple, canned peaches, yogurt, and apple juice (GI 44).

After a low GI breakfast, the women's postmeal glucose and insulin response was noticeably lower than after a high GI breakfast. And when they jogged on a treadmill for sixty minutes three hours later, they used up significantly more fat as a source of fuel after a low GI breakfast than after a high GI breakfast.

Whether you are exercising for health and fitness, for weight loss or control, or for competition, it's a real plus to use more fat as your fuel source during exercise.

What If You Simply Walk for Exercise?

Low GI pre-exercise meals can still work for you even if you aren't an athlete, jogger, or cyclist. The Loughborough team found that women will use up an average of 7.5 grams of fat and 42 grams of carbohydrate walking on a treadmill for sixty minutes after a low GI breakfast (similar to the one described) compared with only 3.7 grams of fat and 52 grams of carbohydrate after a high GI one.

So, if you are counting the calories, the women use up twice as many from fat in the low GI trial compared with the high GI one.

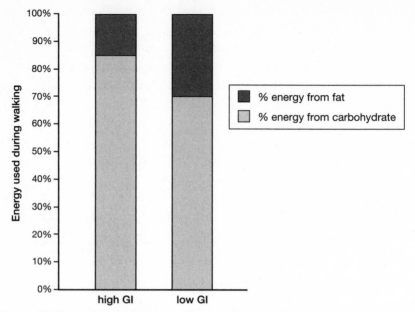

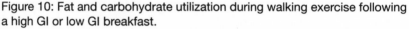

Figure 10: Fat and carbohydrate utilization during walking exercise following a high GI or low GI breakfast.

Low GI Foods: When and How Much?

Let's start with *when*. Generally, low GI foods are best eaten two to four hours before you exercise so that the meal will have left your stomach but remain in your small intestine, slowly releasing glucose energy for hours afterward.

The slow rate of carbohydrate digestion that is a characteristic of low GI foods helps to ensure there is a steady release of glucose into your bloodstream. Most importantly, during prolonged exercise, this steady release of glucose provides an essential energy source when muscle glycogen stores start to become depleted. This is how low GI pre-exercise foods can improve endurance performance.

However, you may need to experiment with different timings— eating two, three, or four hours before exercising—to see what works best for you. It can be difficult to get the right balance between not feeling too full and not feeling hungry before you start your exercise session.

It is also important to experiment with food choices to find ones that suit you and your digestive system best. Some low GI foods, particularly those with a high fiber content, can cause discomfort like stomach cramps and/or flatulence. Luckily, there are many low GI, low-fiber foods to choose from, including pasta (not whole wheat), noodles, rice such as basmati, Uncle Ben's converted long-grain rice, Uncle Ben's long grain and wild rice, and the new low GI white breads (look for the GI Symbol ⒢).

Now, let's decide *how much* to eat. What we know from research is that athletes can substantially improve endurance performance when they consume two hundred to three hundred grams of carbohydrate two to four hours before exercise (that's equivalent to around seven to ten slices of bread).

However, if you are essentially exercising for your health and fitness or for weight loss, or if you are not training on a daily basis, your overall carb requirements before exercise will be much, much less. In the study of recreational exercisers we outlined above, the women ate a breakfast that contained one gram of carbohydrate per 2 pounds of their body mass, i.e., seventy grams if they weighed 154 pounds.

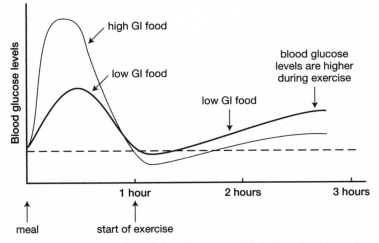
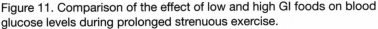

Figure 11. Comparison of the effect of low and high GI foods on blood glucose levels during prolonged strenuous exercise.

What about Carbs During Exercise?

You need to consume carbs while you are exercising only for events lasting ninety minutes or more. Many people—both athletes and weekend warriors—make the mistake of gulping down sports drinks that contain large amounts of glucose during exercise so they end up consuming just as much energy as they are expending!

If you do need to consume carbs during exercise, then this is when high GI carbs come in handy. High GI foods are digested in a flash, and their glucose is released into the bloodstream very quickly. This means the glucose is available to your muscles almost immediately.

Although we don't actually know the ideal amount of carbohydrate intake during exercise, it is generally recommended that athletes consume thirty to sixty grams an hour. This is when sports drinks come into their own, as they are an ideal way of providing fuel to the working muscle as well as helping with vital rehydration.

What other options are there? Well, several sports bars and gels are available; jelly beans or other gummy sweets will also provide a rapid source of glucose.

The Highs and Lows of GI and Recovery

Postexercise recovery is a critical challenge for athletes and recreational exercisers, and one that's all too often overlooked. Good nutrition between training sessions is vital for rapid and effective recovery. This is the time when you need to top up your muscle and liver glycogen stores. And if you are an athlete who trains or competes twice a day, you really need to replenish your glycogen stores fast.

How? Well, you can achieve this by increasing both insulin and glucose concentrations in the bloodstream rapidly during the immediate postexercise period. Did you know that during the first thirty to sixty minutes after exercise, your muscles are particularly sensitive to increases in insulin and there is increased activity of a glycogen-storing enzyme called glycogen synthase. This means that when you eat or drink something, the glucose virtually "speeds" into the muscle cells and is converted to glycogen. Consuming high GI carbs as soon as possible means you can really make the most of this window of opportunity.

Where Do You Get 50 grams of Carbs?

CEREALS	BREADS and CAKES
4 shredded wheat biscuits	3 slices of raisin toast
10 tablespoons cornflakes	2 muffins
14 tablespoons bran flakes	3 English muffins
2 average servings of oatmeal	4 slices white bread
FRUIT	**COOKIES and SWEETS**
2 large bananas	4 mini puff pastries, fruit filled
1 15-oz can fruit	2 Milky Way bars
4 medium apples	8 hard candies
4 oz dried apricots	1 Mars bar
8 tablespoons raisins	3 cereal bars
DRINKS	**GRAINS**
28 fl oz 6 percent carbohydrate sports drink	½ cup rice (uncooked)
34 fl oz diluted orange drink	½ cup pasta (uncooked)
16 fl oz Coca-Cola	1 15-oz can of spaghetti

What does this mean in practical terms? It means having fifty to seventy-five grams of carbs within the first thirty minutes after exercise and then a further fifty to seventy grams every two hours until you have consumed a total of five hundred grams, or until you have eaten a high-carb meal.

When it comes to the GI of your diet, exercise, and recovery, it's very much what suits you. The type of exercise, for example, whether the session is intense or intermittent, can make a difference.

If your recovery period . . .

. . . is longer than a few hours or restoring muscle glycogen after exercise is not your goal, then you don't need to eat large amounts of high GI carbs straight after exercise.

Dr. Stevenson and her colleagues ran another trial in which they asked athletes to run on a treadmill for ninety minutes at 70 percent of their maximum capacity (to reduce their muscle glycogen stores). Then, over the following twenty-four-hour period, they gave the athletes a high GI or low GI diet consisting of eight grams of carbohydrate per kilogram of body mass in mixed meals that would typically form part of an athlete's diet. Back at the lab the following morning, they asked the athletes to run to exhaustion on a treadmill at 70 percent of their maximum capacity.

What they found was that the athletes' endurance capacity was significantly improved after a low GI recovery diet compared with a high GI diet. In the low GI trial, the athletes used more fat as a fuel source, which meant they "spared" their muscle glycogen stores for later in the exercise session.

But, when they repeated this trial with intermittent exercise (typical of soccer, hockey, basketball, and baseball) rather than an intense exercise session, they found no differences in recovery of endurance capacity between high GI and low GI diets. However, if you are exercising primarily for your health and fitness or for weight loss, a low GI postexercise meal may help your body maintain a higher rate of fat burning (oxidation).

Here's what happens. Your body's fat oxidation (a technical term that means fat burning) will be elevated postexercise but will be rapidly suppressed if you eat high GI carbohydrates. This is because your body's higher insulin response to the blood glucose spike after a high GI meal or snack suppresses enzymes that oxidize fat. This basically means you burn less fat and more carbohydrate.

Your body's lesser insulin response after a low GI carb meal or snack suppresses fat oxidation to a lesser extent. What's the benefit? It means your body continues using fat as an energy source long after you have finished exercising. Because weight gain tends to creep up on most of us, every little bit counts!

 If you are exercising primarily . . .

. . . for your health and fitness or for weight loss, a low GI postexercise meal may help your body maintain a higher rate of fat burning (oxidation).

Take the quiz on pages 142–143 to determine if your diet is fit for peak performance.

Tricia's Story

I am a firm believer in the GI because it has changed my life. I am a runner, and I found that as I was training and trying "fad" diets at the same time, I was getting migraines about once a week. I was really tired all the time and often had a nap in the middle of the day. Then one day I found the GI. I started putting it into practice right away. One of the things I love about the GI is it is so simple. I followed the recommendations for athletes and ate low glycemic before a workout and higher after. It has not only meant no more headaches, but it has also increased my endurance in running. I feel healthier and I have so much energy. I tell everyone I know about the GI, because it just makes sense. It has become a healthy lifestyle for me and my family. Tomorrow I am running a half-marathon and the GI helped get me there!

Michael's Story

In the 1990s, I was extremely fit, competing in triathlons of all distances including Ironman. However, since 2000, a back injury and work commitments led to a fairly sedentary lifestyle, and I put on thirty pounds. The back would not heal, and finally a chiropractor advised me to start exercising. By exercising at least once daily, I was able to cure my back injury by strengthening my abdominals. Recently I discovered low GI foods, and last weekend I completed a three-hour run without any after-effects, my longest run in seven years.

I used to eat only white bread and jasmine rice, etc. I have now changed to whole-grain bread and basmati rice. My whole family is benefiting from this. We all eat the same meals, and no one complains about my cooking or my wife's. My wife, who has always been fairly sedentary, is now running and doing triathlons, as are two of my daughters, aged seven and eleven (at twenty months, the youngest is still a bit young). My wife has also lost about fifteen pounds and is working toward her pre-children weight. We are finding more energy to do more activities as a family. I believe this is due to a conscious decision to eat better carbohydrates with a lower GI.

Is Your Diet Fit for Peak Performance?

Take the diet-fitness quiz below and see how well you score. It's a good idea to use this quiz regularly to pick up on areas where you may need to improve your diet.

1. Circle your answer.

- I eat at least 3 meals a day with no more than 5 hours between. Yes/No

EATING PATTERNS

Carbohydrate checker

- I eat at least 4 slices of bread each day (1 roll = 2 slices of bread). Yes/No
- I eat at least 1 cup of breakfast cereal each day or an extra slice of bread. Yes/No
- I usually eat 2 or more pieces of fruit each day. Yes/No
- I eat at least 3 different vegetables or have a salad most days. Yes/No
- I include carbohydrate such as pasta, rice, and potatoes in my diet each day. Yes/No

Protein checker

- I eat at least 1 and usually 2 servings of meat or meat alternatives (poultry, seafood, eggs, dried peas/beans, or nuts) each day. Yes/No

Fat checker

- I spread butter or margarine thinly on bread or use none at all. Yes/No
- I eat fried food no more than once per week. Yes/No
- I use polyunsaturated or monounsaturated oil (canola or olive) for cooking (circle yes if you never fry in oil or fat). Yes/No
- I avoid oil-based dressings on salads. Yes/No
- I use reduced-fat or low-fat dairy products. Yes/No

- I cut the fat off meat and take the skin off chicken. Yes/No
- I eat fatty snacks such as chocolate, chips, cookies, Yes/No
  rich desserts/cakes, etc., no more than twice a week.
- I eat fast or take-out food no more than once Yes/No
  per week.

Iron checker
- I eat lean red meat at least 3 times per week or Yes/No
  2 servings of white meat daily or, for vegetarians,
  include at least 1–2 cups of dried peas and beans
  (e.g., lentils, soybeans, chickpeas) daily.
- I include a vitamin C source with meals based on Yes/No
  bread, cereals, fruits, and vegetables to assist the
  iron absorption in these "plant" sources of iron.

Calcium checker
- I eat at least 3 servings of dairy food or soy milk Yes/No
  alternative each day (1 serving = 8 oz milk or
  fortified soy milk; 1 slice (1½ oz) hard cheese;
  8 oz yogurt).

Fluids
- I drink fluids regularly before, during, and after Yes/No
  exercise.

Alcohol
- When I drink alcohol, I mostly drink no more than Yes/No
  the recommendation for the safe driving blood
  alcohol limit (circle yes if you don't drink alcohol).

2. **Score 1 point for every *Yes* answer.**

Scoring scale

18–20	Excellent	15–17	Room for improvement
12–14	Just made it	0–12	Poor

Note: Very active people will need to eat more breads, cereals, and fruit than on this quiz, but to stay healthy, no one should be eating less.

16

The Latest Findings about the GI

AS WE SAID IN THE INTRODUCTION, research conducted by scientists throughout the world has underscored, not only to us, but to many individual experts and health authorities worldwide, that the GI has implications for everybody. It is truly a glucose revolution, in that a growing mountain of research on the GI has permanently changed the way we understand carbohydrates and their effect on our bodies. The reason is simple: high blood glucose levels are a key—and undesirable—characteristic of many diseases.

In this chapter, we share with you some of the latest scientific findings about carbohydrates, blood glucose levels, and the GI. Some of it gets a bit technical, so bear with us. We have tried to keep it as clear and straightforward as we can. In many of these areas, there's a lot more research to be done. But what's clear is that eating a low GI diet has far-reaching benefits for everybody's long-term health and well-being.

Carbohydrates, GI, and Brain Function

Your brain is the hardest working "muscle" in your body, and it never switches off. Of the many nutrients that make up a diet, glucose is the only one that the brain can use. For this, it draws on glucose circulating in the blood. Star-shaped brain cells called astrocytes also store a little glucose in the form of glycogen that acts as a buffer between glucose in the blood and glucose in the fluid nourishing the brain. But after an overnight fast or a long period of mental activity without food, blood glucose levels gradually decline. And they decline more during a period of intense mental effort, such as doing math versus reading a magazine! When stores of glycogen become limited, your brain benefits greatly from a top-off.

One of the best reasons to include some carbohydrate in every meal is the well-documented effect on mental performance. Studies are showing that intellectual performance, particularly at breakfast time, is improved following the intake of a carbohydrate-rich food. Demanding mental tasks are most improved, while easy tasks are not affected. The tests included various measures of "intelligence," including word recall, maze learning, arithmetic, short-term memory, rapid information processing, and reasoning. The improved mental ability following a carbohydrate meal, especially breakfast, has been demonstrated in all types of people—young adults, university students, people with diabetes, the elderly, and people with Alzheimer's disease.

Several recent studies suggest that low GI carbohydrates may enhance learning and memory better than high GI carbohydrates. In other words, the type of carbohydrate eaten may be just as important as the quantity, with a low GI breakfast such as traditional oatmeal having a better effect on memory function than a high GI breakfast such as cornflakes. The reason may be related to blood glucose stability and the absence of the "overshoot" that often accompanies high GI meals. The stress hormone cortisol appears to be involved.

Cortisol's natural function is to prepare the body for fight or flight, with a small amount improving memory, but too much impairs it. Work by Dr. Clemens Kirschbaum at the Technical University of Dresden has shown that the consumption of high GI carbohydrates increases the production of cortisol in response to stress. This means there is a trade-off between carbohydrates as brain food and their role as magnifiers of the brain-draining stress response.

Older people with type 2 diabetes have significantly greater risk of performing poorly in cognitive function tests such as recalling word lists. Dr. Carol Greenwood at the University of Toronto found that a low GI meal generally results in better verbal memory in the post-meal period, particularly for those who experience the greatest food-induced elevations in blood glucose levels, compared with a high GI meal. In the highly ranked medical journal *Diabetologia* in 2006, she and her colleagues reported their findings of a study involving a group of twenty older adults with type 2 diabetes. Both the GI of the carbohydrate meal and individual differences in response to the meal contributed to the variation in consequent memory recall. They found that performance following the meal of high GI bread was poorer than that following the meal of low GI pasta on measures of working memory, executive function, and auditory selective attention. Sustained attention showed no sensitivity to the type of carbohydrate food consumed.

In Chapter 5 (page 39), we discuss what happens when your diet is low in carbohydrate and the brain makes use of ketones, a by-product of the breakdown of fat.

Did You Eat Breakfast This Morning?

Most of us have been told (countless times) that breakfast is the most important meal of the day. But a lot of us still skip breakfast. We are not good examples, because an alarming number of kids, around 25 percent, are breakfast skippers too. Why? Well, the usual suspects. Too tired. Needed more sleep. Rushed. Not hungry. Don't like breakfast. Dieting.

Writing in the *Journal of the American Dietetic Association* in 2007, Dr. Ruth Striegel-Moore reported that the older a girl gets, the more likely she is to skip breakfast. The study found that only 60 percent of nine-year-old girls regularly ate breakfast, but by age nineteen this had plummeted to less than 30 percent. The diets of the breakfast eaters were consistently higher in calcium and fiber than the skippers, and they had a lower body mass index. As it turns out, skipping breakfast is not such a good idea!

The GI and Dementia

High blood glucose levels are being increasingly linked to dementia, even in its mildest forms. Scientists are already aware that there is a connection between diabetes and cognitive problems. But a four-year study of postmenopausal women found that chronically elevated blood glucose (in technical terms, glycated hemoglobin or HbA1c levels of 7 percent or higher) was linked with an increased risk of developing mild cognitive impairment.

Dr. Kristine Yaffe and her colleagues at the University of California, San Francisco, were interested in the prevalence of mild cognitive impairment in groups of women with and without diabetes. The four-year study looked at 1,983 women whose blood glucose levels were tested at the beginning of the study. Over the course of the study, eighty-six women developed mild cognitive impairment or dementia. For every 1 percent increase in HbA1c, the women had a greater likelihood of developing mild cognitive impairment or dementia. Women with a HbA1c of 7 percent or higher were four times more likely to develop mild cognitive impairment or dementia than women who tested at less than 7 percent. Even when the researchers excluded the women known at the outset to have diabetes, there was still a statistically significant association.

Reducing the Risk of Dementia
Controlling insulin resistance in middle age may help reduce the risk of dementia in later life. Researchers from the Medical University of South Carolina examined over 7,000 healthy adults who were given a series of cognitive tests at the outset and followed up six years later. They reported that those with the highest level of insulinemia, a condition in which insulin levels in the blood are higher than normal, had significantly greater declines in memory and word-recall tests.

The GI and Acne
Most teenagers agonize about their skin, cursing the pimples that appear just before an important social event. Scarring and low self-esteem are sometimes the lifelong products of severe teenage acne. What is not as well known is the fact that many adults also suffer from acne long after they have left adolescence behind. Interestingly, there is an astonishing difference in the incidence of acne in non-Westernized societies. When Dr. Staffan Lindeberg from Sweden studied 1,200 Papua New Guinea islanders in 1990, he found not a single case of acne, even among the 300 who were aged between fifteen and twenty-five years. The same was true among 115 young Ache hunter-gatherers in Paraguay.

Because acne at any age can be a disfiguring and socially restricting disease, it is understandable that people both young and old are constantly searching for "miracle cures." Although diet has been considered in the past a cause of acne, clinical trials showed no effect of eliminating specific foods, including chocolate, fats, sweets, and soft drinks. Dermatologists know that acne results from a combination of three factors:

- Overactive sebaceous follicles (oil-producing glands) causing blockages,
- increased production of oily sebum, and
- colonization of the skin follicle with bacteria that generates inflammation.

Consequently, dermatologists and doctors today generally don't make dietary recommendations to their patients with acne. They commonly prescribe hormone-regulating pills and antibiotics. These are effective treatment options, but, like all drugs, they have side-effects and are not for everyone.

A review published in the dermatology journal *Retinoids* has identified a possible link between diet, high blood insulin levels, and acne. Differences in environmental factors rather than genes are thought to explain these findings. When people migrate from a rural to an urban area, or from one country to another, increased rates of acne are often noted.

However, Professor Loren Cordain from the University of Colorado has suggested that acne may result from the combination of insulin resistance and high insulin levels. His Melbourne colleague Professor Neil Mann has been putting the theory to a test. In the latest of their studies, published in 2006 in the *American Journal of Clinical Nutrition*, Mann and his colleagues (not Cordain) randomly assigned forty-three boys to a conventional, healthy, low-fat diet or a diet with a lower glycemic load.

To reduce glycemic load, they increased protein intake a little at the expense of carbohydrates and replaced high GI carbohydrates with low GI carbs. After twelve weeks, total lesion counts in the boys on the low glycemic load diet had declined by nearly 25 percent compared with only 12 percent in the conventional diet group. They also reported a little unintended weight loss (around six pounds) and greater improvement in insulin sensitivity in the low GI group.

Further research is needed to determine whether it's weight loss or diet composition that makes the difference. But in the meantime, we can be assured that a low GI diet is going to do more for both your skin and your waistline than the traditional fat-reduced diet.

A low GI diet . . .

. . . will do more for your skin and your waistline than a reduced-fat diet.

Low GI for Your Eyesight's Sake

Age-related macular degeneration (AMD) is a terrible name for a devastating disease that affects the central macula of the eye, leaving sufferers with only peripheral vision. The macula is the small, yellowish spot in the middle of the retina that provides the greatest visual acuity and color perception. The macula lets us see fine detail and is critical to central vision, helping us to recognize faces, drive a car, read a newspaper, or do close handwork.

Unfortunately, AMD is now one of the most common causes of blindness among older adults in the Western world. As we age, our risk increases: people in their early fifties have only a 2 percent chance, but it leaps to 30 percent by age seventy-five. *AMD Alliance International* estimates that 25 million to 30 million people are affected worldwide. There's no known cure, but there is something you can do.

Just as there are optimum ways of eating for a healthy heart, liver, skin, brain, and kidneys, so is there one for the eyes. In particular, the red, orange, and yellow colors in foods are actually antioxidants that belong to a large family of more than six hundred carotenoids. Brightly colored vegetables, dark leafy greens (the yellow colors are hiding there), and egg yolks are rich in these protective compounds. You can eat these vegetables in generous amounts, but limit eggs to five to seven a week because their saturated fat content contributes to other risks.

New studies published in the *American Journal of Clinical Nutrition* suggest that a low GI diet could also be a key part of your AMD prevention plans. Why would that be the case? Well, the retina has among the highest supplies of blood and nutrients, including glucose, and is dependent on adequate glucose delivery from the circulation to maintain its function. Because glucose stores in the retina are negligible and there are no glucose transporters in the cell membrane, it appears that glucose levels in the retina reflect whatever level is found in the blood. High levels spell trouble because excessive uptake produces high reactive charged particles called free radicals that damage all the machinery inside the cell.

Researchers from Tufts and Harvard universities were the first to notice the link between GI and vision. They had followed 526 women without previous vision problems from the Nurses Health Study for ten years. At regular intervals, they assessed the nurses' diets using a food-frequency questionnaire. They found that when total carbohydrate intake was constant, consuming a high GI diet was associated with a doubling of the risk of developing AMD.

Similarly, Professor Paul Mitchell, the lead researcher of the Blue Mountains Eye Study in New South Wales, and his colleagues found that a high GI diet, but not a high-carbohydrate diet, was linked to an almost 80 percent higher risk of having age-related macular degeneration within the ten years of the study. They also found the incidence of cataracts was higher among elderly people who chose a high GI diet.

Although "observational" data like these cannot establish that the observed association is "cause and effect," they indicate a new direction for further studies.

Eight Tips for Making Your Eyesight Last

Exactly what causes AMD is still not fully understood. If you have a parent with the condition, you have a 50 percent higher risk of suffering from it yourself. Smokers have a four times greater risk than nonsmokers, and those with high blood pressure, obesity, or high cholesterol are also likely to suffer from it. Looking after yourself in your later years can have a significant impact on how long your eyesight lasts. According to leading Australian nutritionist Catherine Saxelby, you should try to:

■ Avoid smoking.
■ Maintain a healthy weight that's right for you, neither too fat nor too thin.
■ Eat large servings of dark green vegetables and leafy salad greens as often as you can.
■ Enjoy different colored fruits and vegetables for natural antioxidants.

- Make the switch to low GI carbs.
- Use oils rich in monounsaturated fat (olive, canola) or polyunsaturated fat (sunflower, grapeseed); limit intake of saturated fats (full-fat dairy foods, take-out foods, deli meats).
- Enjoy fish twice a week.
- Stay active to help manage your blood pressure and cholesterol.

High GI Diets and Fatty Liver

As the incidence of obesity in adults and children increases, so does a disease of the liver called nonalcoholic fatty liver disease, or NAFL, which we discussed briefly on page 123 in Chapter 14. It is a significant health problem that leaves sufferers feeling tired and unwell. Untreated, the liver cells become inflamed, and NAFL turns into nonalcoholic steatohepatitis, or NASH. In time, NASH may develop into cirrhosis of the liver, a life-threatening condition associated with liver failure. The latest figures suggest fatty liver affects 30 percent of American adults.

Although the origins of the disease are still uncertain, we now know it is strongly linked with insulin resistance and is relatively common in people with type 2 diabetes. In susceptible people, the cells of the liver have accumulated an excessive amount of fat. In the past, the condition was more often than not a sign of excessive alcohol intake, but these days, it's more likely to be associated with a large waist circumference and the metabolic syndrome (see Chapter 12).

Currently, there is no effective treatment other than gradual weight loss, which makes the findings of a new Italian study published in the *American Journal of Clinical Nutrition* timely. Professor Furio Brighenti and colleagues from the University of Parma in Italy suggest that a low GI diet may help people with NAFL, more so than low-carb or high-fiber diets, and could be a complementary tool for preventing or treating it. In their study of 247 apparently healthy individuals, the researchers assessed the degree of liver enlargement by ultrasound measurement, as well as their usual diet, including the quality and quantity of carbohydrate. They found that the GI of the diet was the best marker for fatty liver—the higher the GI, the greater the prevalence of fatty liver, especially in people with insulin resistance. They found no specific effect of total fiber intake, total carbohydrate intake, or glycemic load.

In the meantime, you can take the sensible steps recommended by Dr. Angela Zivkovic and colleagues in a review of diets for management of fatty liver in the July 2007 issue of *American Journal of Clinical Nutrition*.

- Avoid sudden or quick weight loss (it can precipitate liver failure).
- Include omega-3 fats from foods such as salmon.
- Include monounsaturated fats from nuts and olive and canola oils.
- Eat plenty of fruits and vegetables (but go easy on potatoes).
- Eat high-fiber, low GI breads and cereal products.
- Reduce intake of sweet drinks and added sugars, including fructose.
- Reduce intake of saturated fat (fried foods, cakes, and cookies).
- Visit a dietitian who can tailor a good diet to your food preferences.

Researchers have found . . .

. . . that a low GI diet may help people with NAFL, more so than low carbohydrate or high-fiber diets.

Adrian's Story

I was diagnosed in early 2006 with prediabetes and nonalcoholic fatty liver. It's something that has scared me very much. I would start getting tired about 11 a.m. everyday, while working on a morning shift. I would feel so sluggish that I just wanted to sleep. I had to drive about forty minutes to and from work, and some afternoons, I'd get so tired I'd pull over and sleep. Two hours later, I'd wake up and be ready to face the drive home. The change in my blood glucose levels was so noticeable after I went on a low GI eating plan. Each morning I would wake up as if I had been hit by a bus, feeling so lethargic. Things I used to eat/drink while at work would have been McDonald's, Pepsi, iced teas, lots of watermelon. I couldn't believe it when I stopped having these things in my daily routine; everything changed. I developed an eye for looking at the back of food labels and started talking to everyone about my new low GI life. I now know what the difference is and don't want to go back to the way I was before. My liver test results in March 2006 were 68 and then in March 2007, they were 49. This is a dramatic result, and my doctor was happy to see that, with my determination, I changed something that was potentially going to kill me.

The GI and Cancer

There's good evidence from various studies that high blood glucose levels are linked to some types of cancer—colon, breast, prostate, and ovarian. This is because constant spikes in blood glucose that cause the body to release more insulin also increase a related substance called "insulin-like growth factor one" (IGF-1). Both these hormones increase cell growth and decrease cell death, and have been shown to increase the risk of developing cancer. Professor Ed Giovannucci at Harvard University was among the first to make the link between insulin levels and cancer growth.

Obesity, particularly abdominal obesity, is a strong predictor of both colorectal cancer and diabetes. Recent reports from the American Cancer Society Cancer Prevention Study and the Iowa Women's Health Study showed an increased risk of colorectal cancer among people with diabetes. Perhaps more importantly, insulin resistance, or factors linked to insulin resistance, has been associated with an increased risk of colorectal cancer.

If insulin resistance and hyperinsulinemia are risk factors for cancer, and if a high GI or high GL diet increases the risk for insulin resistance, it should follow that such a diet also increases the risk for cancer. Despite the beautiful logic, the scientific findings to date are very mixed.

Some studies support the view that high GI diets increase the risk of cancer. The first study to test the theory found a direct association between dietary glycemic index and colon cancer risk, i.e., the higher the GI in the diet, the greater the risk of colorectal cancer. The researchers found that a sedentary lifestyle in conjunction with a high GI diet magnified the risk. Similarly, an Italian study reported that the dietary glycemic index was related to the risk of colorectal cancer among men and breast cancer among women.

As time passes, however, many studies are *not* positive, i.e., they are finding no relationship between GI or glycemic load and risk of cancer. One reason for the mixed findings could be the lack of validation of the food-frequency questionnaires that have been used to assess dietary intake. Some questionnaires are better than others at estimating carbohydrate intake, and few have been specifically validated to assess the GI. And some studies are smaller and shorter in duration than others.

Recently, Dr. Alan Barclay from the University of Sydney attempted to make sense of all the conflicting findings by conducting a "meta-analysis" that throws all the valid studies together and "weighs" better studies more heavily than smaller studies. When all studies were analyzed in this way, there were statistically significant relationships between GI and the risk of colorectal cancer, breast cancer, endometrial cancer, and all cancers combined. While further studies are necessary, it does no harm to put low GI on your list of cancer prevention strategies.

Sleep and the GI

Tossing and turning at night? You're not alone. Sleep difficulties such as taking a long time to fall asleep, waking up during the night and not falling back to sleep easily, and waking too early are increasingly common. According to the Gallup Organization, nearly 50 percent of adults do not sleep well at least five nights per month. Between 10 and 40 percent say they have intermittent insomnia, and around 15 percent have long-term sleep difficulties. In the United States, it's been reported that 25 percent of women have chronic insomnia.

The current treatment options for insomnia are pharmacological (drugs) and cognitive behavioral therapy. Treatments are considered effective if they shorten sleep onset (the lag time between hitting the pillow and falling asleep) or increase total sleep time by thirty minutes. Popular remedies used to treat sleep difficulties include prescribed sedatives and tranquilizers, herbal extracts and complementary medicines, massage and relaxation techniques, regular physical activity, and avoidance of stimulants such as caffeine before sleeping. Cognitive behavioral therapy for insomnia, however, is considered the best practice.

What about food itself? We already know that both the timing of meals and their nutrients can influence your sleep quality. Consuming a meal too close to bedtime, for example, will disturb sleep for reasons that are not entirely clear. Science has shown that nutrients can influence sleep via their effect on levels of the amino acid, tryptophan, a precursor for brain serotonin and a "feel-good" hormone and sleep-inducing agent.

One factor that promotes the entry of tryptophan into the brain (and therefore serotonin production) is its concentration relative to that of several other amino acids, i.e., the *tryptophan ratio*. This is where the GI comes into the picture.

High GI carbohydrates have the ability to increase the tryptophan ratio under the direct action of insulin. Thus, a high GI meal might be expected to promote sleep via an increase in brain tryptophan uptake and serotonin production. Paradoxically, the sleep experts believe a meal with a high protein content will reduce serotonin production because it supplies relatively more of the other amino acids, thereby reducing the ratio.

A study led by doctors Chin Moi Chow and Helen O'Connor at the School of Exercise and Sport Science at the University of Sydney tested the theory that a high GI meal might aid sleep. In the setting of a sleep laboratory, four hours before bedtime, twelve healthy men between the ages of eighteen and thirty-five were given a meal containing 90 percent of its energy as carbohydrate in the form of either low GI rice or high GI rice. The researchers found that sleep onset was only nine minutes after the high GI meal, considerably shorter than the seventeen minutes taken to fall sleep after the low GI meal. They also showed that the high GI meal was more effective if it was consumed four hours before bedtime rather than one hour before. No effects on other sleep variables were observed.

While any natural, safe therapy that improves sleep is good news, much larger, long-term studies are required before we recommend that people with sleep problems start experimenting with high GI meals. Scientists are also exploring the idea that sleepiness and alertness on the job might be affected by the GI of the lunchtime meal. Stay tuned!

The GI and Gum Disease

Periodontitis, a disease of the gums, is a leading cause of tooth loss in adults—around 30 percent have it. It's a serious infection that destroys the soft bone and tissue that support your teeth, but it is both treatable and preventable. It's long been known that daily brushing and flossing and regular professional cleaning can greatly reduce the chances of developing gum disease.

Findings from the first study to look at whole-grain intake in conjunction with periodontitis risk suggest that eating at least four servings of whole grains a day may reduce the likelihood of periodontitis in healthy people, possibly by improving their insulin sensitivity. In a prospective study, researchers from McMaster University in Canada tracked, over fourteen years, more than 34,000 healthy men (those with diabetes, heart disease, or a history of stroke were excluded) aged forty to seventy-five years at the start of the study.

The men eating the most whole-grain foods (around three or more servings a day), including brown rice, dark breads, oats, whole-grain breakfast cereals, popcorn, wheat germ, bran, and other grains were 23 percent less likely to develop periodontitis than those who ate less than one serving a day. Although they also found that the men who ate the most cereal fiber were less likely to develop gum disease, they found no link between total dietary fiber and periodontitis risk.

There are countless reasons to include more whole cereal grains in your diet, but it's hard to ignore the fact that you are getting all the benefits of their vitamins, minerals, protein, dietary fiber, and protective antioxidants. *Some* whole-grain foods (not all) also have a low or moderate GI, slowing the digestion and absorption of carbohydrates from the gut and keeping blood glucose levels stable. There are a number of studies showing that the management of blood glucose levels reduces the risk of periodontitis in people with diabetes, so it may well be that lower blood glucose levels will reduce the risk of periodontitis in nondiabetics.

Take Steps to Prevent Gum Disease

- Brush your teeth twice a day and floss once a day.
- Visit your dentist every six months for a checkup and cleaning to remove the buildup of tartar from areas your brush can't reach.
- Eat a healthy diet, including plenty of low GI whole grains (see page 199)—at least four servings a day.
- If you have diabetes, manage your blood glucose levels.
- Do not smoke; people who smoke are four times more likely to develop gum disease than people who don't.

Questions & Answers

Fifty Frequently Asked Questions
about the GI, Answered

17
Fifty Frequently Asked Questions about the GI, Answered

SINCE THE FIRST EDITION of this book was published, we've heard from thousands of readers all over the world asking us to clarify or elaborate on many different aspects of the GI, carbohydrates, and diet. Here are the most frequently asked of those questions. The Q&As are grouped into the following subject categories:

- GI values of specific foods and food groups
- Sugar and starch
- GI and mixed meals, portion sizes, and the myth of diet restriction
- GI and diabetes
- GI, blood glucose, and other metabolic processes
- Advanced Q&As especially for health professionals and other researchers

 High, medium, or low GI . . .

- A high GI value is 70 or more.
- A medium/moderate GI value is 56–69 inclusive.
- A low GI value is 55 or less.

Q&As about GI Values of Specific Foods and Food Groups

1. *What's the GI of a caffé latté and a cappuccino?*

Most coffee-and-milk drinks will have a low GI because they are based on milk, a low GI food. Don't sweeten them with more than a teaspoon or so of sugar and say no thanks to the flavored syrups lined up on the counter. In fact, a caffé latté, cappuccino, or café au lait can be an easy way to help you get your two to three daily servings of dairy foods. Regular or skim milk has a low GI (27–34)—a function of the moderate glycemic effect of its sugar (lactose) plus milk protein, which forms a soft curd in the stomach and slows down stomach emptying.

Be aware that some coffee drinks available at coffee shops can be energy dense. For instance, many drinks such as "Frappuccinos" at coffee chains clock in at 500 calories, some even have as many as 730 calories. The more complicated your coffee drink, the greater the chance that it is, in fact, packed with calories.

Regular whole milk is high in saturated fat, but the wide range of reduced-fat milks—including skim, 1 percent, and 2 percent—are readily available alternatives. If you prefer soy milk (GI 36–45), make sure you opt for calcium-fortified *and* reduced fat. We don't recommend rice milk as a suitable substitute; it has a high GI (79).

How much milk are you getting with your coffee? Well, to some extent, it depends on the barista and where you buy it. But here are some standard definitions:

- **Cappuccino** is traditionally equal parts espresso, steamed milk, and frothed milk.
- **Caffé latté** is a single shot of espresso with steamed milk.
- **Café au lait** is a single shot of espresso with steamed milk—approximately a 3:1 ratio of milk to coffee.

2. *Some soft drinks have a low GI. How often should children be allowed to have them?*

Sweetened drinks (including soft drinks and sweetened juices), even if they have a low GI, should not be an everyday beverage. Here's why: liquid calories may be a little stealthier than others, in that they tend to sneak past the satiety center in your brain, which would normally help stop you from overeating. This isn't to say that everyone should avoid soft drinks all the time, but consumption ought to rank as "occasional" or "keep for a treat" if you're trying to lose weight.

An increase in soft-drink intake is contributing to the child obesity problem. Our children are drinking more of these sweetened drinks than we did when we were children. And, of course, the increase in serving size from the old-fashioned eight-ounce bottle and twelve-ounce can to the widely available sixteen-ounce bottle doesn't help. Soft drinks aren't the only problem, either. Too much fruit juice, sweetened or unsweetened, is an easy way for us to gulp down extra calories.

3. *Potatoes, one of my favorite foods, have high GI values. Does this mean I have to avoid them?*

First of all, you don't need to say no to potatoes altogether just because they may have a high GI. They are fat free (when you don't fry them), nutrient rich, and filling. Not every food you eat has to have a low GI. Enjoy them, but in moderation.

Second, look for lower GI varieties or serve them in a way that reduces the glycemic response. University of Toronto researchers found that the GI of potatoes ranged from 65 to 88, depending on the variety and cooking method. Precooking and reheating potatoes or consuming cold cooked potatoes (such as potato salad) reduced the glycemic response. Freshly cooked and mashed potatoes had the highest GI. And researchers at Sweden's University of Lund found that preparing potatoes the day before and serving them cold as potato salad with vinegar or a vinaigrette dressing can lower the GI.

Third, remember that potatoes are a relative newcomer to the Western dinner plate. Although the Spanish brought them to Europe from South America in the mid-sixteenth century, they didn't become a regular part of the European diet until the late-eighteenth century and into the nineteenth century, when they replaced traditional whole-grain staples such as wheat, barley, rye, and oats, which have much lower GI values. So look back for a healthy future and add variety to your meals by enjoying whole-grain foods (see page 199), legumes, pasta, noodles, and basmati rice on a regular basis, and potatoes occasionally. And keep those portions moderate. You'll reduce the overall GI and GL of your diet and your risk of chronic disease.

Low GI Cooking Tips

If potatoes are your favorite food, don't cut them out. Instead, eat them in moderation, cut your usual portion in half, and add a lower GI accompaniment such as sweet corn. Or cook them ahead of time, then cool and reheat before eating (which lowers the GI).

- **Steam** small new potatoes (with their skin on for added nutrients).

- **Bake** a potato and add a tasty, low GI topping, such as sweet corn, beans, or chickpeas.

- **For mashed potatoes,** substitute half the potato with white beans such as cannellini.

- **Boiled potatoes** or a simple potato salad made with a vinaigrette dressing have a lower GI and are a much better choice for weight control than French fries or potato chips, which are far higher in fat and calories.

---

4. *What's the GI of beef, chicken, fish, eggs, nuts, and avocados?*

These foods contain no carbohydrates or so little that their GI can't be tested according to the standard method. Essentially, these types of foods, when eaten alone, won't have much effect on your blood glucose levels. Because we're constantly asked about them, we now include these foods in the tables in Part 5 and have given them a GI value of 0. Likewise, the glycemic load of these foods is 0.

5. *Why is there no GI for blackberries and raspberries?*

Most berries have so little carbohydrate that it's difficult to test their GI (except for strawberries, GI = 40, and blueberries, GI = 53).

Berries' low carbohydrate content means their glycemic load will be low, so you can enjoy them by the bowlful. They are a good source of vitamin C and fiber; some berries also supply small amounts of folate and such essential minerals as potassium, iron, calcium, magnesium, and phosphorus. Eat them fresh, add them to fruit salads and smoothies, use them in a delicious dessert, decorate cakes with them, or make them into jams, fruit spreads, and sauces.

6. *Does the GI increase with serving size? If I eat twice as much, does the GI double?*

The GI always remains the same, even if you double the amount of carbohydrate in your meal. This is because the GI is a relative ranking that compares one source of carbohydrate with another, per unit of carbohydrate.

But if you double the amount of food you eat, you can expect to see a higher blood glucose response; that is, your glucose levels will reach a higher peak and take longer to return to baseline compared with a normal serving size. This is where GL—a measure of the glycemic potency of foods per average serving—comes in handy, because it puts together both the amount of carbohydrate you eat and its GI to help predict how much a serving of food will raise blood glucose. (See pages 18–19 for our full discussion of GL.)

7. *What's the GI of beer?*

Generally, alcoholic beverages contain very little carbohydrate. Most wines and spirits contain virtually none; regular beer contains around ten to thirteen grams of carbohydrate per twelve-ounce bottle, stout around fourteen grams of carbohydrate per twelve-ounce bottle, while a light beer has from three to six grams of carbohydrate per serving (again, a twelve-ounce bottle). A can of regular (not diet) soda, on the other hand, has between thirty-five and forty-five grams of carbohydrate.

Because beer has so little carbohydrate, it's difficult to test its GI, which is why we haven't tested many brands of beer and why we listed its GI and GL as 0 in earlier editions of this book and others in our series. But, eventually, we decided that the valid way to test beer would be by comparing responses to a ten-gram carbohydrate portion of beer (about 300 ml) with a ten-gram carbohydrate portion of glucose (as we explain on pages 12–13, in Chapter 2, in GI testing, a fifty-gram carbohydrate portion is normally used). In this test, beer's GI is 66. Its glycemic load can be calculated as follows:

$$66 \times 10 \div 100 = 6.6 \text{ (or, rounded up, GL = 7)}$$

Thus, beer will raise glucose levels a little, but not a lot. If you drink beer in large volumes (not a good idea anyway, from an overall health perspective), then you could expect it to have a significant effect on blood glucose.

8. *Why do most varieties of rice have such a high GI value?*

It's true that most varieties of rice are high GI; over 70 is typical, even in brown rice and imported varieties from Thailand. The reason can be traced back to the state of gelatinization of the starch in the cooked grains (see page 21). Despite rice's "whole-grain" nature, complete gelatinization takes place during cooking, meaning millions of microscopic cracks and fissures in the grains allow water to penetrate right to the middle of the grain during cooking, allowing the starch granules to swell and the starch to hydrate.

Nonetheless, some varieties of white rice, such as basmati, have substantially lower GI values. The reason: they have more amylose starch, which resists gelatinization. If you are a big rice eater, we recommend choosing basmati, Uncle Ben's converted, long-grain, or wild rice, or, alternatively, rice noodles (rice vermicelli is low GI). If you like sushi, you're also in luck. The vinegar used in making sushi as well as in *nori* (seaweed) helps to lower sushi's GI to 48.

9. *I have read in some GI lists that fresh coconut is low GI. Is this true?*

Coconut is a nut (not a fruit) and can't be GI tested. It contains very little carbohydrate per serving—just one gram in a fifteen-gram portion—but it is high in fat (five grams in a fifteen-gram portion), and the fat it contains is nearly 90 percent saturated. So when cooking, use very small amounts of coconut milk, flaked (desiccated) coconut, or other products made from coconut. Tip: some health-conscious cooks use light evaporated milk flavored with coconut essence.

10. *Why has the GI value of carrots changed from 92 to 41?*

When carrots were first tested in 1981, their GI was 92, but only five people were included in the study, and the variation among them was huge. This was in the early days of GI testing, and the reference food was tested only once. When carrots were assessed more recently, ten people were included, the reference food was tested twice, and a mean value of 41 was obtained, with narrow variation. It was clear that this result was more accurate and that the other value should be ignored.

Unfortunately, one of the most repeated criticisms of the GI approach was the fact that carrots were being excluded from diets simply because of their high GI. This demonstrates the need for a reliable, standardized methodology for GI testing. It is also another case for not using the GI in isolation when creating a healthy diet plan.

11. What's the GI of cornstarch?

We're often asked about the GI of thickeners such as arrowroot, corn-starch, and instant tapioca. These starchy powders thicken sauces, soups, gravies, and pie fillings without adding fat or going lumpy. All you do is mix about a tablespoon of cornstarch in a tablespoon of water, whisk that into the liquid you are thickening, and cook for about a minute, stirring constantly to remove the slightly starchy flavor. These proportions will make about one cup (eight ounces) of a medium-thick sauce. As far as we know, none of these thickeners has been GI tested (at least, we haven't seen any published results). Our estimate is that their GI would be about 70. In small amounts (one teaspoon per serving), their GL will be only 3–4.

Low GI Cooking Tips

Here are some alternative ideas for thickening sauces and soups:

- **Sauces:** Reducing the sauce will thicken it and intensify the flavor.
- **Soups:** For vegetable soups, using a blender, food processor, or food mill, purée some of the cooked vegetables, then stir them back into the soup to thicken. Adding grated starchy vegetables like sweet potato or yams will thicken a vegetable soup, or stale bread crumbs (sourdough or grainy, of course) in a mushroom soup. For a creamy soup, you can stir in a little light evaporated milk or low-fat yogurt. Puréed cooked or canned white beans will also thicken a vegetable soup.

12. *A high-fat food may have a low GI. Doesn't this make these foods sound healthy, even when they're not?*

The GI is a measure of carbohydrate quality, not an all-in-one index of a food's nutritional worth. We don't recommend jelly beans simply because they are low in fat, and the same goes for foods that are low GI but "nutritionally challenged." It's important to think about all of the different nutritional qualities of a food, and not only its GI.

For example, potato chips and French fries are lower GI than baked potatoes. Corn chips are lower GI than sweet corn. The reason: large amounts of fat in food tend to slow the rate of stomach emptying and therefore the rate at which foods are digested. Yet the saturated fat in these foods makes them less healthful and contributes to a greatly increased risk of heart disease.

If we were to weigh the health benefits of a high GI but low-fat food (e.g., potatoes) versus one high in saturated fat but low GI (e.g., some cookies), then we would vote for the potatoes. Again, the GI was never meant to be the sole determinant of what foods you choose to eat. It's essential to base your food choices on the overall nutrient content of a food, including fiber, fat, and salt. This is where the GI Symbol Program helps consumers identify nutritious sources of low GI carbs (see www.gisymbol.com) with its distinctive logo Ⓖ (for more on the GI symbol, see page 168).

Another important point to stress here: not all high-fat foods are unhealthy. Foods that contain heart-healthy fats—avocados, nuts, and legumes—are excellent foods.

Save foods that contain saturated fats, even if they're low GI—such as candies, cakes, and cookies—as treats for special occasions.

13. *Why are many high-fiber foods high GI?*

Dietary fiber is not one chemical constituent; rather, it's composed of many different sorts of molecules. As we explained in Chapter 3 (see "The Effect of Fiber on the GI," page 27), fiber can be divided into soluble and insoluble types. Soluble fiber is often viscous (thick and jellylike) in solution and remains viscous even in the small intestine. It slows down digestion, making it harder for enzymes to digest the food. Foods with more soluble fiber, like apples, oats, and legumes, are low GI as a result.

Insoluble fiber, on the other hand, is not viscous and doesn't slow digestion, especially if it's finely milled. This is why whole-meal bread and white bread have similar GIs, and why whole-wheat pasta and brown rice have values similar to those of their white counterparts.

14. *I'm an avid cook, and I often make my own bread, pancakes, muffins, cookies, and other baked goods. Which flours, if any, are low GI?*

To date, there are no GI values for any raw flours of any kind, whether milled from wheat, soy, rice, or other grains. This is because the GI rating of a food must be determined physiologically (in real people). So far we haven't had volunteers willing to consume fifty-gram portions of raw flour! What we do know, however, is that many bakery products such as scones, pastries, and cakes made from fine flours, whether white or whole wheat, are quickly digested and absorbed. However, some products also made with fine flours, such as crackers and noodles, are often low GI. The final GI of products made with flour is unpredictable.

With your own baking, try to increase the soluble fiber content by partially replacing flour with oat bran, rice bran, or rolled oats. The recipes in Part 4 of this book include a variety of low and moderate GI baked goods.

15. *Will GI values ever be included on food labels?*

Food manufacturers are increasingly interested in having the GI of their products measured. In fact, some are already testing for research purposes only and consequently withholding the data; others are going so far as to include the GI on labels. As more and more research highlights the benefits of low GI foods, consumers and dietitians alike are asking food companies and diabetes organizations for GI information. The GI symbol Ⓖ, a trademark of the University of Sydney in Australia and in other countries (including the United States), is a public health initiative that provides consumers with a guide to healthy foods that have been reliably GI tested. Unfortunately, some manufacturers make low GI claims on products that are probably not. Look for the official symbol whenever you shop.

How Do You Know If It's Truly Low GI?

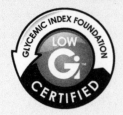

The GI symbol makes healthy shopping easier. This symbol means that the food has been assessed by the experts. And it's your guarantee that the GI value stated near the nutrition information table is reliable.

Foods that carry the certified GI symbol have also been judged against a range of nutrient criteria so you can be sure that the food is a healthy nutritional choice for its food group. In the tables in Part 5, you'll see that we have added a ⓖ beside the products that carry the GI symbol.

Why Put the GI Symbol on Food Labels?

Until now, people have had to rely on published lists of the glycemic index of foods to help them decide which carbohydrate foods to eat. Placing the GI value directly on the labels of foods makes it much easier for you to choose foods on the basis of their GI.

Which Foods Carry the GI Symbol?

Even though only low GI foods carry the symbol at present, medium and high GI foods can also carry the symbol, provided they meet the nutrient criteria. The symbol identifies foods that have had their GI tested properly and that are a healthy choice for their food category. The GI ranking (low/medium/high) is stated beneath the symbol, and the GI value is specified near the nutrition information panel. To carry the GI symbol, the food has to be independently tested following a standardized international method.

16. *When I don't see GI information on a food product, can I estimate a food's GI by looking at the ingredients or the nutrition label?*

A packaged food's nutrition information panel will tell you the carbohydrate content, but it won't indicate the GI of that food. If it contains at least ten grams of carbohydrates per serving, you can be sure it will have at least some effect on your blood glucose, but there's no way of telling whether it will be a little or a lot. Similarly, you can't estimate the GI of a food by looking at its ingredient list, because it won't tell you the final state of the starches in the food, which ultimately determines the GI value.

That said, we can make some generalizations about the GI of different food categories that you can keep in mind when choosing foods that haven't been GI tested. Legumes, for example, have some of the lowest GI values. Most pasta and noodle products tend to be low GI foods (a fact that seems to surprise many, but, again, it comes down to the way these products are made). Most fresh fruits are low GI, as are carbohydrate-rich dairy foods like milk, yogurt, ice cream, pudding, and custard. In contrast, most bread, bakery products, rice, and cereals are high GI, although a select few will be lower GI. As we mentioned above, protein-rich foods—cheese, meat, eggs, and poultry—don't have measurable GI values, because they contain little if any carbohydrates. The same is true for salad vegetables. The most comprehensive list of GI values now available appears in the tables in Part 5.

17. *Should I add up the GI each day?*

No. GI values are not like calories and grams of fat. You don't add them up to get a final value for the day. That's because the GI is a measure of carbohydrate quality, not quantity. The overall GI value for the day is a bit like mixing paints; the final color will reflect the dominant colors used. In practice, researchers can "add up" the final GI for the whole day (or whole diet) by using a "weighting" factor for each of the carbohydrate-containing foods that make up the diet. The weighting is a percentage value that represents the proportion of total carbohydrate contributed by each food. Consumers don't need to worry about this. All that's needed is a decision to eat at least one low GI food in each meal. This will reduce the overall GI of your diet.

Q&As about Sugar and Starch

18. *Is there a difference between naturally occurring sugars and refined sugar?*

Not in GI terms. Naturally occurring sugars are those found in milk and other dairy products and fruits and vegetables, including their juices. Refined sugar means added sugar, table sugar, honey, maple syrup, or corn syrup. Both sources include varying amounts of sucrose, glucose, fructose, and lactose. Some nutritionists make a distinction between them, because natural sugars are usually accompanied by micronutrients such as vitamin C.

The rate of digestion and absorption of naturally occurring sugars is no different, on average, from that of refined sugars. There is, however, wide variation within food groups, depending on the food. The GI of fruits varies, from 25 for grapefruit to 76 for watermelon. Similarly, among the foods containing refined sugar, some are low GI, some high. The GI of sweetened, low-fat yogurt is only 26 to 28, while a Milky Way bar has a GI of 62 (lower than bread).

19. *Why do nutritionists recommend starchy foods over sugary foods?*

Sugar has an image problem that stems largely from research with rodents using unrealistic amounts of pure sugar. It's also seen as a source of "empty calories" (energy without vitamins or minerals) and concentrated energy. But much of the criticism doesn't stand up to actual research findings.

Most starchy foods have the same energy density as sugary foods (see page 60), and even a soft drink has the same calorie content per gram as an apple. Starchy foods, such as whole-grain cereals (see page 199), can be excellent sources of vitamins, minerals, and fiber, but some pure forms of starch and modified starches are added to foods that are "empty calories."

So there really isn't a big difference between sugars and starches, either in nutritional terms or in terms of the glycemic index. Our advice is to use sugar to your advantage by adding it to nutritious foods (such as brown sugar on oatmeal or jam on low GI bread) to make them taste even better.

20. *GI and fructose: what's the story?*

Fructose is one of the four main sugars in our diet (sucrose, glucose, and galactose are the other three). It occurs naturally in large amounts as a component of fruit and honey. Apples, for example, contain around 12 percent sugar, of which 50 percent is fructose.

Table sugar (refined sucrose from sugar cane) and naturally occurring sucrose in fruit also release fructose when digested. Every molecule of sucrose yields one molecule of fructose and one of glucose. Thus ten grams of sucrose (two teaspoons) yields five grams of fructose and five grams of glucose.

In the United States, the food industry uses a great deal of high-fructose corn syrup (HFCS) as the source of sweetness for soft drinks and other foods. (Among other reasons, it is cheaper than sugar and the use of HFCS in baked goods gives them a better appearance than using sugar. The effect on the body of eating HFCS is virtually identical to that of consuming sugar.) These syrups contain fructose and glucose in roughly equal quantities. After digestion, however, there is very little to separate table sugar from high-fructose corn syrups.

Even during normal storage in the pantry, much of the sucrose in manufactured foods breaks down into equal proportions of glucose and fructose. A solution of fructose alone is not well absorbed and may cause gastrointestinal discomfort and loose stools, if consumed in sufficient quantities. In total, people in the Western world probably eat between twenty and fifty grams of fructose "equivalents" a day, about half their total intake of sugars.

Because humans evolved on a diet rich in fruit, berries, and honey, we have a long history of consuming fructose as a significant source of energy. Nonetheless, there are concerns about the effect of consuming it in excessive amounts. Whether present levels of fructose consumption pose a risk to health is the subject of ongoing debate among scientists.

Sugar and Obesity—Is There a Link?

A scientific expert workshop in Europe recently reviewed the controversial role of sugars in relation to obesity and human health. They paid particular attention to the quality of the scientific evidence and identifying gaps in our knowledge. They concluded that higher intake of carbohydrates, including dietary sugars was often associated with a *lower* (yes, lower) body weight. But they also stressed that more trials were necessary to determine the optimal amount of sugars vs. starches in diets for weight loss. They warned that sugar sweetened drinks, including soft drinks and fruit juices, may be specifically associated with excess weight gain in children and young adults but larger and longer trials were needed to settle the score. Surprisingly, Australians have reduced their intake of added sugars by 25 percent yet rates of obesity continue to climb.

Q&As about the GI and Mixed Meals, Portion Sizes, and the Myth of Diet Restriction

21. *Can you use the GI to predict the effect of a meal containing a mixture of foods with very different GI values?*

Yes, the GI can predict the relative glycemic effect of different mixed meals containing foods with very different GI values. In a major study we published in the June 2006 edition of the *American Journal of Clinical Nutrition,* we found that the GI works just as predictably whether people eat a single portion of one item, or a normal meal. In total, we studied thirteen different breakfasts that varied widely in fat, protein, carbohydrate, fiber, and energy content, as well as the GI of the individual foods. Just two things predicted the final glycemic effect— the amount of carbohydrate and the GI of the carbohydrate. All other factors were of minor importance.

You may have heard otherwise and read about studies in which the GI was of "no value." Unfortunately, not all studies are designed well, and some investigations don't know the GI of the foods they are including in their studies—they guess! That's not good science, and it's not appropriate to draw conclusions from flawed studies. (See also "Can the GI Be Applied to Everyday Meals?" on pages 16–17).

22. *What size portion does a food's GI refer to? For example, the GI of bananas is 52. Does this correspond to one banana?*

A food's GI value doesn't refer to a specific quantity of food; instead, it's a measure that reflects the quality of the carbohydrate in that food, specifically, its ability to raise blood glucose levels, gram for gram, or weight for weight, of carbohydrate. So for your example, this would mean that 52 is the GI for one banana, small or large. The glycemic load (GL) takes into account both the quantity and quality of carbohydrate (see pages 18–20).

23. *I haven't been able to find a reference to what GI number a person should aim for when trying to diet. Is there a formula?*

The simple answer is, no, there's no formula. You don't need to add up the GI each day. In fact, there's no counting at all, as there is with calories. The basic technique for eating the low GI way is simply, "this for that"—swapping the high GI carbs in your diet for quality, low GI carbs. This could mean eating oatmeal at breakfast instead of a high GI breakfast cereal, low GI bread instead of normal white or whole-wheat bread, or sparkling apple juice in place of a soft drink. We've found that many people who do just this reduce the overall GI of their diet, manage their blood glucose better, and lose weight.

24. *Opponents of the low GI approach say that low GI diets are too restrictive, that they narrow the range of foods that can be eaten. Is this true?*

It's absolutely a myth that you have to narrow the range of foods you eat on a low GI diet. In fact, most people who take a low GI approach to eating say the exact opposite: unlike many other diet plans, the glycemic index has actually *expanded* their range of foods, because they've been encouraged to try things they have never eaten before (e.g., Indian dhals, Asian noodles, lentil soups). Plus, they say they're relieved to finally have "permission" to consume foods containing sugar, such as jams and ice cream.

The idea that all low GI foods are high in fiber and not very tasty is also a myth. All-Bran and chickpeas may not be everyone's favorite foods, but many people enjoy low GI foods like pasta, noodles, oats, legumes, and a huge variety of fruits and vegetables. For delicious, low GI menu ideas and recipes, see Part 4 of this book.

25. *Do I need to eat low GI foods at every meal in order to benefit from a low GI diet?*

Not necessarily. The good news is that the effect of a low GI food carries over to the next meal, reducing the glycemic impact of higher GI foods. This applies to a breakfast eaten after a low GI dinner the previous evening. It also applies to lunch eaten after a low GI breakfast. This unexpected beneficial effect of low GI meals is called the "second meal" effect. Don't take this too far, however; on the whole, we recommend that you aim for at least one low GI food per meal.

26. *I am about to introduce my baby to solids and have been advised to start with rice cereal. I worry about giving my baby rice cereal as her first food. What is the current guidance on GI for babies and young children?*

Chapter 14, The GI and Children, gives our full thinking and recommendations with regard to children and the GI. Regarding rice cereal specifically, Dr. Heather Gilbertson, a dietitian and educator with many years' experience in the management of children with diabetes, advises: "Introduction of rice cereal for infants should not cause any problems. I would generally recommend mixing it with expressed breast milk to reduce its glycemic effect. Rice cereal is an important introductory food for babies, as it is iron-fortified. Infants need additional iron intake at six months of age to meet their requirements." Deliberately avoiding or limiting carbohydrate-containing foods will also cause the blood glucose levels to drop low in an infant with a diagnosed metabolic disorder.

Mothers need to encourage their babies to try a wide range of tastes and textures of the fruit and vegetable variety (focusing on either low GI or a combination of low with high to modify the effect). As children get older, mothers can introduce dairy foods, which all have a low GI, plus baked beans, oatmeal, and other low GI breads and cereals.

27. *Is there a GI plan for breast-feeding mothers who want to get back to their prepregnancy weight?*

Joanna McMillan Price, our coauthor of *The Low GI Diet Revolution* and *The Low GI Diet Revolution Cookbook,* advises, "A low GI diet is ideal while you are breast-feeding, which requires a lot of energy—and, theoretically, this additional energy comes from the body fat laid down during pregnancy. Of course, in reality, many women have to make a concerted effort to work off the baby weight. To do this, though, it is important that you don't go on a restrictive diet or take any sort of extreme measures.

"This is what makes the low GI approach so successful—you can forget about trying to count calories or even your portions of food. Make low GI foods the mainstay of your meals, and trust your appetite and eat to satisfaction while you are breast-feeding.

Also, do some exercise, even if it's just a daily walk with the stroller. You should then find that the weight slowly starts to shift—but, realistically, give yourself at least that first six months to get back to your prepregnancy weight."

Q&As about the GI and Diabetes

28. *Does sugar cause diabetes?*

No. There is absolute consensus that sugar in food does not cause diabetes. Type 1 diabetes (insulin-dependent diabetes) is an auto-immune condition triggered by unknown environmental factors, such as viruses. Type 2 diabetes (noninsulin-dependent diabetes) is strongly inherited, but lifestyle factors, such as lack of exercise and being overweight, increase the risk of developing it. In the past, when the dietary treatment of diabetes involved strict avoidance of sugar, many people wrongly believed that sugar was in some way implicated as a cause of the disease. While sugar is off the hook, high GI foods are not. Population studies have shown that high GI diets increase the risk of developing both type 2 diabetes and gestational diabetes (diabetes during pregnancy).

29. *Why are people with diabetes now allowed sugar?*

For a long time, people with diabetes were advised to avoid all sugar. That's because health-care professionals were taught that simple sugars were uniquely responsible for high blood glucose levels. But research has proved that people with diabetes can eat the same amount of sugar as the average person, without compromising diabetes control.

It's important, however, to remember that "empty calories"—whatever the source, be it sugar, starch, fat, or alcohol—won't keep your body operating optimally. The clichéd expression "moderation in all things" has withstood the test of time for obvious reasons. Research shows that moderate daily consumption of refined sugar (thirty to fifty grams or six to ten teaspoons) doesn't compromise blood glucose management. Keep in mind that this refers not only to the sugar you add to coffee or cereal but also to the sugar already contained in the foods you eat—jams, ice cream, yogurt, and so on.

30. *Can GI values obtained from tests on healthy people be applied to people with diabetes?*

Yes. Several studies show a strong correlation between values obtained in healthy people and people with diabetes (type 1 and type 2). By its very nature, GI testing takes into account differences in glucose tolerance between people. High GI foods are still digested quickly, and low GI foods are still digested slowly. Some people with diabetes have *gastroparesis,* a disorder in which the emptying of the stomach slows down. The ranking of foods according to their GI values is still applicable.

31. *Some vegetables, such as pumpkin, appear to have higher GI values. Does this mean people with diabetes shouldn't eat them?*

People with diabetes can eat pumpkin (GI 66), parsnip (GI 52), turnip and rutabaga (GI 72), whatever their GI value. Unlike potatoes and cereal products, these vegetables are low in carbohydrate. So their glycemic load is low. Other low-carbohydrate vegetables are carrots, broccoli, tomatoes, onions, and salad greens, which contain only a small amount of carbohydrate but are packed with micronutrients. They should be considered "free" foods for everyone. Eat them to your heart's content. See the vegetables section in the tables in Part 5.

32. *If additional fat and protein cause lower glycemic responses, shouldn't you advocate higher protein or higher fat diets for people with diabetes?*

Yes and no. It's a matter of degree and quality, rather than quantity. This type of diet shouldn't be taken to extremes because very low-carb diets have little to recommend them; they are difficult to sustain and they don't reduce the risk of chronic disease. If your preference is to eat more protein and fat and moderately reduce carbohydrate intake, then go ahead. The Joslin Diabetes Center recommends a diet with 40 percent of energy from carbohydrates (that's lower than is typical), with a greater proportion of protein and good fats. The emphasis should be on quality—good fats, low GI carbs, and nutritious protein sources such as fish, poultry, lean red meat, tofu, and legumes. If your preference is for higher carbohydrate intake, then that's okay too, but the quality of those carbs is of paramount importance.

33. *Would someone with diabetes need to reduce their insulin dose if they changed to low GI foods?*

In theory, yes, but in practice, no. Most studies have not shown a need for a significantly reduced insulin dose when consuming a low GI diet. This is probably because the insulin dose is dictated not just by carbohydrates in the diet but by protein and fat as well. Preliminary studies of people using insulin pumps have suggested that they could reduce their insulin dosage and maintain the same blood glucose levels, but further research is needed to confirm this.

34. *How can I feed a big family with cost-effective, no-hassle, low GI foods?*

Feeding a big family on a budget can be hard. But low GI eating often means making a move back to the inexpensive, filling, and healthy staple foods that your parents and grandparents may have enjoyed: traditional oats in oatmeal for breakfast; legumes such as beans, chickpeas, and lentils (all available dry or, for expediency, in cans); cereal grains like barley; and plenty of fresh fruits and vegetables, which have a naturally low GI.

Some of these foods may take a little more time to prepare than high GI processed, packaged, and more expensive convenience foods, but you will save money and reap immeasurable health benefits, and many of these foods will keep you and your family firing with energy all day. In the GI tables in Part 5, you'll find plenty of low GI foods to choose from that won't break your budget. Your diabetes dietitian or educator will also have plenty of ideas for low-cost, low GI meals that the whole family will enjoy.

35. *I have diabetes, but I enjoy an occasional drink. Is that a problem?*

Enjoying a small amount of alcohol with food will have little effect on your blood glucose levels. Indeed, recent research from the University of Sydney suggests that a glass or two of wine with or before a meal may reduce glucose levels by 25 percent. But the amount and kind of carbohydrate you eat with the alcohol is much more important than the alcohol itself. This is because there's very little carbohydrate in most alcoholic drinks: on average, a ten-ounce glass of regular beer contains only five grams (or one teaspoon) of sugar; low-alcohol beer has four grams; a three-and-a-half ounce glass of wine has a mere two grams; and a standard shot of spirits has less than one gram of sugar.

Moderate drinking is the amount that has been linked with the least risk and greatest benefits. The good news is that research indicates that, in general, the level of alcohol consumption associated with the least risk for people with diabetes is the same as that for the rest of the adult population. That is, men are advised to drink no more than two standard drinks on any day, women no more than one, and both men and women should aim to have at least two alcohol-free days each week.

However, if you are overweight, have poorly managed blood glucose levels, high blood pressure, high triglycerides, or other diabetic complications, your diabetes health-care team may advise you to drink less or not drink at all.

What Is a Standard Drink?

A standard drink is less than you think! Technically, it's an amount that contains 15 grams of pure alcohol and is equal to:

- 12 ounces of regular beer
- 5 ounces of wine
- 1½ ounces of distilled spirits

It's easy to underestimate the amount you drink, so if you want to stick to the guidelines, learn how much is in a standard drink of whatever type of alcoholic drink you like before you start drinking. A simple way of doing this is:

- Check the number of standard drinks listed on the label of the bottle, and
- Measure out a standard drink with a measuring cup so you know exactly what it looks like.

When you do this, you will probably be surprised by how much your favorite glass actually holds. For example, most wine glasses, when full, can hold almost two standard drinks!

Q&As about GI, Blood Glucose, and Other Metabolic Processes

36. *I understand that low GI foods help keep blood glucose stable. What's wrong with high blood glucose levels?*

High blood glucose levels pose a threat to your health even if you don't have diabetes. In fact, elevated blood glucose levels within the "normal" range can damage the blood vessels and circulatory system, increasing the risk of a heart attack, type 2 diabetes, weight gain, and even certain types of cancer. It does so by increasing the production of damaging free radicals and creating oxidative stress and inflammation.

Over time, the effects of high blood glucose levels become even more noticeable. In people with poorly controlled diabetes, problems may occur with the skin, leading to bacterial infections, fungal infections, and itching. Nerves may be damaged, causing numbness, prickling, tingling, burning, and aching sensations. There may even be a loss of nerve function, so that a process like digestion is impaired. The narrowing of large blood vessels will slow blood flow and cause heart disease, stroke, and the loss of circulation, which can lead to amputation. Small blood vessels may become damaged, which can cause problems that may include blurry vision, blindness, and kidney disease.

For all of these reasons, we advise that eating a diet rich in low GI foods helps to control blood glucose levels in people with and without diabetes, and can ward off both short- and long-term health problems.

37. *What is the effect of extra protein and fat on blood glucose response?*

Eaten alone, protein and fat have little effect on blood glucose levels. So a steak or a piece of cheese, for example, won't produce an increase in blood glucose. It's the *carbohydrate* in foods that is primarily responsible for the rise and fall in glucose after meals.

Both protein and fat will reduce your blood glucose response when they're eaten along with carbohydrate. Both cause a delay in stomach emptying, thereby slowing the rate at which carbohydrate can be digested and absorbed. So a high-fat meal may have a lower glycemic effect than a low-fat meal, even if they both contain the same amount and type of carbohydrate. This doesn't make the GI less important.

You can expect to see a lower glycemic response to meals that incorporate low GI carbs even if you add fat and protein. Moreover, if you lower glycemic responses by ADDING fat or protein you be consuming 2 to 3 times more calories, which completely outweighs any benefit one might obtain from the reduced glucose response.

Exchanging low GI starchy foods like pasta for high GI ones like high GI bread doesn't add any calories.

38. *Does low carb automatically mean low GI?*

No. Here's why: low carb is only about *quantity;* it simply means that a food or meal does not contain much carbohydrate. It says nothing about the *quality* of the carbs in the food or the meal on your plate. You could be eating a low-carb meal, but the carbs could have a high GI. Low GI, on the other hand, is all about quality of carbohydrates.

Whether you are a moderate- or high-carb eater, low GI carbs offer significant health benefits, as we detail throughout this book: promoting weight control, reducing your blood and insulin levels throughout the day, and increasing your sense of feeling full and satisfied after eating. We suggest that you make the most of quality carbs and reap the health benefits, such as:

- Vitamin E from whole-grain cereals
- Vitamin C, beta-carotene, and potassium from fruits and vegetables
- Vitamin B6 from bananas and whole-grain cereals
- Pantothenic acid, zinc, iron, and magnesium from whole grains and legumes
- Antioxidants and phytochemicals from all plant foods
- Fiber, which comes from all of the above and is not found in any animal food

39. *If carbohydrates increase my blood glucose level, wouldn't a low-carbohydrate diet make sense?*

In theory, a low-carbohydrate diet seems a logical choice if your aim is simply to reduce blood glucose levels. But presumably your goal is optimum health, with not just good glycemic control, but reduced risk of chronic disease. If so, low-carbohydrate diets have little to offer. In practice, they are difficult to sustain over the long term because carbohydrates are part and parcel of our Western diet. In fact, as we mention throughout this book, there is strong evidence to suggest that moderate- to high-carbohydrate diets are better for your health and easier to sustain.

Some popular diets are based on the concept of avoiding carbohydrate-based foods—even fruits and vegetables are restricted—while fatty meat and dairy foods laden with saturated fat, cholesterol, and calories form the basis of the diet. We should be wary of these diets. Chances are they are high in saturated fats and a recipe for ill-health in the long term.

Low-carb diets come in many forms, however. Some are not as extreme as that just described. The South Beach Diet, for example, recommends less carbohydrate (about 30–40 percent instead of 55 percent) and more protein (25–30 percent instead of 15 percent) and good fats such as olive oil. It includes advice about quality of carbohydrate (low versus high GI) and type of fat (unsaturated versus saturated). If you enjoy this way of eating, then there's nothing really wrong with it. But over time, you may find yourself yearning for higher carb foods like bread and potatoes. More research is needed before we can be sure that diets such as this are safe over the long term.

40. *The GI has been criticized because of variability in blood glucose responses between people and in the same person from day to day. How much variation should we expect? How much is okay?*

When we measure the GI of a food in a group of individuals, not everyone produces the same GI. For example, if we test apples (average GI = 38), then one individual might produce a GI of 20 and another 60. This is a natural biological variation that has been traced back to day-to-day variability in glucose tolerance in the same individual. One of the reasons we test the reference food three times in any one person is to obtain a reliable indication of this variability. The apple itself is not variable. Its carbohydrate remains unchanged, and the GI is a characteristic of the apple, not the person.

There is nothing crude about GI testing. At a minimum, 240 datapoints are needed to generate one published GI value (at the University of Sydney, 640 datapoints are collected). The bottom line is that foods classified as being high, medium, or low GI will show the same ranking in different individuals (as shown in Figure 12 on page 182).

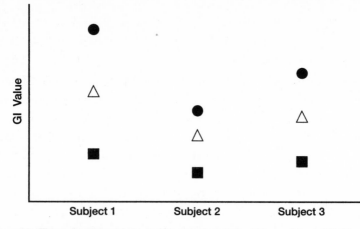

Figure 12. Three foods with high (●), intermediate (▲), and low (■) GI values will follow the same ranking in different individuals.

This natural variability in blood glucose response has been a major source of criticism of the glycemic index. But it is illogical to criticize the glycemic index on these grounds, because the variability applies to *every* dietary approach, whether it be carbohydrate exchanges, carbohydrate counting, or a lower carbohydrate diet. Indeed, the diagnosis of diabetes is based on only two to three blood glucose readings. You can rely on the published GI value as a reliable ranking of foods, reflecting how you as an individual will respond to different foods most of the time.

41. *Does it matter if you eat carbs after 5 p.m.?*

No scientific evidence supports the idea of avoiding carbohydrates— or any foods, for that matter—after 5 p.m., 8 p.m., or any other time. People with diabetes who are taking insulin or other blood glucose-lowering medication, in particular, should *definitely* not practice a "carb curfew." If you want to reduce your total energy intake, the better strategy, beyond exercising and eating fewer calories, is to eat low GI carbohydrates, which will make you feel fuller longer and reduce hunger pangs.

42. *I have recently been diagnosed with celiac disease on top of diabetes. It's extremely hard to find both low GI and wheat-free foods. Any suggestions?*

Good news: finding such foods may not be as hard as you think (or as it once was). Our publication *The New Glucose Revolution Low GI Gluten-free Eating Made Easy* is a practical guide to diet and recipes for people with celiac disease. Many Far East and Southeast Asian foods—Indian dhals or stir-fries served with rice, sushi, and noodles—are all low GI. Vermicelli noodles prepared from rice or mung beans and low GI rices, such as basmati, also meet your needs. Feel free to eat as many vegetables as you choose, while picking low GI fruits. If you can eat dairy products without a problem, then take advantage of their universal low GI values. On the other hand, if you are lactose intolerant, try yogurt with active cultures and lactose-free milk. Even ice cream can be enjoyed if you ingest a few drops of lactase enzyme (Lactaid) first. The GI tables in Part 5 include a section on gluten-free foods (see page 324).

43. *I've read that dairy products cause an increase in insulin secretion. Their GI is around 30–50, but their insulin index is three times higher.*

All proteins stimulate insulin secretion; they are said to be insulinogenic. The proteins in milk may be more insulinogenic than others because they are meant to stimulate the growth of young mammals. Insulin is a growth hormone designed to drive nutrients into cells, not just glucose but also amino acids, the building blocks of new tissue. Milk may contain a unique combination of amino acids that together are more insulin stimulating than any alone. This disparity between glucose and insulin response is not unique to dairy products. We've found that certain sweets and baked products also do this. Chocolate may also contain amino acids that stimulate insulin secretion.

44. *How relevant is the GI for athletes?*

"The glycemic index is a useful tool to help athletes select the right type of carbohydrates to consume both before and after exercise," says Dr. Emma Stevenson from Loughborough University in the U.K. Several studies have investigated the effect on fuel usage, during prolonged endurance exercise, of changing the GI of carbohydrates eaten before exercise. Studies have consistently reported that a low GI pre-exercise meal results in better maintenance of blood glucose concentrations during exercise and a higher rate of fat burning. This is likely to reduce reliance on muscle carbohydrate stores during prolonged exercise and possibly improve endurance performance. Eating a high GI meal before exercise may result in a glucose spike before the onset of exercise and then hypoglycemia occurring within the first thirty minutes of exercise. Unfortunately, there is little information on the effect of the GI of carbohydrates eaten before intermittent, power, or strength-related sports.

During recovery from exercise, replenishing muscle stores of carbohydrate is of high metabolic priority. Eating high GI carbohydrates after exercise increases plasma glucose and insulin concentrations, and this facilitates muscle glycogen resynthesis. If, however, you are exercising for weight-loss purposes or are involved in weight-restricted sports, low GI carbohydrates after exercise may be more beneficial because the lower glucose and insulin concentrations will aid in fat burning.

Advanced Q&As, Especially for Health Professionals and Other Researchers

45. *Does the area under the curve give a true picture of the blood glucose response? What about the shape of the curve and the size of the glycemic spike?*

The area under the curve (see "How Scientists Measure a Food's GI Value" on pages 12–15) may not be perfect, but it's thought to give the best summary measure of the overall degree of hyperglycemia experienced after eating. In our GI-testing database (containing tests on thousands of foods), we've been able to show that the GI correlates with the absolute blood glucose level at the peak and at sixty and ninety minutes after the start of the meal. In population studies, the GI of the overall diet correlates with measures such as glycated hemoglobin (HbA1c) that are related to average glucose levels and the risk of complications. In fact, recent studies have surprised even the experts, because postprandial glycemia influences overall control much more than fasting or premeal blood glucose levels. Glycemic spikes appear to be important, too, but there is a close relation between the area under the curve and the peak response. If one is high, the other is high; conversely, if one is low, the other is low.

46. If testing were continued long enough, wouldn't you expect the areas under the curve to become equal, even for very high and very low GI foods?

Many people assume that if the amount of carbohydrate in two foods is the same, then the areas under the curve will ultimately be the same. This isn't the case, though, because the body is not only absorbing glucose from the gut into the bloodstream, but also *extracting* glucose from the blood. Just as a garden can utilize a gentle rain better than a sudden deluge, the body can metabolize slowly digested food better than quickly digested carbohydrate. Fast-release carbohydrate causes "flooding" of the system, and the body cannot extract the glucose from the blood fast enough. Just as water levels rise quickly after a torrential rain, so do glucose levels in the blood. But the same amount of rain falling over a longer period can be absorbed into the ground, and water levels do not rise.

47. Isn't the insulin response more important than the GI value? Wouldn't it be better to have an insulin index of foods?

The insulin demand exerted by foods is indeed important for long-term health, but it doesn't necessarily follow that we need an insulin index of foods instead of a glycemic index. When they have been tested together, the glycemic index is extremely good at predicting a food's insulin index. (In other words, a low GI food has a low insulin index value and a high GI food has a high insulin index value.) There are some instances, however, in which a food has a low GI but a high insulin index value. This applies to dairy foods and to some highly palatable, energy-dense "indulgence foods." Some foods (such as meat, fish, and eggs) that contain no carbohydrate, just protein and fat (and have a GI of essentially zero), still stimulate significant increases in blood insulin.

We don't currently know how to interpret this type of response for long-term health. It may be a good outcome, because the increase in insulin has contributed to the low level of glycemia. On the other hand, it may be less than ideal, because the increased demand for insulin contributes to beta-cell "exhaustion" and the development of type 2 diabetes. Until studies are carried out to answer these types of questions, the glycemic index remains a proven dietary tool for predicting the effects of food on health.

48. Why are glucose and white bread used as test foods in GI testing? Why not only glucose?

In the past, some scientists used a fifty-gram carbohydrate portion of white bread as the reference food, because it is more typical of what we actually eat. On this scale, where the GI value of white bread is set at 100, some foods will have a GI value of over 100, because their effect on blood glucose levels is higher than that of bread.

The use of two standards has caused some confusion, so the glucose = 100 scale is now recommended. It is possible to convert from the bread scale to the glucose scale using the factor 0.7 (70 ÷ 100). This factor is derived from the fact that the GI value of white bread is 70 on the glucose = 100 scale.

To avoid confusion throughout this book, we refer to all foods according to a standard whereby glucose equals 100.

49. How low should a low GI diet go?

We believe there's a real need to define the difference between a low GI *diet* and a low GI *food*. Because a low GI food is defined as 55 or less, people have made the reasonable assumption that a whole diet that averages less than 55 is "low enough." In fact, the average Australian and American diets already have a GI of 56 to 58, because we all eat low GI fruits and dairy products, and, of course, sugar has a medium GI (68). To reduce the risk of chronic disease, we believe that a low GI eating pattern/diet must have a much lower number.

What we now know from observational/cohort studies is that the GI of the diet of people in the lowest quintile (20 percent of the population) is about 40–45. Since this reduces the risk of chronic diseases like diabetes and heart disease, and people can achieve it in real life, we think it's a reasonable definition of a low GI diet or low GI meal (i.e., 45 or less).

50. Does retrograded starch ever revert back to regular starch?

Yes, retrograded starch will revert back to normal starch if it's reheated, perhaps not all of it, but much of it. That's the basis of making stale bread into "fresh" bread by heating it up in the oven. So twice-cooked potatoes will remain high GI. Even cold potatoes have a high GI because only 10 percent of the starch is retrograded. Some critics debate the fact that cooking makes a difference to the GI of potatoes, but the effect is relatively small and the overall message is that potatoes usually have a high GI. Having said that, we are discovering that some varieties have a lower GI—in the high 50s. These are usually called waxy potatoes, and they are recommended for making a potato salad because they keep their firm shape.

Your Guide to Low GI Eating

Making the Change to a Low GI Diet

Putting It on the Plate

Weekly Low GI Menu Ideas

The Low GI Shopper

Fifty Recipes for Low GI Living

18
Making the Change to a Low GI Diet

EATING A LOW GI DIET IS EASY. The crux of it is to be smart with your carbohydrate choices. Replace highly refined carbohydrates such as white bread, sugary treats, and crispy puffed cereals with less processed carbohydrates such as grainy bread, pasta, legumes, fruit, and vegetables.

While this sounds simple, it has science on its side. There's no measuring, no numbers, just eating the foods your body is designed for.

With low GI eating:

- You won't go hungry.
- You'll feel better.
- You'll look better.
- You'll have more energy.

One of our most frequently received requests is "just tell me what to eat!" So, in this section of the book, we focus on food and give you some simple guidelines for making the switch to everyday low GI eating. There's no specific order in which you have to do things and no strict week-by-week list of diet dos and don'ts.

Exactly how you incorporate low GI eating into your life is up to you. Some people want to eat low GI foods all the time; others some of the time. That's OK. There's room for both approaches—and, in reality, that's how most of us eat anyway.

Claire's Story

When I was twenty-six weeks into my first pregnancy, I visited the pathologist's for a second glucose test (GTT), having had a slightly abnormal reading previously. There was no history of diabetes in my family and despite having reactive hypoglycemia, I assumed I'd be in the clear. Little did I know that this fairly routine visit to the pathologist would end up changing my life. I was diagnosed with gestational diabetes.

*I consulted a dietitian and saw my endocrinologist, but the real turning point came when my mother, my healthy eating mentor, found a book that became my bible—*The New Glucose Revolution. *It changed my life and showed me that while it seemed like I had a well-balanced diet, I ate too many high GI foods. By making simple changes, I was able to manage my blood glucose levels with a balanced, low GI diet for the rest of the pregnancy.*

After giving birth, I was diagnosed with impaired glucose tolerance (IGT or prediabetes). This was despite losing somewhere between twenty and forty pounds (depending on whether you read my scales or my doctor's). I was told that if I wanted another child and a healthy life without type 2 diabetes, I had to lose weight and get fit. I took it very seriously. Within six months, I was cleared of IGT.

I have since had another child and despite doing all the right things, I was diagnosed with gestational diabetes again, from week twenty-eight. After the birth, I made a big effort to get back to my prepregnancy weight, and I was given the all-clear within three months and have continued to stay healthy since.

While it was all very stressful, I am so thankful that I had the wake-up call early enough. Not only am I living a healthy life, but so is my family. The knowledge I have gained about the GI has proven invaluable in starting to teach healthy eating habits to my kids—despite the sugar marketers' minefield in the supermarket. In retrospect, I am so positive about my experience that I hope other people can perhaps catch my enthusiasm and realize the benefits I have brought not only to my family but to my friends and others around me.

This for That

Everyday low GI eating is easy, a fact that may surprise you if you've struggled to follow other nutrition programs. Simply substituting high GI foods with low GI alternatives will give your overall diet a lower GI and deliver all the benefits of low GI eating. This could mean eating granola for breakfast instead of corn flakes, whole-grain bread (see page 199) instead of white, or fruit in place of cookies, for example. Whatever your usual diet, use the table on page 194 to help you identify the low GI choices.

Ten Steps to a Healthy Low GI Diet

The best way for any of us to eat is to choose from a wide variety of fresh foods that we enjoy and that satisfy us. Of course, we need to have sufficient protein and moderate amounts of carbohydrate and fats and a whole host of vitamins and minerals as well. So how can you be sure you'll meet all your nutritional needs? Along with incorporating your low GI carbohydrate choices, the following ten steps will give you a blueprint for eating a healthy and low GI diet for life.

1. Eat regularly.
2. Eat seven or more servings of fruit and vegetables (at least five servings of vegetables and two of fruit) per day.
3. Eat low GI forms of breads and cereals.
4. Eat more legumes (beans, chickpeas, lentils).
5. Use low-fat dairy foods and calcium-enriched soy products.
6. Include fish, seafood, or an alternative source of omega-3.
7. Eat nuts regularly.
8. Choose lean red meats, skinless chicken, and eggs or plant proteins like tofu.
9. Minimize your salt intake.
10. If you drink alcohol, keep it moderate.

"This for That": Substituting Low GI for High GI Foods

HIGH GI FOOD	LOW GI ALTERNATIVE
Cookies	A slice of whole-grain (see page 199) low GI bread with jam, fruit spread or nut spread or a slice of fruit bread
Breads such as soft white or whole wheat	Dense breads with whole grains, stoneground flour, sourdough, and commercial breads with the GI symbol ⓖ
Breakfast cereals—most commercial processed cereals	Traditional rolled oats, muesli, and commercial, low GI brands listed in the tables in Part 5; look for the GI symbol ⓖ
Cakes and pastries	Raisin toast, fruit loaf, and fruit buns, particularly whole-grain varieties
Chips and packaged snacks such as Twinkies, Pop-Tarts, pretzels	A handful of fresh grapes or cherry tomatoes, dried fruit or nuts
Doughnuts and croissants	Try a skim-milk cappuccino or smoothie instead.
French fries	Leave them out! Have salad or extra vegetables instead. Corn on the cob, coleslaw, or bean salad are better fast-food options.
Candy	Chocolate is lower GI but high in fat. Healthier options are nuts, raisins, dried apricots, and other dried fruits.
Granola bars	Make a homemade version or try dried fruit and nuts instead; look for low GI labeling.
Potato	Prepare small amounts of potato and add some sweet potato or sweet corn. You can also try sweet potato, yam, taro, or baby new potatoes—or just replace with other low GI or no GI vegetables.
Rice	Longer grain varieties such as basmati, or Uncle Ben's converted long-grain rice, Japanese sushi rice, barley, cracked wheat (bulgur), quinoa, pasta, or Asian rice noodles.
Soft drinks and fruit juice drinks	Use a "diet" or low-calorie variety, if these are a regular part of your diet. Juice has a lower GI but isn't lower in calories. Water is best.
Sugar	Moderate the quantity; consider pure floral honey, apple juice, fructose, agave syrup, and stevia as alternative sweeteners.

Simply substituting high GI foods . . .

. . . with low GI alternatives will give your overall diet a lower GI and deliver all the benefits of low GI eating.

1. Eat Regularly

Remember the basics: three meals a day is a must, but eating as often as every three hours is regular eating for some. It depends on your level of hunger. The main thing is that you don't skip meals. Going a long time between meals (more than about five hours) can trick your body into starvation mode. This gives the signal that food is in short supply, and your body responds by slowing down its metabolic rate (the rate at which it burns energy). In this state, when you do eat, your food will be metabolized differently. It will be directed to storage to enhance survival. What's more, when the next mealtime arrives, you may be absolutely famished and tend to gorge.

Eating regularly appears to have a connection with body weight. Studies have found that people who eat on four to six occasions in a day have healthier body weights than those who eat only two to three meals, even if the total amount of food is similar. Even three meals a day is better than one or two when it comes to blood fat levels, too. Eating regularly tends to give structure to your eating habits, allowing you to become more aware of what you eat. This in turn makes it easier to establish good habits and identify problem eating.

- Eat a good breakfast. Fire up your engine with low GI carbs. A good breakfast recharges your brain and speeds up your metabolism after an overnight fast. Choosing a low GI cereal is one of the most important things you can do to start your day; a bowl of traditional oatmeal in winter or muesli in the summer will sustain you through the morning.
- Give priority to eating. Think about where you'll be at your next meal or snack time. Be prepared to let eating take precedence over other activities. Carry a snack with you (e.g., a piece of fruit, a nut bar, a small pack of dried fruit and/or nuts). Make meals a time to relax and enjoy eating; you are more likely to feel satisfied if you do.

- Refuel at lunchtime to maintain energy levels right through the afternoon. Hold back on the high GI carbs to minimize that post-lunch energy dip. And take time over one main meal every day to make sure you aren't missing out on the vital vegetables you need.
- Eat small: think of the size of your fist. The bigger the portion in front of you, the more you'll end up eating, so serve small and eat more often if you need to. Don't let fast-food chains upsize your serving for a little extra money. If it's not in front of you, you won't eat it.
- Plan meals ahead. Cook and freeze for when you come home tired. Take some time on the weekend to think about meals for the week ahead. Write a shopping list. Take food with you when you will be away from home for a meal. Avoid grabbing food on the run.
- Listen to your stomach. Stop eating when you are comfortably full, not stuffed. And if you're unsure whether you've eaten enough, stop anyway and wait. It takes twenty minutes for your stomach to signal fullness to your brain, so give the message a chance to get through. If you don't feel hungry when mealtimes come around, just eat a very small portion.
- Eat a little of whatever you really feel like. Be mindful when you eat it. Take the time to enjoy it fully, free of other distractions. Denying yourself can create cravings and lead to a binge.

Studies have shown . . .

. . . that people who weigh themselves nearly every day gain less weight over time than people who weigh themselves less often.

2. Eat Seven or More Servings of Fruit and Vegetables (at Least Five Servings of Vegetables and Two of Fruit) per Day

Fruit and vegetables are a pivotal part of a healthy low GI diet. Nutrient rich and low in calories, they are the sort of foods you can't really overdo. A high fruit and vegetable intake has consistently been linked with protection from cancer, obesity, heart disease, macular degeneration, and other age-related diseases. Unique combinations of vitamins and antioxidants in fruit and vegetables keep your skin and eyes healthy and function like personal bodyguards, protecting cells throughout the body from the damage that occurs as a natural part of aging and from pollutants in the environment.

There are myriad ways to incorporate fruit and vegetables in your diet.

- Increase your ALA (the plant form of omega-3) with broccoli, Swiss chard, spinach, cabbage, Asian greens, and green beans.
- Throw some vegetables on the barbecue along with the meat. Try zucchini, sweet corn, red peppers, mushrooms, eggplant, or thick slices of parboiled sweet potato.

Which Spud?

Potatoes are one of the most popular vegetables, and their GI varies depending on the variety and cooking method. Precooking and reheating potatoes or eating cold, cooked potatoes (such as potato salad) reduces the glycemic response. The highest GI values are found in potatoes that have been freshly cooked and in instant mashed potatoes.

- Potatoes, red, cubed, boiled, then stored overnight in the fridge. Consumed cold (GI 56), 1 medium.
- Canned new potatoes, eaten hot (GI 65). These are the "tiny taters" whose lower GI is probably linked to their small size and compact starch. Serve two or three with an ear of corn to lower the glycemic impact.
- New potatoes, unpeeled, boiled whole (GI 78). The smaller these are, the lower the GI is likely to be. Cook them with the skin on for extra nutrients.
- Potatoes, baked, Russet Burbank, boiled without fat, 1 medium (GI 76).
- Potatoes, red, boiled, with skin on, consumed hot, 1 medium (GI 89). Note that cooked, cooled and consumed cold (as in potato salad), the GI is 56.

Potatoes are fat-free and contain a host of vitamins and minerals, especially potassium and vitamin C. To retain the most nutrients in your potatoes, scrub them well and steam or boil them in their skins. The thinnest layer of skin can be easily rubbed off once cooked, if you wish.

- Include salad ingredients in a sandwich or bread roll.
- When eating out, order a side salad (and pass on the chips).
- Wash apples when you first bring them home and place in a bowl in the fridge so they are ready to grab and go.
- Prepare vegetables with a little healthy oil, lemon juice, balsamic vinegar, garlic, or black pepper to make them tastier.
- Chop fresh pineapple or melon into large chunks and keep on hand in the refrigerator for snacks during the day.
- Put a plate of sliced apple or a bowl of grapes beside you to nibble on as you work, read, or watch TV as an alternative to chips or ice cream.
- Serve a fruit platter after a meal as dessert.

3. Eat Low GI Forms of Breads and Cereals

Cereal grains including rice, wheat, oats, barley, rye, and their products (bread, pasta, breakfast cereal, flour) are the most concentrated sources of carbohydrate in our diet. Because of this, the form in which we eat these foods has a major impact on the GI of our diet. Breads and cereals with a low GI are:

- Densely grained breads, traditional sourdough, or commercially made low GI breads
- Barley—e.g., pearl barley in soup, casseroles, salads, or a barley risotto
- Whole-wheat or cracked wheat such as bulgur in tabbouleh
- Low GI rice such as basmati, Uncle Ben's converted long-grain rice, and Uncle Ben's long-grain and wild rice blend
- Traditional rolled oats for breakfast as oatmeal or in muesli
- Pasta and noodles. If you have to eat a gluten-free diet, then wheat, rye, barley, oats, and triticale and foods made from these grains are off the menu.

The good news is that there are now low GI gluten-free breads and breakfast cereals on the supermarket shelves (see the tables in Part 5). And you can also make the most of other low GI cereal grains and products, including:

- Corn, a great standby on its own or added to soups, salads, and casseroles

- Quinoa, to make cereals, salads, or tabbouleh or serve as an accompaniment
- Buckwheat, which can be added to soups and casseroles or used to make tabbouleh
- Rice noodles and vermicelli, which can be added to Thai salads, rice paper rolls, or Asian soups
- Buckwheat and bean thread noodles (check to see if they are completely gluten-free), which can be used in place of rice

Are All "Whole-grain" Foods Low GI?

"Whole-grain" is one of the latest buzzwords in nutrition. You'll see it on everything from corn-flake packets to rice crackers. Unfortunately, "whole-grain" and "low GI" have been used as though they are interchangeable terms. This is not the case.

Food labeling legislation requires that a food that is labeled "whole-grain" contains all the components of whole cereal grains, present in their natural proportions. It doesn't mean that the grains are in their natural form and doesn't even hint at whether the food has a low GI. In fact, many processed whole-grain foods such as whole-wheat bread and toasted bran flakes have a high GI. Why? It all comes down to the physical state of the fiber and the starch in the food (see pages 21–23).

When we use the term "whole-grain," we are referring to grains that are eaten in nature's packaging, or close to it: traditional rolled oats, cracked wheat, and pearl barley, for example. The slow digestion and absorption of these foods will trickle fuel into your engine at a slower rate, keeping you satisfied for longer. We like to say that your body is doing the processing, not the manufacturer.

When we use the term "whole-grain" . . .

. . . we are referring to grains that are eaten in nature's packaging, or close to it: traditional rolled oats, cracked wheat, and pearl barley, for example.

4. Eat More Legumes

Legumes, including lentils, chickpeas, soybeans, and kidney beans are one of nature's lowest GI foods. Include them at least twice a week (more often, if you are a vegetarian). They are easy on the budget, versatile, filling, and packed with nutrients, providing a valuable source of protein, carbohydrate, B vitamins, folate, iron, zinc, magnesium, and fiber.

Whether you buy dried beans, lentils, and chickpeas and cook them yourself at home, or opt for the convenient, time-saving canned varieties, you are choosing one of nature's lowest GI foods.

A bean meal doesn't always have to be vegetarian; try using beans in place of grains or potatoes. You could serve a bean salsa with fish or cannellini bean purée with grilled meat. Butter beans can also make a delicious potato substitute.

Because they are high in protein, legumes are an ideal substitute for meat. Introduce them to your family gradually by incorporating them in meals with meat, as chili con carne or a filling for tacos or burritos, for example. You could also try:

- Three-bean mix with a salad
- Canned kidney beans in a bolognaise sauce
- Hummus dip or spread
- Dhal (lentils or split peas cooked with spices) as an accompaniment to curry
- Pea and ham soup
- Potatoes baked with onions, beans, and lean bacon
- Firm tofu cubed, marinated, and added to stir-fries

 Of all foods eaten . . .

. . . by populations around the world, legumes are associated with the longest lifespan.

The Special Benefits of Soy

Soybeans and soy products such as tofu and tempeh have been a staple in Asian diets for thousands of years and are an excellent source of protein. They are also rich in fiber, iron, zinc, and vitamin B. They are lower in carbohydrate and higher in fat than other legumes, but the majority of the fat is polyunsaturated. Soy is also a rich source of phytochemicals.

Foods based on soybeans also have a beneficial role in your defense against heart disease. There are two components of soybeans with the potential to reduce heart disease risk: soy protein and antioxidant substances called isoflavones. Soy foods improve blood fats, lowering the bad (LDL) cholesterol and increasing the good (HDL) cholesterol. Studies suggest that one to two servings of soy-protein–rich food each day may be sufficient to provide long-term health benefits. Just one cup of soy milk constitutes a serving and can be used as a nutritionally balanced replacement for dairy milk, providing it is low fat and calcium enriched. Try:

- Soy milk on your breakfast cereal
- A soy banana smoothie
- Soy yogurt for a snack

5. Use Low-Fat Dairy and Calcium-Enriched Soy Products

Dairy products provide energy; protein; carbohydrate; vitamins A, B, and D; calcium; phosphorous; and magnesium. Virtually all dairy foods have low GI values, largely thanks to lactose, the sugar found naturally in milk, which has a low GI of 46. By choosing low-fat varieties of milk, yogurt, ice cream, and custard, you will enjoy a food that provides you with sustained energy, boosting your calcium intake but not your saturated fat intake. Low-fat milk supplies as much (and usually more) calcium than full-cream milk:

- 1 cup (8 oz) of low-fat milk contains about 415 mg calcium and only 0.5 grams fat
- 1 cup (8 oz) of regular milk contains about 295 mg calcium and 9.7 grams fat.

Calcium is the most abundant mineral in our bodies. It builds our bones and teeth and is involved in muscle contraction and relaxation, blood clotting, nerve function, and regulation of blood pressure. Research shows that calcium-rich low-fat dairy products:

■ Can help lower high blood pressure
■ May protect against cancer, particularly cancer of the bladder, bowel, and colon, and possibly against breast, ovarian, pancreas, and skin cancers
■ Can favorably influence blood fat levels and reduce the risk of stroke
■ Can reduce the risk of kidney stones
■ Can assist in weight regulation

If you eat only plant foods or want to avoid dairy products, soy products such as soy drinks, yogurts, and desserts are the answer. Soy products are not naturally high in calcium, so look for calcium-fortified products if you are relying on them as a source of calcium. And choose the reduced-fat ones, of course. Sesame seeds, dried apricots and figs, Asian greens, and the edible bones of fish also contain calcium.

To meet our calcium requirements, we recommend that adults eat two to three servings of dairy products every day. Good low-fat dairy choices include skim, no-fat, or low-fat milk and no-fat or low-fat yogurts. A serving is: 1 cup (8 oz) milk, 1.5 ounces of low-fat cheese, or 1 small container (7 oz) of yogurt.

What If You Are Lactose Intolerant?

Some people are lactose intolerant because the enzyme lactase is not active in their small intestines. If you are lactose intolerant, you should still be able to enjoy cheese, which is virtually lactose-free, and yogurt. The microorganisms in yogurt are active in digesting lactose during passage through the small intestine. Alternatively, try lactose-reduced or lactose-free milk and milk products, or low GI, low-fat, calcium-enriched nondairy alternatives such as soy milk. Note that rice milk has a high GI value (92).

6. Include Fish, Seafood, or an Alternative Source of Omega-3

Eating fish regularly is associated with a reduced risk of heart disease, improvements in mood and lower rates of depression, better blood fat levels, and enhanced immunity. It is likely that the protective components are the very long-chain omega-3 fatty acids. Exactly how they work is a topic of much research. They can reduce inflammation in the body, iron out irregularity in heart beat, reduce blood fat levels, and might play a valuable role in treating depression and Alzheimer's disease. Modern Western diets almost certainly do not provide enough of the polyunsaturated omega-3 fats. Our bodies make only small amounts of these unique fatty acids, so we rely on dietary sources, especially fish and seafood, for them.

While the very long-chain omega-3 fats are also found in some other animal foods, seafood contains ten to a hundred times more than other food groups. For this reason, we suggest you have at least one to two fish meals per week.

Which Fish Is Best for Omega-3?

Oily fish, which tend to have darker-colored flesh and a stronger flavor, are the richest source of omega-3 fats. Fresh fish that contain the highest amounts of omega-3 fats include:

- Swordfish
- Atlantic salmon
- Southern bluefin tuna*
- Gemfish*
- Atlantic, Pacific, and Spanish mackerel

* Species identified by the Australian Bureau of Rural Sciences as overfished.

Sustainable Fish Facts

Shopping for fish can be a bit of a minefield. For up-to-date facts and information on sustainable fish, visit:

www.montereybayaquarium.org/cr/seafoodwatch.aspx

You can download a printable pocket guide as well.

Eastern and Pacific oysters and squid (calamari) are rich sources of omega-3. Canned fish such as salmon, sardines, mackerel, and, to a lesser extent, tuna are rich sources. Look for canned fish packed in water, canola oil, olive oil, tomato sauce, or brine, and drain well.

Alternative Sources of Omega-3 fats

The very long-chain omega-3 fats can also be found in:

- Lean red meat, kidney, and liver
- Regular and fish oil-enriched eggs
- Some manufactured products that have encapsulated tuna oil added to them as a source of long-chain omega-3, for example, high omega-3 bread

Mercury in Fish

Due to the risk of high levels of mercury in certain species of fish, the U.S. Food and Drug Administration (FDA) has advised that pregnant women, nursing mothers, women planning pregnancy, and young children should avoid consuming certain species but can continue to consume a variety of fish as a part of a healthy diet. Shark, swordfish, king mackerel, and tilefish should not be consumed, because these long-lived, larger fish contain the highest levels of mercury. Pregnant women should select a variety of other kinds of fish—shellfish, canned fish such as light tuna, smaller ocean fish, or farm-raised fish. The FDA recommends two three-ounce servings per week, but says you can safely eat up to twelve ounces of cooked fish per week.

Plant Sources of Omega-3

A shorter chain form of omega-3, alphalinoleic acid (ALA for short), is found in plants. Our bodies can convert this to a longer chain form but to support conversion, it is important you avoid eating too much of the omega-6 class of fats (found especially in sunflower, safflower, soybean, and corn oils).

Good sources of ALA are:

- **Flaxseed oil.** This is the richest plant source of ALA. However, it is extremely prone to turning rancid with heat and time and (ironically) develops a fishy odor and taste. Purchase it in very small quantities and store carefully. It is best used in salad dressings. Alternatively, flaxseeds themselves can be freshly ground and sprinkled on cereal or added to cakes and muffins.

- **Canola oil.** This oil is high in monounsaturated fat but also contains significant amounts of ALA. Margarines are available based on canola oil, and these are also a source of ALA.

- **Walnuts and pecans.**

- **Soybeans and soy beverages enriched with omega-3.** Soybean oil is a source of omega-3, but its high omega-6 content makes it less desirable as a source of ALA.

- **Green leafy vegetables.** Particularly broccoli, cabbage, spinach, Swiss chard, kale, and parsley.

Note: Olive oil is not a rich source of omega-3 but is considered "omega neutral" because the fatty acids it contains do not oppose the action of omega-3s.

7. Eat Nuts Regularly

People who eat nuts once a week have lower levels of heart disease than those who don't eat any nuts. There are probably several reasons for this. Nuts contain a variety of antioxidants that keep blood vessels healthy; arginine, an amino acid that helps keep blood flowing smoothly; and folate and fiber, both of which can lower cholesterol levels. Nuts have even been shown to help blood glucose control in people with diabetes.

Although nuts are high in fat (averaging around 50 percent), the fat is largely unsaturated, so they make a healthy substitute for foods such as cookies, cakes, pastries, potato chips, and chocolate. Because they are so nutrient and energy dense, a little goes a long way. We suggest you have about thirty grams most days (or the equivalent). They also contain relatively little carbohydrate, so most do not have a GI value.

- Nuts are perfect for staving off hunger as a between-meal snack. Enjoy a small handful on their own or with a little dried fruit.
- Use nuts in food preparation. For example, use toasted cashews in a chicken stir-fry, sprinkle walnuts or pine nuts over a salad, top fruity desserts with almonds, or add chopped nuts to muesli.
- Use hazelnut spread on bread or try peanut, almond, or cashew butter rather than butter or margarine.
- Sprinkle a mixture of ground nuts and flaxseeds over cereal or salads, or add to baked goods such as muffins.

Chestnuts

Chestnuts are something of an anomaly in the nut family—they are very low in fat and are a great source of carbs (GI 54 for crushed, uncooked chestnut kernels). They are also high in dietary fiber and rich in B-group vitamins and minerals. They are versatile. You can roast them in an open fire and enjoy hot, or add them to soups, stir-fries, stuffings, casseroles, vegetable dishes, pasta, risotto, and desserts. You'll find fresh chestnuts in your supermarket or produce store from autumn to early winter.

8. Choose Lean Red Meats, Skinless Chicken, and Eggs

Reducing your intake of saturated fat doesn't mean you need to avoid meat. Red meat is the best dietary source of iron, the nutrient used in carrying oxygen in your blood, and the main source of zinc, which is a part of over a hundred enzymes active in the body. A good iron and zinc status can improve energy levels and exercise tolerance. A chronic shortage of iron leads to anemia, with symptoms including pale skin, excessive tiredness, breathlessness, and decreased attention span. Even mild iron deficiency can cause unexplained fatigue.

Although chicken contains about one-third the iron of red meat, it is readily absorbed, as it is from red meat, and provides a versatile, nutrient-rich alternative.

If you enjoy meat, we suggest eating lean red meat two to three times a week, accompanying it with salad and vegetables. Trim all visible fat from meat and remove the skin (and the fat just below it) from chicken. Game meats such as rabbit and venison not only are lean but are also good sources of omega-3 fatty acids. So are organ meats such as liver and kidney. Leaner deli meat products are pastrami, roast beef, leg ham, and rolled turkey breast.

Eggs also contain valuable amounts of the nutrients found in meat, although the iron is not as well absorbed. It used to be thought that eggs should be limited because of their high cholesterol content, but studies have found recently that our bodies compensate for an increased cholesterol intake by reducing the liver's cholesterol production. This means that most people (adults and children) can eat an egg a day, for example, without harming their hearts. However, a small percentage of people have an inherited condition called familial hypercholesterolemia, which impairs this self-regulation. To enhance your intake of omega-3 fats, you might use omega-3-enriched eggs. These are produced by feeding hens a diet (including canola and flaxseeds) that is naturally rich in omega-3s.

9. Minimize Your Salt Intake

An estimated 75 percent of the salt we eat is from salt already existing in foods, not salt we voluntarily add. Bread and butter or margarine, for example, contribute much of the salt in our diets. Low-salt breads take some adjusting of the taste buds, but low-salt margarines, which are easy to find on supermarket shelves, are not noticeably different in taste.

Salt causes the body to hold onto fluid, which then increases blood pressure. High blood pressure, or hypertension, is a serious health problem, particularly for those with heart disease or diabetes. Even children eating a high-salt diet are at risk of an increase in blood pressure. Lowering salt intake lowers blood pressure, although some people will respond more than others. A high salt intake has other consequences:

■ The more salt we eat, the more calcium we excrete, so a high salt intake is a risk for osteoporosis (calcium is leached from our bones).

- Bronchial reactivity (the chance of our bronchial tubes going into spasm) is linked to sodium balance, so there is some evidence that the severity of asthma is related to salt intake.
- Meniere's disease, which causes vertigo, tinnitus, and intermittent hearing loss, although the cause is uncertain, is partially treated with a low-salt diet.
- Risk of stroke, gastric cancer, and kidney stones is also increased, according to some studies.

Foods high in salt include:

- Canned, bottled, and packaged soups, sauces, gravy bases, and stock cubes
- Sausages, ham, bacon, and other cured meats
- Pizza, burgers, fried chicken, and other take-out foods
- Pickles, chutneys, olives
- Snack foods such as potato chips

We recommend that you minimize the frequency with which you eat salty foods. Once your taste buds adapt to a lower salt intake—over three to four weeks—you will find it easier to eat less salt and harder to eat salty foods.

Check food labels for the salt content (listed as "sodium"). A low-salt food contains less than 120 mg sodium per 100 grams. Aim for less than 450 mg per 100 grams in convenience and ready-to-eat foods. Don't routinely add salt to your food at the table or when cooking and ensure that any salt that you do use in the home is iodized (as an additional dietary source of iodine).

10. *If You Drink Alcohol, Keep It Moderate*

Of everything we drink, alcohol can be considered the most fattening, not simply because of its calorie content, but because it has priority as a fuel over other nutrients: as long as there's alcohol in your system, anything else is surplus until the alcohol is burned up—and surplus calories are stored largely as body fat. Looking at it another way, just one can of beer replaces all the calories burned by twenty minutes of brisk walking.

There is no doubt that large quantities of alcohol should be avoided, but several studies have suggested that a moderate alcohol intake can have a protective effect against heart disease in some people. People who drink one or two standard drinks per day, but not necessarily every day, show a reduced risk of heart disease, with the effect being greatest among those with other risk factors for heart disease. It is important to note the finding that having three or more drinks per day actually increases the risk of death!

Taking Control

The current guidelines for low risk to health from drinking alcohol are that men consume no more than two standard drinks and women consume no more than one standard drink per day.

A standard drink is:

- 5 oz wine
- 12 oz beer
- 1.5 oz spirits

All contain .6 fluid oz of alcohol.

For information, counseling, or other assistance to help moderate your alcohol intake, contact the drug and alcohol service in your area.

Who Shouldn't Drink Alcohol?

If you have a fatty liver, high triglycerides, pancreatitis, advanced neuropathy, or any form of liver disease, you should not drink any alcohol.

Also, if you are pregnant, planning to have a baby, or breast feeding, we recommend you do not drink any alcohol.

Tips for Drinking Less

If you think you are drinking too much, try some of the following ideas to help reduce your alcohol intake:

- Drink some water or a diet soft drink before you drink any alcohol, so you are not thirsty when you start.
- Order a glass of wine and a glass of water at the same time.
- Sip your alcoholic drink slowly.
- Drink a nonalcoholic drink after every alcoholic drink (e.g., water or a diet soft drink).

19
Putting It on the Plate

THERE ARE THREE SIMPLE STEPS to putting together a balanced, low GI meal.

1 is for carbs—the low GI ones

Carbs are an essential although sometimes forgotten part of a balanced meal. They are going to satisfy your appetite and ensure a steady trickle of fuel to keep you energized. Think about what you feel like having: rice, pasta, noodles, bread, beans?

We want you to eat at least one low GI carb at each meal.

2 is for protein

Another part of the satisfaction equation, protein will help to keep you going between meals, and it lowers the glycemic load by replacing some of the carbohydrate, but not all! Think lean meat, skinless chicken, fish, seafood, eggs, cheese, tofu, nuts, or legumes.

3 is for fruits and vegetables

Do a double-check: did your last meal include some fruit or vegetables? If anything, they should have the highest priority in a meal. Nonetheless, a meal based *solely* on fruit or low-carb vegetables won't be sustaining for long. A sandwich made with just lettuce, tomato, cucumber or other low-calorie vegetables and without a source of protein is a recipe for hunger.

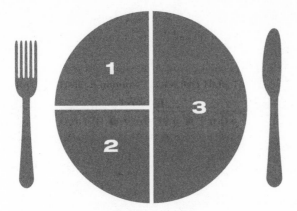

1 = carbs, 2 = protein, 3 = fruits and vegetables

A plate model like this can be adapted to any serving sizes. The bigger your body, the bigger your plate, but keep the food in these proportions! On the following pages, you'll discover how these proportions work in daily meals.

Low GI Breakfasts

1 | Low GI carbs—
for example,
breakfast cereal,
bread, rice, oats,
toast, muesli, etc.

3 | Fruit and/or
vegetables—
for example, fruit
juice, tomato,
mushrooms,
dried fruit,
grapefruit,
strawberries,
banana, etc.

2 | A source of
protein—for
example, low-fat
milk, yogurt,
eggs, cheese

What's for Breakfast?

A Cooked Breakfast

1   Top whole-grain (see page 199) toast with

+

2   scrambled egg and

+

3   spinach, sautéed mushrooms, or steamed asparagus.

Oatmeal

1   Cook traditional or steel-cut oats with water and

+

2   low-fat milk or soy milk, plus a dollop of low-fat Greek-style
yogurt, and

+

3   top with fresh or frozen berries.

Ricotta Fruit Toast

1 Spread toasted low GI fruit bread with

+

2 fresh ricotta cheese and

+

3 top with tomato slices, fruit spread, or slices of stone fruit in season.

Mixed-Grain Oatmeal

1 Cook a combination of rolled oats, rolled barley, and roasted buckwheat in

+

2 low-fat or soy milk. Stir in flaxseeds and sunflower seeds and

+

3 top with chopped, dried apricots.

Pita Bread with Cheese and Vegetables

1 Pita bread with

+

2 *labneh* (Arabic-style soft yogurt cheese) and

+

3 sliced tomato, cucumber, and olives.

Bircher Muesli

1 Soak a cup of oats and a tablespoon of honey with

+

2 low-fat or soy milk in the refrigerator overnight; then

+

3 stir in a grated apple and a tablespoon of raisins before serving.

Rice with Egg and Vegetables

1   Steamed low GI rice, e.g., basmati, served with

+

2   egg and

+

3   steamed spinach.

Corn Fritters

1   Combine the kernels from an ear of sweet corn with ¼ cup plain flour,

+

2   2 beaten eggs, fresh herbs, and seasoning and pan-fry spoonfuls in a nonstick pan about 2 minutes on each side; and

+

3   serve with grilled or slow-roasted tomatoes.

French Toast

1   Dip 4 slices of sourdough bread into

+

2   a mixture of 2 eggs, ¼ cup of skim milk, and a teaspoon of pure vanilla extract, and

+

3   cook in a greased pan for 2–3 minutes on each side, then top with pan-fried pear or apple slices, a drizzle of maple syrup, and a sprinkling of cinnamon.

Low GI Lunches

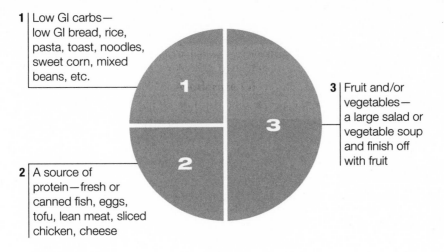

1 | Low GI carbs—low GI bread, rice, pasta, toast, noodles, sweet corn, mixed beans, etc.

2 | A source of protein—fresh or canned fish, eggs, tofu, lean meat, sliced chicken, cheese

3 | Fruit and/or vegetables—a large salad or vegetable soup and finish off with fruit

What's for Lunch?

Salmon Wrap

1 Spread flat, unleavened bread (e.g., lavash or pita) with a blend of ricotta and light cream cheese, then

+

2 top with slices of smoked trout or salmon,

+

3 drizzle with lemon juice, add baby spinach leaves, and roll up tightly in plastic wrap and refrigerate before serving.

Asian Noodle Salad

1 Toss soaked and drained mung bean vermicelli with

+

2 strips of lightly browned chicken breast or rump steak

+

3 and very thin strips of raw salad vegetables such as red onion, red pepper, carrot, cucumber, and fresh mint. Dress with mixture of two tablespoons each of lime juice, sweet chili sauce, and canola oil, with a teaspoon each of fish sauce, brown sugar, sesame oil, and white vinegar.

Salmon with New Potato Salad and Creamy Lemon Dressing

1 Combine cooked and cooled, diced new potatoes with

$$+$$

2 drained canned salmon and

$$+$$

3 chopped shallots and celery. Dress with a mixture of low-fat natural yogurt, lemon juice, whole-grain mustard, salt, and pepper.

Pasta with Bacon and Zucchini

1 Take some fresh cooked pasta and toss in

$$+$$

2 a few strips of lean bacon,

$$+$$

3 zucchini, fresh asparagus, and crushed garlic, all stir-fried in a little olive oil. Add a diced, fresh ripe tomato and stir into the pasta, garnishing with fresh basil leaves if desired.

Vietnamese Noodle Soup

1 Mung bean vermicelli with

$$+$$

2 wafer-thin slices of beef fillet,

$$+$$

3 spring onions, ginger, peppercorns, bean shoots, and soy sauce in a boiling beef stock.

Easy Pilaf

1 Combine red lentils cooked in chicken stock with low GI rice,

$$+$$

2 toasted pine nuts,

$$+$$

3 sautéed chopped onion, garlic, and tomatoes and serve hot or cold.

Stir-fried Noodles
1 Stir-fry noodles

+

2 with tofu, scrambled egg,

+

3 onion, bok choy, bean shoots, and soy sauce.

Chicken and Noodle Soup
1 Add rice noodles or mung bean vermicelli and

+

2 shredded chicken to a clear soup with

+

3 shallots and minced ginger.

Quick and Easy Fried Rice
1 Combine cooked and cooled low GI rice and sweet corn kernels with

+

2 diced lean bacon, small cooked prawns, and strips of omelette and stir-fry with

+

3 peas, shallots, and bean sprouts. Dress with oyster sauce or reduced-salt soy sauce.

Chili Bean Fajitas
1 In corn tortillas, wrap warmed chili beans with

+

2 grated reduced-fat tasty cheese

+

3 and avocado and serve with extra lettuce or greens.

Low GI Main Meals

1 | Low GI carbs—basmati, Uncle Ben's converted long grain rice or long grain and wild rice blend, pasta, noodles, sweet corn, chickpeas, lentils, baby potatoes, mixed beans, etc.

2 | A source of protein— fish or seafood; lean beef, pork, or veal; trim lamb; skinless chicken

3 | Fruit and/or vegetables— fill half the plate with vegetables or accompany the meal with a large salad; again, fruit makes a perfect finish

What's for Dinner?
Fish and Salad
1   Serve diced baby potatoes roasted in garlic, cumin, and olive oil with

+

2   a fish fillet dressed with herbs and lemon alongside

+

3   mixed vegetables or salad.

Country Chicken Casserole
1   Include chunks of sweet potato, sweet corn, and butter beans

+

2   in a chicken casserole with

+

3   onions, carrots, celery, and mushrooms.

Tomato Tortellini

1 Top spinach and ricotta tortellini with

+

2 shaved parmesan

+

3 and a tomato pasta sauce; serve a salad on the side.

Roast Chicken with Rosemary on Pesto and Tomato Pasta

1 Serve ribbon (tagliatelle, fettucine) pasta tossed in pesto and sundried tomatoes with

+

2 bite-sized chunks of roasted chicken flavored with rosemary and garlic and

+

3 steamed broccoli alongside.

Cabbage Rolls

1 Use a mixture of cooked basmati rice, tomato, onion, and pepper with

+

2 lean minced beef

+

3 to make cabbage rolls. Serve with a tomato, onion, and black olive salad.

Asian Snapper

1 Serve steamed low GI rice with

+

2 a baked or steamed whole snapper

+

3 served on a bed of stir-fried vegetables with green mango salad dressing.

Tandoori Chicken

1 Try turmeric-flavored basmati rice with

$+$

2 tandoori chicken,

$+$

3 cucumber, lettuce, onion, lemon wedges, and natural yogurt.

Salad Niçoise

1 Cooked and cooled new potatoes, cut into wedges and combined with

$+$

2 fresh or canned tuna and quartered hard-boiled eggs with

$+$

3 lettuce, blanched green beans, olives, spring onions, and tomatoes, all drizzled with olive oil and lemon juice.

Chili Mint Lamb and Tomato Salad

1 Prepare bulgur wheat with boiling water and the juice and zest of a lemon; then

$+$

2 combine with slices of char-grilled lamb fillet,

$+$

3 slices of Lebanese cucumber, a handful of torn mint leaves, halved cherry tomatoes, red pepper strips, and finely chopped red chili. Dress with a mixture of olive oil and lemon juice.

Spaghetti with Tomato, Olives, and Feta

1 Toss spaghetti or your favorite pasta with

$+$

2 cubes of fat- and salt-reduced feta and

$+$

3 tomato, red onion, basil, olives, and arugula.

Quick and Easy Low GI Desserts

Stuffed Baked Apples

Remove the cores from large green Granny Smith or Golden Delicious apples and stuff with a combination of dried fruits (e.g., raisins, chopped apricots, and pears), walnuts or pecans, cinnamon, and brown sugar. Bake in a moderately hot oven for 15 minutes. Serve with low-fat plain yogurt or vanilla custard.

Fruit Plate

Place a selection of sliced fresh fruits on a platter (e.g., mango, pineapple, strawberries, kiwi, and cantaloupe). Add a bowl of low-fat plain yogurt combined with a tablespoon of floral honey for dipping.

Baked Stone Fruit

Bake whole stone fruit in a syrup of 1 cup white wine, ½ cup water, and ½ cup floral honey flavored with vanilla and cinnamon in a moderately hot oven until tender (about 15 minutes) and serve with light vanilla ice cream.

Fruit Crumble

Spoon cooked apple and rhubarb, fresh or canned peaches, plums, and strawberries into a wide, casserole-type dish. Top with a crumble topping made by combining equal parts of rolled oats, brown sugar, and whole-wheat flour with a little margarine. Bake in a moderately hot oven for 15–20 minutes.

Chocolate Sauce

Place 5 ounces dark chocolate, chopped into small pieces, 1 tablespoon canola oil, and 3 tablespoons cold water into a small saucepan and heat gently, stirring occasionally until combined. Pour it over low-fat ice cream or baked pears or offer as a dipping sauce.

Mango Lassi

Combine 1½ cups diced mango with ½ cup of fresh orange juice, ice cubes, 1 tablespoon floral honey, and 1 teaspoon rosewater (optional). Process until just mixed, then add 1½ cups low-fat natural yogurt and blend until frothy. Makes 4 cups.

20
Weekly Low GI Menu Ideas

THE FOLLOWING MENUS ILLUSTRATE a healthy low GI diet with everyday foods. You can use them for ideas for your own meals or follow them closely to try out a low GI diet.

Beverages have been included only where they make a significant nutrient contribution, so supplement the menus with a range of fluids such as water, tea, coffee, herbal teas, and mineral or soda water with lemon or lime slices.

And remember to allow yourself a treat occasionally. Indulge in a little of whatever you fancy, but only when you really feel like it. Savor it! For example:

- 3–4 squares of dark chocolate
- 1–2 scoops of your favorite ice cream
- 1 oz of a favorite cheese
- A glass of dessert wine

A Low GI Summer Menu

	MONDAY	TUESDAY	WEDNESDAY
Breakfast	Toasted sour-dough with mozzarella or baked ricotta cheese, seasonal fruit and a low-fat latté	Natural muesli topped with strawberries and low-fat vanilla yogurt	Whole-grain toast spread with peanut butter and topped with sliced banana
Lunch	Tabbouleh* and hummus on flat bread Fresh fruit	A sourdough or grainy bread roll with lean prosciutto, chopped black olives, and sliced fennel	Salmon with New Potato Salad and creamy lemon and yogurt dressing
Dinner	Glazed chicken with mashed sweet potato and stir-fried greens*	Quick and Easy Fried Rice	Spinach and ricotta cannel-loni with pine nuts and tomato sauce, and mixed green salad and vinaigrette
Snack	Fresh strawber-ries dipped in dark chocolate	Chopped pine-apple, melon, and passion fruit with yogurt and crushed nuts	Baked summer fruits (peach, apricot, plums and berries) served with light vanilla fromage frais

Note: Underlined meal ideas detailed in Chapter 19.
* See recipe in Chapter 22.

How Can the Sweet Fruits of Summer Be Low GI?

Not only are summertime grapes, peaches, mangoes, and melons sweet and juicy, they are highly nutritious. People who eat three or four serv-ings of fruit a day, particularly apples and oranges, have the lowest overall GI and the best blood glucose control.

Naturally sweet and filling, fruit is widely available, inexpensive, portable, and easy to eat—just like other snack foods, but without the

THURSDAY	FRIDAY	SATURDAY	SUNDAY
Fresh fruit salad with a dollop of low-fat yogurt and a sprinkle of toasted muesli or a dried fruit/nut mix	High-fiber low GI cereal with low-fat milk and a glass of orange juice	Corn fritters with slow-roasted tomatoes	Sourdough toast with poached egg, sautéed mushroom and lean bacon
Pasta with Bacon and Zucchini Sliced fruit	Asian Beef Noodle Soup	Salmon Wraps	Barbecued sweet corn Chicken drumsticks with apricot glaze
Barbecued fish, roasted baby potatoes with garlic and rosemary, and fresh asparagus with lemon and pepper	Stuffed eggplant with mixed green salad and an herb sourdough roll	Fresh oysters with mango and pepper salsa Barbecued steak with roast vegetable salad and balsamic vinaigrette	Spaghetti tossed with tuna, tomato, garlic, olives, and herbs A glass of red wine
Summer berries with ricotta cream	Cantaloupe, honeydew, and watermelon fruit salad	Fresh Fruit Cheesecake*	Grapes, sliced pear, a small piece of cheese, and a few crackers

added fat and sugar. In fact, the sugars in fruits and berries have provided energy in the human diet for millions of years. It shouldn't come as too much of a surprise, therefore, to learn that these sugars have low GI values. Fructose, in particular—a sugar that occurs in all fruits and in floral honeys—has the lowest GI of all. Fruit is also a good source of soluble and insoluble fibers, which can slow digestion and provide a low GI. And as a general rule, the more acidic a fruit is, the lower its GI value.

A Low GI Winter Menu

	MONDAY	TUESDAY	WEDNESDAY
Breakfast	Fresh grapefruit, whole-grain toast with baked beans	Raisin-Studded Oatmeal*	Grainy English muffins spread with margarine and orange marmalade and a glass of fruit juice
Lunch	<u>Stir-fried Noodles</u>	Roasted Butternut Squash and White Bean Soup* with a whole-grain roll	Roast beef sandwich on low GI bread with mustard and salad
Dinner	Spicy Beef Ragout*	Pork and Noodle Stir-fry with Cashews*	Easy Tuna Bake*
Snack	Hot low-fat milk and honey	Fresh fruit plate with honey yogurt dipping sauce	Pan-fried pears with pecan nuts and ice cream

Note: <u>Underlined</u> meal ideas detailed in Chapter 19.
* See recipe in Chapter 22.

The Ideal Low GI Winter Food

Winter is a perfect time to experiment with cooking legumes—beans, peas, chickpeas, and lentils—which reign supreme as low GI foods. "Eat more legumes" is Step 4 of our "Ten Steps to a Healthy, Low GI Diet" on page 193. We suggest you include them in your meals at least twice a week (more, if you are vegetarian). Canned legumes are a quick and easy way to begin trying them out, but preparing dried legumes yourself is the cheapest, most traditional, and lowest GI way of using them. When time is short, split red lentils can be cooked in twenty to twenty-five minutes. Simply simmer gently in 1⅓ times as much vegetable stock flavored with a bay leaf until all the stock is absorbed and serve

THURSDAY	FRIDAY	SATURDAY	SUNDAY
Scrambled egg with sautéed pepper and onion on grainy toast	Sourdough toast topped with herrings or sardines and a squeeze of lemon	French toast topped with pan-fried apple slices and maple syrup	Savory omelette with shallots, mushrooms, tomatoes, and parsley with reduced-fat tasty cheese
Sweet corn, mushrooms, and sliced cheese on grain muffins	Toasted cheese and tomato sandwich on grainy bread	Minestrone Soup* with sourdough bread	Asparagus, Arugula, and Lemon Barley "Risotto"*
Spaghetti Bolognaise with green salad and vinaigrette	Roast Chicken with Rosemary on Pesto and Tomato Pasta	Baked lamb with roasted root vegetables	Grilled blue-eye cod with lemon and oven-baked sweet potato or potato wedges
Apple Cranberry Crisp*	Stuffed Baked Apples with vanilla custard	Low-fat ice-cream with syrupy orange slices and toasted almonds	Poached or canned apricots and low-fat custard

in place of mashed potato. You'll find lots of recipes using legumes, such as lentil and barley soup, black bean soup, and spicy pilaf with chickpeas, on pages 252, 256, and 281.

A Week of Low GI Vegetarian

	MONDAY	TUESDAY	WEDNESDAY
Breakfast	Peach Mango Raspberry Shake*	Mixed-Grain Oatmeal with dried apricots	Buttermilk Pancakes with Glazed Fruit*
Lunch	Whole-grain sandwich with egg salad, lettuce, snow pea sprouts, and cucumber	Tofu, avocado, and cucumber sushi	Lentil burger with salad, tomato, and chutney on a bread roll
Dinner	Roast vegetable couscous with garlic yogurt dressing	Vegetable Lasagna*	Winter Vegetarian Stew*
Snack	Fruit Crumble with soy custard	Banana split with soy ice cream	Fresh fruit

Note: Underlined meal ideas detailed in Chapter 19.
* See recipe in Chapter 22.

The Importance of the GI to Vegetarians

A vegetarian or vegan diet is naturally high in carbohydrate, which is traditionally healthy; however, as discussed earlier, industrialization and modernization have meant that the nature of the carbohydrate in a vegetarian diet is different now. High GI types of rice, modern breads, bakery products, processed breakfast cereals, and crispbreads make it all the more important to recognize and incorporate the right type of carbs in a vegetarian diet. To ensure your vegetarian diet is low GI, include plenty of the traditional, low GI forms of carbohydrate—truly whole-grain bread (see page 199), fruit, oats, cracked wheat, bulgur, barley, dried peas, beans, and lentils.

For more information and recipes for a low-GI vegetarian diet, see *The New Glucose Revolution Low GI Vegetarian Cookbook*.

You can get all the nutrients you need on a vegetarian diet; however, a little knowledge of the best plant sources is helpful.

THURSDAY	FRIDAY	SATURDAY	SUNDAY
Whole-grain toast with baked beans and a glass of fruit juice	Tofu and spinach soup with rice noodles	Bircher muesli with mango and passion fruit	Scrambled egg and grilled tomato or spinach on sour-dough toast
Pita bread with hummus, falafel, and tabbouleh	Baked potato with baked beans and grated cheese	Roasted veg-etable frittata with salad and a whole-grain bread roll	Spicy Pilaf with Chickpeas*
Red lentil dhal with spiced basmati rice	Lentil and Barley Soup* with sour-dough bread	Pasta with basil pesto and a tossed salad	Barbecued veg-etable kebabs with peanut sauce
Fresh fruit salad with low-fat ice cream	Poached pears with Chocolate Sauce	Apricot, Honey, and Coconut crunch*	Hot cocoa

For iron:

- Eat legumes, tofu, dark-green leafy vegetables, and whole grains (see page 199) regularly.
- Include a vitamin C-rich fruit or vegetable at each meal.
- Limit your intake of tea and coffee and drink them between meals rather than with meals.

For zinc:

- Eat legumes, tofu, nuts, seeds, and whole grains regularly.

For vitamin B12:

- Select a variety of foods every day, including eggs, dairy products, and B12-fortified foods.
- If you don't eat these foods regularly, you will need to take a B12 supplement.

A Week of Low GI Gluten-free

	MONDAY	TUESDAY	WEDNESDAY
Breakfast	Gluten-free muesli with strawberries and yogurt	Honey Banana Smoothie*	Quinoa porridge with poached peaches and low-fat yogurt
Lunch	Chili Bean Fajitas made with corn tortillas, with salad	Roasted Butter-nut Squash and White Bean Soup*	Asian noodle salad
Dinner	Sirloin steak with pasta and kidney bean salad	Gluten-free Spaghetti with Tomato, Olives, and Feta*	Cabbage Rolls with tomato, onion, and black olive salad
Snack	Fresh fruit salad with yogurt	Yogurt Berry Jello*	Nuts, dried fruit, and a half-inch cube of cheese

Note: Underlined meal ideas detailed in Chapter 19.
* See recipe in Chapter 22.

How Can a Gluten-free Diet Be Low GI?

So many gluten-free foods—such as rice cakes, potatoes, and puffed-rice cereals—are high GI that it might seem impossible to eat both low GI and gluten-free. However, there is an increasing selection of gluten-free breads, cereals, pastas, and cookies on the market that have a low GI (see page 322 in the GI tables where gluten-free products are listed). Look for ingredients such as chickpea or other flours based on legumes, psyllium, soy, and rice bran in breads and cereals. Buckwheat noodles (soba), cellophane (bean thread) noodles, and rice noodles are all low GI. Quinoa is a supernutritious gluten-free, low GI grain. Legumes are an essential component of a low GI gluten-free diet. Fruit and dairy products that are naturally gluten-free also help to lower the GI of the diet.

THURSDAY	FRIDAY	SATURDAY	SUNDAY
Rice cooked with low-fat milk, diced pear, and maple syrup	Boiled egg, gluten-free toast, and orange juice	Gluten-free toast with peanut butter and low-fat hot chocolate	Gluten-free corn fritters with tomato and lean bacon
Salmon and cranberry bean salad	Rice paper rolls with chicken, bean thread noodles, carrot, snow peas, and chives with dipping sauce	Tacos with lean ground beef, lettuce, tomato, reduced-fat cheese, and avocado	Niçoise salad
Chicken, vegetable, and cashew nut stir-fry with rice noodles	Asian Snapper with low GI rice on stir-fried vegetables with green mango dressing	Warm Lamb and Chickpea Salad*	Sweet Chili Chicken with Mashed Sweet Potatoes and Stir-fried Greens*
Low-fat, gluten-free hot chocolate	Handful of almonds	Low-fat Mango Lassi	Fresh fruit

21
The Low GI Shopper

TO MAKE IT EASY TO COOK the low GI way every day, at every meal, you need to stock the right foods. Here are some ideas for what to keep in your pantry, fridge, and freezer.

What to Keep in Your Pantry

Asian sauces: Hoisin, oyster, soy, and fish sauces are a good basic range.

Barley: One of the oldest cultivated cereals, barley is very nutritious and high in soluble fiber. Look for products such as pearl barley to use in soups, stews, and pilafs.

Black pepper: Buy freshly ground pepper or grind your own peppercorns.

Bread: Low GI options include grainy, stone-ground whole-grain, pumpernickel, sourdough, flat bread, and pita bread. Choose breads that are made with intact kernels.

Breakfast cereals: These include traditional rolled or steel-cut oats, natural muesli, and low GI packaged breakfast cereals.

Bulgur wheat: Use it to make tabbouleh, or add to vegetable burgers, stuffings, soups, and stews.

Canned beans: Canned beans of all varieties; chickpeas, and lentils are widely available, are convenient to use, and a great time saver. See also dried beans, below.

Canned evaporated skim milk: Makes an excellent substitute for cream in pasta sauce.

Canned fish: Keep a good stock of canned tuna packed in spring water, plus canned sardines and salmon.

Canned vegetables: Sweet corn kernels and tomatoes can help boost the vegetable content of a meal. Tomatoes, in particular, can be used freely, because they are rich in antioxidants, as well as having a low GI.

Couscous: Ready in minutes; serve it with casseroles, stews, or stir-fries.

Curry pastes: A tablespoon or so makes a delicious curry base.

Dried beans and lentils: Lentils, split peas, beans, chickpeas, and beans of all varieties (cannellini, butter, kidney, pinto, lima, mixed, baked).

Dried fruits: Dried apricots, fruit medley, raisins, prunes, and berries.

Dried herbs and spices: Oregano, basil, thyme, parsley, rosemary, marjoram, ginger, garlic, and hot peppers are most commonly used.

Honey: Try to avoid the commercial honeys or honey blends and use the "pure" honey, locally harvested, if possible. These varieties naturally have a much lower GI.

Jam: A tablespoon of good-quality jam (with no added sugar) contains fewer calories than lightly spreading butter or margarine on toast.

Mustard: Seeded or whole-grain mustard is useful as a sandwich spread and in salad dressings and sauces.

Noodles: Many Asian noodles, such as hokkien, udon, and rice vermicelli, have low to intermediate GI values because of their dense texture, whether they are made from wheat or rice flour.

Nuts: Try adding soy "nuts" (dry roasted soybeans) and/or Chick Nuts (see recipe on page 269) to a nut mix.

Oils: Try olive oil for general use; some extra-virgin olive oil for salad dressings, marinades, and dishes that benefit from its flavor; and sesame oil for Asian-style stir-fries. Canola or olive oil cooking sprays are handy, too.

Pasta: A food to be eaten as often as desired—just remember to stick with moderate portions. Fresh or dried, the preparation is easy.

Quinoa: This whole grain cooks in about ten to fifteen minutes and has a slightly chewy texture. It can be used as a substitute for rice, couscous, or bulgur. It is very important to rinse the grains before cooking.

Rice: Low GI varieties (see page 194).

Rolled oats: In addition to their use in oatmeal, oats can be added to cakes, cookies, breads, and desserts.

Sea salt: Use in moderation.

Spices: Most spices, including ground cumin, turmeric, cinnamon, paprika, and nutmeg, should be bought in small quantities because they lose pungency with age and incorrect storage.

Stock: Make your own stock or buy ready-made low-salt products that are available in long-life cartons in the supermarket.

Tomato paste: Can be used with great versatility in soups, sauces, and casseroles.

Vinegar: White wine vinegar, red wine vinegar, and balsamic vinegar are excellent for salads. A vinaigrette dressing (1 tablespoon of vinegar and 2 teaspoons of oil) with your salad can lower the blood glucose response to the whole meal by up to 30 percent. You may use lemon juice instead of vinegar.

Making Sense of Food Claims

Often, the claims on the front of the package don't mean quite what you think.

Here are some prime examples:

- **Cholesterol free**—be careful: the food may still be high in fat.

- **Reduced fat**—but is it *low* fat? Compare fat per 100 grams between products.

- **Low in trans fat**—but check the ingredient list for "hydrogenated" or "partially hydrogenated" oil. FDA regulations allow up to .5 grams to count as zero trans fat; the servings can add up.

- **No added sugar**—do you realize the product could still raise your blood glucose?

- **Lite or light**—light in what? FDA regulations specify that these can mean that a nutritionally altered product contains one-third fewer calories or half the fat of the standard version—and if the food derives 50 percent or more of its calories from fat, the reduction must be 50 percent of the fat. They could also mean simply light in color or texture—in which case qualifying information needs to be included, though exceptions are made for foods like light brown sugar that have a long history of use.

What to Keep in Your Refrigerator

Bacon: Bacon is a flavorful ingredient in many dishes. You can make a little bacon go a long way by trimming off all fat and chopping it finely. Lean ham is often a more economical and leaner way to go. In casseroles and soups, a ham or bacon bone imparts a fine flavor without much fat (but it's also fine to leave out of a recipe that calls for one, if you're vegetarian).

Bottled vegetables: Sundried tomatoes, olives, grilled eggplant, and peppers are handy to keep as flavorful additions to pastas and sandwiches.

Capers, olives, and anchovies: These can be bought in jars and kept in the refrigerator once opened. They are tasty (but salty) additions to pasta dishes, salads, sauces, and pizzas.

Cheese: Any reduced-fat cheese is great to keep handy in the fridge. A block of Parmesan is indispensable and will keep for up to a month. Reduced-fat cottage and ricotta cheeses have a short life, so are best bought as needed; they can be a good alternative to butter or margarine in a sandwich.

Condiments: Keep jars of minced garlic, chili, or ginger in the refrigerator to spice up your cooking in an instant.

Eggs: To enhance your intake of omega-3 fats, we suggest using omega-3–enriched eggs. Although the yolk is high in cholesterol, the fat in eggs is predominantly monounsaturated and is therefore considered a "good fat."

Fish: Today, most fish stores sell a wide variety of fresh fish, which you can use immediately or freeze for later use.

Fresh herbs: Even if you have a cupboard full of dried herbs and spices, fresh herbs are available in most supermarkets (or are easily grown at home in pots, window boxes, or gardens); there really is no substitute for the flavor they provide. For variety, try parsley, basil, mint, chives, thyme, oregano, rosemary, and coriander.

Fresh fruit: Almost all fruits make an excellent low GI snack.

Lemons/lemon juice: Instead of butter, try a fresh squeeze of lemon with ground black pepper on vegetables. The lemon juice's acidity slows gastric emptying and lowers the GI value of a food. Bottled juice is also widely available in the refrigerated section at supermarkets.

Meat: Lean varieties are better; try lean beef, lamb fillets, pork fillets, chicken (breast or drumsticks), and minced beef.

Milk: Skim or low-fat milk is best, or try low-fat, calcium-enriched soy milk.

Vegetables: Keep a variety of seasonal vegetables on hand, such as spinach, broccoli, cauliflower, Asian greens, asparagus, zucchini, and mushrooms. Pepper, shallots, and sprouts (mung bean and snowpea sprouts) can be used to enhance a salad. Sweet corn, sweet potato, and yam are essential to your low GI food store.

Yogurt: Low-fat natural yogurt provides the most calcium for the fewest calories. Have vanilla or fruit versions as a dessert, or use natural yogurt as a condiment in savory dishes.

What to Keep in Your Freezer

Frozen berries: Berries can make any dessert special, and by using frozen ones, you don't have to wait until berry season to indulge. Try blueberries, raspberries, and strawberries.

Frozen yogurt: This is a fantastic substitute for ice cream; some products even have a similar creamy texture, but with much less fat.

Frozen vegetables: Keep a package of peas, beans, corn, spinach, or mixed vegetables in the freezer; these are handy to add to a quick meal.

Ice cream: Reduced- or low-fat ice cream is ideal for a quick dessert, served with fresh fruit.

Making Sense of Nutrition Information Labeling

To get the hard facts on the nutritional value of a food, look at the Nutrition Information table on the package. Here you'll find the details regarding the fat, calories, carbohydrate, fiber, and sodium content of the food. These are the key points to look for:

- Calories—this is a measure of how much energy we get from a food. For a healthy diet, we need to eat more foods with a low-energy density and combine them with smaller amounts of higher-energy foods. To assess the energy density, look at the calories per 100 grams. A low-energy density on solid foods is less than 120 calories per 100 grams.

- Fat—we want a low saturated fat content, ideally less than 20 percent of the total fat. This means that if the total fat content is 10 grams, you want saturated fat less than 2 grams. Strictly speaking, a food can be labeled as low in saturated fat if it contains less than 1.5 grams saturated fat per 100 grams.

- Total carbohydrate—this is the starch, fiber, and any naturally occurring and added sugars in the food. The available carbohydrate is the total carbohydrate fiber. (There's no need to look at the sugar figure separately since it's the total carbohydrate that affects your blood glucose level.) You can use this figure if you are monitoring your carbohydrate intake and to calculate the glycemic load (GL) of your serving of the food. The GL = grams of available carbohydrate per serving × GI ÷100.

- Fiber—most of us don't get enough fiber in our diet, so it's better to look for high-fiber foods. A high-fiber food contains more than 3 grams of fiber per serving.

- Sodium—this is a measure of the nasty part of salt in our food. Our bodies need some salt, but most people consume much more than they need. Canned foods in particular tend to be high in sodium. Check the sodium content per 100 grams next time you buy; a low-sodium food contains less than 120 milligrams sodium per 100 grams.

22
Fifty Recipes for Low GI Living

THE FOLLOWING RECIPES are quick, delicious, low GI, and extremely easy to make. They are full of healthy ingredients, such as whole grains, lean meats, fish and seafood, legumes, and fresh fruits and vegetables. The recipes reflect our low GI eating approach and emphasize:

- Low GI carbs
- Monounsaturated and omega-3 fats
- A moderate to high level of protein.

A Note About the Recipes

All the recipes in this section have been analyzed using computerized nutrient-analysis programs,* and the energy, protein, carbohydrate, fat, and fiber content per serving are shown.

The following information will help put this nutritional profile into context for you. Where a range of servings is given for the recipe, the nutritional information relates to the higher number.

GI. We have given each recipe a GI rating, which is our best estimate of the range in which the GI value falls. A calculated GI value is not

---

* Foodworks, Xyris Software (Australia) Pty. Ltd., and ESHA Food Processor SQL.

realistic for all recipes, because the carbohydrate may be used in the recipe in a different form from that in which the original GI value of the food was tested.

Energy. This is a measure of how many calories a serving provides. A moderately active woman aged eighteen to fifty-four years requires about 1,900 calories a day; a man, about 2,400 calories. Those who burn lots of energy through exercise need a higher calorie intake than those who live more sedentary lives.

Carbohydrate. It is not necessary to calculate how many grams of carbohydrate you eat on a daily basis; however, if you're an athlete or you have diabetes, you may find this information useful.

To consume around 50 percent of energy from carbohydrate, on average, women need about two hundred grams a day, while men need about three hundred grams.

Athletes can consume anywhere from three hundred to seven hundred grams of carbohydrate a day, providing 50 to 60 percent of their energy needs.

To have an idea of the impact the carbohydrate in the recipe may have on your blood glucose level and insulin response, multiply the carbohydrate content per serving of the recipe by its GI value to give you the glycemic load. See pages 18–20 for a discussion of the glycemic load and the tables in Part 5 for glycemic load values.

Fat. We have aimed to keep our recipes low in fat, in particular, low in saturated fat. For this reason, we have used mono- and polyunsaturated margarines and oils. Omega-3 fatty acids from fish and seafood have many health benefits, so we have included a number of recipes containing these foods and used omega-3–enriched eggs.

The amount of fat that is appropriate in your diet depends on your calorie intake and the overall composition of your diet. A low-fat diet for most people could contain somewhere between thirty and sixty grams of fat per day. If you are not trying to lose weight, there is no harm in consuming larger amounts of fat, so long as it is predominantly unsaturated and has no added trans fat.

Fiber. Most of the recipes are high in fiber, both soluble and insoluble. Dietary guidelines recommend a daily fiber intake of at least thirty grams.

People with diabetes should aim for forty grams of fiber. A slice of whole-wheat bread provides two grams of fiber, an average apple four grams. The average American consumes only about fifteen grams of fiber a day.

So, that's the nutrition part of it. Now it's time to start cooking and embark on the low GI road to fitness and good health. Enjoy!

Breakfasts and Brunches

■

Honey Banana Smoothie

Peach Mango Raspberry Shake

Raisin-Studded Oatmeal

Muesli with Mixed Fresh Fruit

Buttermilk Pancakes with Glazed Fruit

Blueberry Muffins

Bran Muffins with Apples and Walnuts

Blueberry, Oatmeal, Cornmeal Quick Bread

Spanish Tortilla with Red Pepper

HONEY BANANA SMOOTHIE

The smoothie is a quick but sustaining breakfast. Many variations are possible using different combinations of fruits, milks, and yogurts. The evaporated milk must be chilled to froth up well in this recipe.

PREPARATION TIME: 5 minutes   COOKING TIME: None   SERVES 2

Low GI

Per serving: Cal 190 ■ Carb 35 g ■ Fat 0.5 g ■ Fiber 2 g

1 large, ripe banana
1 tablespoon All-Bran breakfast cereal
1 cup low-fat milk, chilled
½ cup evaporated low-fat milk, well chilled
2 teaspoons honey
few drops vanilla extract

1. Peel banana and coarsely chop.
2. Combine with remaining ingredients in a blender and blend for 30 seconds or until smooth and thick. Serve immediately.

PEACH MANGO RASPBERRY SHAKE

Peaches, mangoes, and raspberries are all low GI fruits, making this a great choice for breakfast.

PREPARATION TIME: 5 minutes   COOKING TIME: None   SERVES 1

Low GI

Per serving: Cal 170 ■ Carb 39 g ■ Fat 0 g ■ Fiber 5 g

¼ *cup chopped fresh or frozen peaches*
¼ *cup chopped fresh or frozen mango*
¼ *cup fresh or frozen raspberries*
¼ *cup no-fat plain yogurt*
½ *cup apple juice*

1. Combine all ingredients in a blender and purée until smooth. Serve immediately.

RAISIN-STUDDED OATMEAL

A quick and easy breakfast with a lot of stick-to-your-ribs character.

PREPARATION TIME: 5 minutes   COOKING TIME: 10 minutes   SERVES 2

Low GI

Per serving: Cal 210 ■ Carb 38 g ■ Fat 3 g ■ Fiber 3 g

⅔ cup traditional rolled oats
1 cup low-fat milk
1 small ripe banana, mashed
1 heaping tablespoon raisins

1. Place the oats in a saucepan or large microwavable bowl. Add enough water to cover, plus about ⅔ cup of the milk.

2. Bring to a boil and boil for 2 minutes or microwave on high for 1 to 2 minutes.

3. Add the banana and cook for an additional 1 to 2 minutes.

4. Add the remaining milk to make a smooth consistency and stir in raisins.

MUESLI WITH MIXED FRESH FRUIT

Creamy rolled oats, plump raisins, and crunchy almonds combined with plain yogurt, milk, and fresh fruit.

PREPARATION TIME: 5 minutes   SOAKING TIME: overnight
COOKING TIME: None   SERVES 2

Low GI

Per serving: Cal 365 ■ Carb 50 g ■ Fat 11 g ■ Fiber 6 g

1 cup traditional rolled oats
⅔ cup low-fat milk
1 tablespoon raisins
½ cup (4 oz.) low-fat plain yogurt
¼ cup whole almonds, chopped
1 apple, grated
lemon juice (optional)
mixed fresh fruit, such as strawberries, pear, plum, blueberries, cherries

1. Combine the oats, milk, and raisins in a bowl. Cover and refrigerate overnight.

2. Add the yogurt, almonds, and apple; mix well.

3. To serve, adjust the flavor with lemon juice. Serve with fresh fruit.

BUTTERMILK PANCAKES WITH GLAZED FRUIT

Golden light pancakes served with warm, soft summer fruits.

PREPARATION TIME: 1 hour 20 minutes   COOKING TIME: 25 minutes
SERVES 4

Low GI

Per serving: Cal 420 ■ Carb 60 g ■ Fat 12 g ■ Fiber 6 g

1 cup instant oatmeal or unprocessed oat bran
2 cups buttermilk
½ cup dried-fruit medley, chopped
½ cup white flour, sifted
2 teaspoons sugar
1 teaspoon baking soda
1 egg, lightly beaten
2 teaspoons mono- or polyunsaturated margarine, melted
low-fat milk (optional)

Glazed Fruit
1 tablespoon mono- or polyunsaturated margarine
1 tablespoon brown sugar
6 medium peaches, apricots, or nectarines, sliced

1. Combine the oats and buttermilk in a bowl and let stand 10 minutes.

2. Stir in the dried fruit, flour, sugar, baking soda, egg, and margarine and mix thoroughly. Let stand for about 1 hour.

3. After standing, add a little low-fat milk if the mixture is too thick.

4. Heat a nonstick frying pan or griddle and spray with oil or grease lightly with margarine. Pour in about 3 tablespoons of batter, cook over medium-high heat until bubbly on top and lightly browned underneath. Turn pancake to brown on other side.

5. Repeat with remaining batter.

6. Set aside to keep warm.

7. To make the glazed fruit, melt the margarine and sugar together over medium heat in frying pan. Stir until sugar is dissolved. Add the sliced fruit and cook over medium heat for 2–3 minutes until softened. Serve warm over the pancakes.

BLUEBERRY MUFFINS

You can replace the blueberries with any berries, such as raspberries. These muffins freeze well and make a great snack to take to work or school.

PREPARATION TIME: 10 minutes   COOKING TIME: 20 minutes
MAKES 12 muffins

Moderate GI

Per serving: Cal 93 ■ Carb 34 g ■ Fat 5 g ■ Fiber 4 g

1 cup blueberries
1½ cups traditional rolled oats
½ cup unprocessed oat bran
1½ cups whole-wheat flour
2½ teaspoons baking powder
¼ teaspoon salt
1 cup apple juice
3 tablespoons canola oil
⅓ cup honey
1 egg

1. Preheat oven to 350°F. Coat a 12-cup muffin pan with cooking spray or line with paper baking cups.

2. In a large mixing bowl, mix together the blueberries, oats, oat bran, flour, baking powder, and salt.

3. In another bowl, combine the apple juice, oil, honey, and egg. Add the flour mixture to the liquid mixture and stir until just combined.

4. Spoon the muffin mixture into the prepared pan, filling the cups three-quarters full. Bake for 15–20 minutes or until golden and cooked through. Cool for 10 minutes on a wire rack before removing from the pan.

BRAN MUFFINS WITH APPLES AND WALNUTS

Chopped fresh apples flavor these moist muffins. They are high in fiber and much lower in fat than traditional bran muffins.

PREPARATION TIME: 20 minutes   COOKING TIME: 15 minutes
MAKES 12 muffins

Moderate GI

Per serving: Cal 148 ■ Carb 26 g ■ Fat 5 g ■ Fiber 4 g

2½ tablespoons mono- or polyunsaturated margarine, softened
½ cup packed brown sugar
⅓ cup fat-free plain yogurt
3 tablespoons honey
1 egg
1 teaspoon grated orange peel
1¼ cups wheat bran
1 cup whole-wheat pastry flour or unbleached flour
1½ teaspoons baking soda
½ teaspoon salt
¼ teaspoon grated nutmeg
¼ teaspoon ground cinnamon
1 small apple, peeled, cored, and diced
¼ cup finely chopped walnuts

1. Preheat oven to 375°F. Coat a 12-cup muffin pan with cooking spray or line with paper baking cups.

2. Place the margarine in a large bowl and beat with an electric mixer until smooth. Add the brown sugar and beat until creamy. Add the yogurt, honey, egg, and orange peel, beating after each addition.

3. In another bowl, combine the wheat bran, flour, baking soda, salt, nutmeg, and cinnamon.

4. Fold the flour mixture into the yogurt mixture, stirring just enough to incorporate the ingredients. Fold in the apples and walnuts.

5. Spoon the batter into the prepared muffin pan. Bake for 15 minutes, or until a toothpick inserted into the center of a muffin comes out clean. Remove from the pan and cool on a wire rack.

BLUEBERRY, OATMEAL, CORNMEAL QUICK BREAD

New York cookbook author and former innkeeper of Crescent Dragon-wagon developed this tender quick bread, which brings together in one bread ingredients familiar to every baker but unusually combined here (one doesn't often see cornmeal and rolled oats in the same recipe). This is wonderful served as part of breakfast or brunch.

PREPARATION TIME: 25 minutes   COOKING TIME: 40–50 minutes   SERVES 16

Moderate GI

Per serving: Cal 120 ■ Carb 21 g ■ Fat 3 g ■ Fiber 1 g

1½ cups unbleached, all-purpose flour	¼ cup old-fashioned rolled oats
1 teaspoon baking powder	2–4 tablespoons walnuts, toasted
½ teaspoon baking soda	and chopped
⅓ cup stone-ground cornmeal	3 tablespoons canola oil
½ teaspoon salt	2 eggs
2 cups fresh blueberries, washed	½ cup plus 2 tablespoons buttermilk
and picked over, or thawed frozen	¾ cup sugar
blueberries	finely grated zest of 1 lemon or orange

1. Preheat oven to 350°F. Coat 4 mini-loaf pans with cooking spray. We like to bake the bread in mini-loaf pans, but you can also use 2 medium loaf pans.

2. Sift the flour, baking soda, baking powder, and salt together in a large bowl. Add the cornmeal.

3. In a small bowl, combine the blueberries, oats, and walnuts. Sprinkle 1 tablespoon of flour mixture over them to coat and add to the bowl of dry ingredients.

4. In a medium-sized bowl, beat together the oil, eggs, buttermilk, sugar, and zest.

5. Stir the wet mixture into the dry mixture using as few strokes as possible until a batter is formed.

6. Spoon batter into the prepared pans. Bake until lightly browned, about 40 to 50 minutes. Check two-thirds of the way through the baking period; if loaves are browning excessively, tent loosely with aluminum foil.

7. Let breads cool for 10 minutes in the pan, then run a knife around the edges of the pan and turn loaves out on a wire rack to cool completely.

SPANISH TORTILLA WITH RED PEPPER

*Don't be confused by the name; Spanish tortillas are much closer to frit-
tatas than to a flour tortilla (though, unlike frittatas, they're not finished in
the oven). This dish's higher GI potatoes, a classic ingredient in a Spanish
tortilla, are married here with fresh or roasted red pepper, which has negligible carbohydrate. A green side salad with vinaigrette will help reduce the
glycemic impact of the potatoes.*

PREPARATION TIME: 10 minutes   COOKING TIME: 45 minutes   SERVES 8

Moderate GI

Per serving: Cal 126 ■ Carb 11 g ■ Fat 11 g ■ Fiber 2 g

4 tablespoons extra-virgin olive oil
2 large fresh or roasted red peppers, thinly sliced
1 onion, thinly sliced
6 small red potatoes, sliced
6 eggs, beaten
2 tablespoons chopped parsley
½ teaspoon salt
¼ teaspoon freshly ground black pepper

1. Heat 1 tablespoon of the oil in a large, nonstick frying pan over
   medium heat. Add the pepper and onion and sauté, stirring
   often, for 10 minutes, or until browned and tender. Remove to
   a larger bowl.

2. Add 1 tablespoon of the remaining oil to the pan, then add the
   potatoes. Cook, turning often, for 15 minutes, or until browned
   and tender. Remove to the bowl with the onion and red peppers.

3. Add the eggs, parsley, salt, and pepper to the bowl. Toss to mix
   well.

4. Wipe the pan and add 2 tablespoons of the remaining oil. Pour
   the egg mixture into the pan. Place the pan over medium heat
   and cook, covered, for 15 minutes, or until the eggs start to set
   and the bottom browns.

5. Place a plate on top of the pan and invert the tortilla onto the
   plate. Add the remaining 2 tablespoons of oil to the pan and
   slide the tortilla back into the pan. Cook, covered, for 5 minutes
   longer, or until browned. Allow to cool at room temperature and
   cut into 8 wedges to serve.

Soups, Salads, and Vegetarian Fare

∎

Lentil and Barley Soup

Roasted Butternut Squash and White Bean Soup

Minestrone Soup

Black Bean Soup

Spinach Salad with Garlic Yogurt Dressing

Split Pea, Watercress, and Goat Cheese Salad

Pasta and Kidney Bean Salad

LENTIL AND BARLEY SOUP

Both lentils and barley are low GI, and each, with their distinctive flavors, contributes to make this zesty, satisfying winter soup.

PREPARATION TIME: 15 minutes   COOKING TIME: 1 hour   SERVES 4 to 6

Low GI

Per serving: Cal 180 ■ Carb 25 g ■ Fat 5 g ■ Fiber 5 g

1 tablespoon oil
1 large onion, finely chopped
2 cloves garlic, crushed, or 2 teaspoons minced garlic
½ teaspoon turmeric
2 teaspoons curry powder
½ teaspoon ground cumin
1 teaspoon minced hot peppers
6 cups water
1½ cups vegetable or chicken stock
1 cup red lentils
½ cup pearl barley
1 15-oz. can chopped tomatoes, undrained and crushed
salt and freshly ground black pepper
chopped fresh parsley or cilantro, to serve

1. Heat the oil in a large saucepan. Add the onion, cover, and cook gently for about 10 minutes or until beginning to brown, stirring frequently.

2. Add the garlic, turmeric, curry powder, cumin, and hot peppers and cook, stirring, for 1 minute.

3. Stir in the water, stock, lentils, barley, tomatoes, and salt and pepper to taste. Bring to a boil, cover, and simmer for about 45 minutes or until the lentils and barley are tender.

4. Serve sprinkled with parsley or coriander.

ROASTED BUTTERNUT SQUASH AND WHITE BEAN SOUP

This is a quintessential autumn low GI soup—perfect for gatherings of all types. The roasted squash and white beans readily soak up stock, so have plenty on hand to add as you need it. If you're not serving a crowd, this yields multiple lunches or dinners, and it freezes beautifully (freeze it in single-portion containers, which thaw more quickly than larger containers).

PREPARATION TIME: 45 minutes SOAKING TIME: overnight
COOKING TIME: 2½ hours SERVES 8

Low GI

Per serving: Cal 252 ■ Carb 43 g ■ Fat 5 g ■ Fiber 12 g

1 cup dry white beans, soaked overnight in large bowl of water, covered
2–4 bay leaves
1 medium butternut squash (about 2–3 lbs.)
1 head of garlic
olive oil
salt and freshly ground pepper
3 medium yellow onions
3 stalks celery
3 medium carrots
1 tablespoon olive oil
3 teaspoons dried thyme
6–8 cups vegetable stock
3 teaspoons ground cumin
¼ cup chopped fresh parsley and/or cilantro
¼ cup grated Parmesan cheese

1. Drain the beans, then bring to a boil in a medium-sized saucepan, covered with water by about an inch. Once they boil, simmer partly covered for about an hour, or however long it takes for the beans to cook through. Keep an eye on the pot and add hot water as the beans absorb the water. Cook just until the beans begin to fall apart. Add the bay leaves and set aside.

2. Slice the butternut squash in half lengthwise. Scoop out the pulp and seeds, scraping away only as much flesh as you need to clean out the pulp and seeds.

3. Fill each of the two cavities with whole, unpeeled garlic cloves; generally, the number of cloves in one medium head of garlic are just the right amount to fill, almost but not to overflowing, the

two cavities. Lightly oil a heavy roasting pan (or heavy tray). Season the pan and the squash halves with salt and freshly ground pepper. Carefully flip the halves, with the garlic cloves in the cavities, face down into the roasting pan (a metal spatula held over the cavities can help keep the cloves from spilling out in the flip).

4. Roast in a 400°F oven for about an hour, or until the skin is browned and crinkly and the flesh is soft and easily pierced. Allow the squash to cool in the pan. Once it's cool, scoop out the flesh and pop the garlic cloves (which will soften and cook through perfectly) and purée in a food processor. Set aside.

5. Finely dice the onions, celery, and carrots. Sauté in a large stockpot or soup pan over medium heat, starting first with the onions (about 10–15 minutes), then add the celery (for about 5 minutes), and then the carrots (about 10 minutes). Season with salt, pepper, and thyme. Add the squash purée and the cooked white beans. Add about 4 cups of vegetable stock, or however much is necessary to cover the contents of the pot. Reduce the heat to low and simmer. Add stock as necessary if the soup gets too thick. The soup can simmer on very low heat for 2–3 hours, but requires only about an hour or so if you don't have that much time. Shortly before serving, taste for seasoning and add, if necessary, a bit more salt, freshly ground pepper, a bit more thyme, and ground cumin. Serve with a sprinkle of Parmesan and parsley or cilantro garnish.

MINESTRONE SOUP

Serve this hearty soup with whole-grain bread and a green salad for a balanced and delicious low GI meal.

PREPARATION TIME: 15 minutes   COOKING TIME: 1 hour 25 minutes
SERVES 6

Low GI

Per serving: Cal 120 ■ Carb 18 g ■ Fat 2 g ■ Fiber 7 g

1 teaspoon olive oil
2 medium onions, chopped
2 cloves garlic, crushed
10 cups water
5 vegetable or beef stock cubes
1 15-oz. can cannellini beans, rinsed and drained
3 carrots, diced
2 sticks celery, sliced
2 small zucchini, chopped
4 tomatoes (approximately 1 lb.), diced
⅓ cup small macaroni pasta
2 tablespoons fresh parsley, chopped
freshly ground black pepper
grated Parmesan cheese, to serve (optional)

1. Heat a little oil in a large heavy-based saucepan. Add the onions and garlic and cook for about 5 minutes or until soft. Add the water, stock cubes, and drained beans. Bring to a boil.

2. Add the carrots, celery, zucchini, and tomatoes to the stock. Reduce heat and simmer, covered, for 1 hour.

3. Add the macaroni and stir. Continue to simmer uncovered for 10 to 15 minutes or until the macaroni is tender.

4. Stir in the parsley and add pepper to taste. Serve with Parmesan cheese if desired.

BLACK BEAN SOUP

Beans are naturally a low GI food and one of nature's nutritional power packs. They are considered good sources of protein, fiber, B vitamins, iron, zinc, and magnesium. Served with whole-grain bread and a salad, this makes a satisfying meal for a small crowd.

PREPARATION TIME: 25 minutes   SOAKING TIME: overnight
COOKING TIME: 1 hour 15 minutes   SERVES 6

Low GI

Per serving: Cal 140 ■ Carb 27 g ■ Fat 0.5 g ■ Fiber 5 g

1 cup dry black beans, soaked overnight in large bowl of water, covered
½ cup diced onions
½ cup peeled and diced carrots
¼ cup diced celery
1 large red pepper, roasted
1 tablespoon minced fresh garlic
6–8 cups vegetable stock
¼ teaspoon ground cumin
½ teaspoon salt
1 teaspoon chopped fresh oregano
2 teaspoons chopped fresh parsley
2 teaspoons chopped fresh coriander

1. Rinse the soaked beans in a colander with fresh water and drain.

2. Lightly spray a large saucepan with olive oil. Sauté the onions, carrots, celery, roasted pepper, and garlic. Add vegetable stock and black beans. Bring to a boil, reduce the heat, and simmer for 1 hour.

3. When the beans are tender, pour into a food processor and purée. Add the cumin, salt, oregano, parsley, and coriander and serve.

SPINACH SALAD WITH GARLIC YOGURT DRESSING

This makes delicious use of one of the classic salad greens and comes from Jane Frank's Eating for Diabetes, *which, like our recipes, provides GI ratings for its 125 recipes; this salad is low GI. Serve it with a low GI wholegrain bread.*

PREPARATION TIME: 15 minutes   COOKING TIME: none   SERVES 4

Low GI

Per serving: Cal 124 ■ Carb 11 g ■ Fat 8 g ■ Fiber 4 g

1 lb. fresh English or baby spinach
2 tomatoes, peeled and diced
6 green onions, thinly sliced on the diagonal
5 tablespoons plain yogurt
2 tablespoons extra-virgin olive oil
2 garlic cloves, peeled and finely chopped
1 tablespoon fresh oregano leaves
sea salt and freshly ground pepper, to taste

1. Wash the spinach well in several changes of water. Dry the leaves carefully and place in a salad bowl together with the tomatoes and spring onions.

2. Whisk together the yogurt, olive oil, chopped garlic, and oregano, and season to taste.

3. Toss the salad with the dressing and serve.

SPLIT PEA, WATERCRESS, AND GOAT CHEESE SALAD

Created by Kate Tait for Delicious *magazine, this salad is a deliciously complete meal in itself and can be prepared, cooked, and served in around 30 minutes. You can buy roasted red pepper prepared in a jar; goat cheese is now available just about everywhere cheese is sold.*

PREPARATION TIME: 15 minutes   COOKING TIME: 30 minutes   SERVES 4

Low GI

Per serving: Cal 273 ■ Carb 37 g ■ Fat 7 g ■ Fiber 13 g

1 cup green split peas, dry
1 tablespoon olive oil
juice of 1 lemon
2 teaspoons ground coriander
½ teaspoon ground ginger
1 red onion, very finely chopped
1 bunch watercress, stalks trimmed (3 cups sprigs)
2 roasted red peppers, cut into strips
¼ cup goat cheese

1. Cook the split peas in a saucepan of boiling water for 15–18 minutes until tender, but firm to the bite.

2. Meanwhile, make the dressing by placing the oil, lemon juice, spices, and onion in a large bowl and whisking until combined.

3. Drain the peas well and add to the dressing. Season to taste if desired, and toss to combine. Let stand for 10 minutes so the flavors absorb, then toss with the watercress sprigs and red pepper strips.

4. Divide evenly among four plates and top with goat cheese.

PASTA AND KIDNEY BEAN SALAD

A summer salad full of flavor, this is easy to prepare with canned beans.

PREPARATION TIME: 15 minutes   COOKING TIME: 15 minutes   SERVES 4

Low GI

Per serving: Cal 130 ∎ Carb 15 g ∎ Fat 5 g ∎ Fiber 4 g

1 cup cooked pasta (e.g., shells or spirals)
1 cup canned red kidney beans, well drained
3 green onions, finely chopped
1 tablespoon fresh parsley, finely chopped

Dressing
1 tablespoon olive oil
1 tablespoon wine vinegar
1 teaspoon Dijon mustard
1 clove garlic, crushed
freshly ground black pepper, to taste

1. Combine the pasta, beans, onions, and parsley in a serving bowl.
2. For the dressing, combine the oil, vinegar, mustard, garlic, and pepper in a screw-top jar; shake well to combine.
3. Pour the dressing over the pasta mixture and toss well.

Light Meals, Lunches, and Savory Snacks

■

Sweet Corn and Crab Hotcakes with Arugula and Oven-Roasted Tomatoes

Tabbouleh

Asian-style Scrambled Tofu

Asparagus, Arugula, and Lemon Barley "Risotto"

Whole-Wheat Penne with Arugula and Edamame

Spicy Noodles

Pasta with Tangy Tomatoes

Chick Nuts

SWEET CORN AND CRAB HOTCAKES WITH ARUGULA AND OVEN-ROASTED TOMATOES

Inspired by Sydney, Australia, restauranteur Bill Granger, whose numerous restaurants have legions of fans, this recipe turns one of the sweetened breakfast staples of his original Bill's restaurant into a savory dinner dish. With its combination of crab and sweet corn, paired with tomatoes, it's perfect as an all-in-one, height-of-summer lunch or light supper.

PREPARATION TIME: 20 minutes   COOKING TIME: 55 minutes   SERVES 6
Moderate GI
Per serving: Cal 286 ■ Carb 31 g ■ Fat 13 g ■ Fiber 3 g

1 cup all-purpose flour
1 teaspoon baking powder
¼ teaspoon salt
¼ teaspoon paprika
2 eggs
½ cup milk
1 cup fresh corn kernels
1 cup canned lump crabmeat
⅔ cup roasted red pepper
½ cup chopped shallots
¼ cup chopped cilantro and parsley, combined
4 tablespoons vegetable oil

To serve
1½ cups roasted tomatoes
1 bunch arugula
olive oil

1. Sift the flour, baking powder, salt, and paprika into a large bowl. Make a well in the center. In a separate bowl, combine the eggs and milk. Gradually add the egg mixture to the dry ingredients and whisk until you have a smooth, stiff batter.

2. Place the corn, crabmeat, red pepper, spring onions, coriander, and parsley in a mixing bowl and add the flour batter to lightly bind the corn-crabmeat mixture.

3. Heat 2 tablespoons oil in a large, nonstick frying pan over medium heat. Drop ¼ cup of the batter into the pan, and repeat, making 2 fritters at a time. Cook for 3–4 minutes, until the underside of each fritter is golden. Turn over and cook on

the other side. Transfer to a plate to keep warm while cooking the remaining fritters.

4. To serve, place two fritters on each plate and top with ¼ cup of roasted tomatoes, a small handful of arugula, and finish with a drizzle of olive oil.

Oven-Roasted Tomatoes
1½ cup cherry tomatoes
4 tablespoons extra-virgin olive oil
sea salt
freshly ground black pepper

1. Preheat oven to 350°F. Place tomatoes in a skillet or roasting pan in which they fit snugly, and drizzle with olive oil. Sprinkle with sea salt and pepper. Roast in the oven about 20 minutes.

TABBOULEH

Tabbouleh is best if you make it ahead, allowing time for the flavors to develop. It keeps for a couple of days in the refrigerator.

Variations include the addition of a chopped cucumber, a crushed clove of garlic, or 2 tablespoons of chopped fresh mint. In the dressing, you can use half lemon juice and half vinegar if preferred.

PREPARATION TIME: 15 minutes   COOKING TIME: 30 minutes   SERVES 4

Low GI

Per serving: Cal 160 ■ Carb 15 g ■ Fat 10 g ■ Fiber 5 g

½ cup cracked wheat (bulgur)
1 cup fresh flat-leaf or continental parsley, finely chopped
1 small onion or 3–4 green onions, finely chopped
1 medium tomato, finely chopped

Dressing
2 tablespoons fresh lemon juice
2 tablespoons olive oil
pinch salt
½ teaspoon freshly ground black pepper

1. Cover the bulgur with hot water and soak for 20–30 minutes to soften. Drain well and roll in a clean, lint-free kitchen towel to squeeze out excess water.

2. Combine the bulgur, parsley, onion, and tomato in a bowl.

3. For the dressing, combine all the ingredients in a screw-top jar; shake well.

4. Add the dressing to the bulgur mixture and toss lightly to combine.

ASIAN-STYLE SCRAMBLED TOFU

Tofu is an easy way of using soy. It contains very little carbohydrate, so it doesn't have a GI value.

PREPARATION TIME: 5 minutes COOKING TIME: 10 minutes SERVES 4
Low GI
Per serving: Cal 239 ■ Carb 18 g ■ Fat 14 g ■ Fiber 7 g

1 lb. firm tofu, patted dry with a paper towel
2 tablespoons olive oil
2 tablespoons sweet chili sauce
2 tablespoons salt-reduced soy sauce
⅓ cup chopped cilantro
4 thick slices low GI whole-grain bread
cilantro and parsley, chopped, for garnish

1. Crumble the tofu into small pieces. Heat the oil in a large wok over high heat, carefully swirling around to coat the side of the wok.
2. Add the tofu and stir-fry for 3–4 minutes or until heated through. Remove the wok from the heat and toss in the sweet chili sauce, soy sauce, and cilantro.
3. Toast the bread and serve topped with the scrambled tofu. Garnish with chopped cilantro and parsley.

ASPARAGUS, ARUGULA, AND LEMON BARLEY "RISOTTO"

Classic risotto is made with arborio rice, but this creamy variant, made with lower GI barley, is an unusual twist—and incredibly delicious. It's terrific either paired with a side salad, or as a bed for grilled fish.

PREPARATION TIME: 10 minutes   SOAKING TIME: overnight
COOKING TIME: 30 minutes   SERVES 4

Low GI

Per serving: Cal 337 ■ Carb 47 g ■ Fat 8 g ■ Fiber 11 g

1 tablespoon olive oil
1 white onion, finely chopped
2 large garlic cloves, finely chopped
1 cup pearl barley, soaked overnight, drained
½ cup white wine
finely grated zest of 1 lemon
3 cups hot vegetable stock
1 bunch asparagus, trimmed, sliced diagonally
1 bunch arugula, trimmed, leaves shredded
¼ cup lemon juice
⅓ cup finely grated Parmesan cheese

1. Heat the olive oil in a large heavy-based pan over medium to low heat. Add the onion and cook, stirring occasionally for 5 minutes or until soft. Add the garlic and cook, stirring, for 30 seconds longer.

2. Increase the heat to medium, add the barley, and cook, stirring, until the barley is evenly coated in the oil. Add the white wine and let it bubble until reduced by half.

3. Add the lemon zest and start adding the stock a ladleful at a time. Cook, stirring, until almost all the stock has evaporated before adding more stock.

4. When you have added all the stock and the barley is almost tender (this will take about 15–20 minutes), add the asparagus and cook for 3–4 minutes.

5. Remove the risotto from the heat, add the arugula, lemon juice, and Parmesan. Cover and let stand for 3–4 minutes.

WHOLE-WHEAT PENNE WITH ARUGULA AND EDAMAME

Like traditional pasta made from durum wheat, whole-wheat pasta is also low GI and a high-fiber choice. Most supermarkets and specialty grocers now carry a variety of sizes and shapes of whole-wheat pasta, alongside the durum choices, so be creative, and enjoy! Edamame, which are young soybeans, can be found in the freezer section of most Asian produce stores and some supermarkets.

PREPARATION TIME: 15 minutes   COOKING TIME: 20 minutes   SERVES 4

Low GI

Per serving: Cal 435 ■ Carb 52 g ■ Fat 16 g ■ Fiber 7 g

2 cups shelled edamame
8 ounces whole-wheat penne (or other shape pasta)
1 tablespoon extra-virgin olive oil
2 cloves garlic, minced
4 cups coarsely chopped arugula
½ cup freshly grated Parmesan

1. Cook the edamame in boiling salted water until they are crispy but tender. Remove them to a bowl with a slotted spoon.

2. Add the pasta to the same water, and cook according to package directions. Drain it in a colander, drizzle with ½ teaspoon of the oil, and set aside.

3. In a large nonstick pan, heat the remaining oil over medium to high heat. Add the garlic and cook 15 seconds. Mix in the arugula, coating it with the oil, and cook until wilted, about 1–2 minutes. Mix in the edamame and remove the pan from the heat. Add the drained pasta, stirring until it is warmed through, and season to taste with salt and pepper.

4. Divide among 4 bowls and top with equal amounts of Parmesan.

SPICY NOODLES

Delicious and good for you, too. Serve as a side dish, or add strips of stir-fried chicken or meat and Asian-style mixed vegetables for a complete meal.

PREPARATION TIME: 10 minutes   COOKING TIME: 15 minutes   SERVES 4

Low GI

Per serving: Cal 280 ■ Carb 45 g ■ Fat 6 g ■ Fiber 4 g

8 oz. dried, thin egg noodles
2 teaspoons oil
2 cloves garlic, crushed, or 2 teaspoons minced garlic
1 teaspoon minced ginger
1 teaspoon minced hot peppers
6 green onions, sliced
1 tablespoon smooth peanut butter
2 tablespoons soy sauce
1 cup prepared chicken stock

1. Add the noodles to a large saucepan of boiling water and boil, uncovered, for about 5 minutes or until just tender.

2. While the noodles are cooking, heat the oil in a nonstick frying pan, add the garlic, ginger, hot peppers, and onions and stir-fry for 1 minute. Remove from the heat.

3. Stir in the peanut butter and soy sauce and gradually add the stock, stirring until smooth. Stir over heat until simmering, and simmer for 2 minutes.

4. Drain the noodles and add to the spicy sauce, stirring to coat. Serve immediately.

PASTA WITH TANGY TOMATOES

A simple, light pasta dish that can be on the plate in about 15 minutes.

PREPARATION TIME: 15 minutes   COOKING TIME: 15 minutes   SERVES 2

Low GI

Per serving: Cal 415 ■ Carb 65 g ■ Fat 10 g ■ Fiber 7 g

5 oz. spaghetti or other pasta
3 medium tomatoes
1 tablespoon olive oil
1 tablespoon capers, drained
1 clove garlic, crushed, or 1 tablespoon minced garlic
juice of 1 lemon
1 tablespoon hot sauce (or to taste)
black pepper
fresh basil leaves, shredded

1. Cook the spaghetti according to package directions.
2. Meanwhile, dice the tomatoes. Combine in a bowl with the olive oil, capers, garlic, lemon juice, hot sauce, pepper, and basil.
3. Drain the spaghetti and return to the saucepan. Add the tomato combination and stir in. Serve hot or warm.

CHICK NUTS

Toasted chickpeas make a terrifically healthy, low GI snack. Spice them up with the flavorings suggested or use your own combinations. All you need is some chickpeas.

PREPARATION TIME: 10 minutes   SOAKING TIME: overnight
COOKING TIME: 45 minutes   MAKES 6 cups

Low GI

Per ½ cup: Cal 320 ■ Carb 45 g ■ Fat 6 g ■ Fiber 15 g

1 1-lb. package dry chickpeas

1. Soak the chickpeas in water overnight. Next day, drain and pat dry with paper towels.
2. Spread the chickpeas in a single layer on a baking tray. Bake at 350°F for about 45 minutes or until completely crisp. (They will shrink to their original size.)
3. Toss with one of the two flavoring options below while hot, or cool and serve plain. After seasoning, allow them to air-dry for a few days to ensure all residual moisture has evaporated.

Chick Devils Sprinkle a mixture of cayenne pepper and salt over the hot chick nuts.

Red Chicks Sprinkle a mixture of paprika and garlic salt over the hot chick nuts.

Main Dishes

■

Vegetable Lasagna

Spinach Pasta with Broccoli Rabe and Scallops

Moroccan Chicken over Couscous

Spicy Beef Ragout

Steamed Mussels over Ratatouille and Basmati Rice

Fish Fillets over Sweet Potato Wedges with
Oven-Roasted Tomatoes

Pork and Noodle Stir-fry with Cashews

Glazed Chicken with Mashed Sweet Potato and
Stir-fried Greens

Warm Lamb and Chickpea Salad

Spicy Pilaf with Chickpeas

Moroccan Kebabs

Winter Vegetarian Stew

Easy Tuna Bake

Lamb Curry with Spinach Rice Pilaf

VEGETABLE LASAGNA

Soft layers of spinach, cheese, and lasagna noodles with a luscious vegetable sauce—this is a fabulous all-in-one-pan meal that's perfect for a cool evening. Dipping the lasagna sheets briefly in hot water before use helps to soften them prior to cooking.

PREPARATION TIME: 35 minutes   COOKING TIME: 1 hour 30 minutes
SERVES 4–6

Low GI

Per serving (for 6): Cal 340 ■ Carb 44 g ■ Fat 10 g ■ Fiber 9 g

1 bunch spinach, washed and stalks removed
8 oz. instant lasagna sheets
2 tablespoons grated Parmesan cheese or low-fat cheddar cheese

Vegetable Sauce
2 teaspoons oil
1 medium onion, chopped
2 cloves garlic, crushed, or 2 teaspoons minced garlic
8 oz. mushrooms, sliced
1 small green pepper, chopped
1 6-oz. can tomato paste
1 15-oz. can beans, any variety, rinsed and drained
1 15-oz. can tomatoes, undrained and mashed
1 teaspoon mixed herbs

Cheese Sauce
1½ tablespoons poly- or monounsaturated margarine
1 tablespoon white flour
1½ cups low-fat milk
½ cup grated low-fat cheese
pinch ground nutmeg
freshly ground black pepper, to taste

1. Blanch or lightly steam the spinach until just wilted; drain well.

2. For the vegetable sauce, heat the oil in a nonstick frying pan. Add the onions and garlic and cook for about 5 minutes or until soft. Add the mushrooms and pepper and cook for a further 3 minutes, stirring occasionally. Add the tomato paste, beans, tomatoes, and herbs. Bring to a boil and simmer partly covered for 15 to 20 minutes.

3. Meanwhile, for the cheese sauce, melt the margarine in a saucepan or a microwave bowl. Stir in the flour and cook 1 minute, stirring (for 30 seconds on high, in microwave).

4. Remove from the heat. Gradually add the milk, stirring until smooth. Stir over medium heat until the sauce boils and thickens, or in microwave on high until boiling, stirring occasionally. Remove from the heat, stir in the cheese, nutmeg, and pepper.

5. To assemble, pour half the vegetable sauce over the base of a lasagna pan (about 6½ x 10½ inches). Cover with a layer of lasagna sheets, then half the spinach. Spread a thin layer of cheese sauce over the spinach. Top with the remaining vegetable sauce and remaining spinach. Place over a layer of lasagna sheets and finish with the remaining cheese sauce. Sprinkle with Parmesan or cheddar cheese.

6. Cover with aluminum foil and bake in a moderate oven (350°F) for 40 minutes. Remove foil and bake for a further 30 minutes or until the top is beginning to brown.

SPINACH PASTA WITH BROCCOLI RABE AND SCALLOPS

This is a beautifully balanced and easy-to-prepare low GI pasta dish—a delicious and not-too-time-consuming midweek meal.

PREPARATION TIME: 15 minutes   COOKING TIME: 30 minutes   SERVES 4

Low GI

Per serving: Cal 551 ■ Carb 65 g ■ Fat 8 g ■ Fiber 4 g

1 lb. broccoli rabe
pinch of salt
8 oz. spinach rotini (spirals) or penne
1 tablespoon olive oil
2 medium yellow onions, finely diced
3 cloves garlic, crushed, or 1½ tablespoons minced garlic
1 lb. shiitake or cremini mushrooms
1 lb. fresh scallops
red pepper flakes, to taste
salt and freshly ground black pepper
¼ cup freshly grated Parmesan cheese
¼ cup chopped fresh parsley

1. Bring a large pot of water to a boil and add the salt. Meanwhile, discard the lower stems of the broccoli rabe and chop into roughly 3-inch pieces. Wash and drain thoroughly, then cook for 2–3 minutes in the boiling water. Remove from the water with tongs, saving the water for the pasta. Immediately plunge the broccoli rabe into ice-cold water, then drain and set aside.

2. Add the pasta to the same pot of boiling water and boil, uncovered, until just tender. Drain and keep warm, reserving ½ cup of the pasta water.

3. While the pasta is cooking, begin the sauce. Heat the oil in a non-stick frying pan. Add the onions, garlic, and mushrooms and cook for about 5 minutes, until softened. Add the broccoli rabe and cook for about 5 minutes, then add the scallops, and cook for about 5 more minutes, until cooked through.

4. Season to taste with red pepper flakes, salt, and freshly ground black pepper.

5. Combine the sauce with the pasta, adding reserved pasta water to thin the sauce.

6. Sprinkle with the Parmesan and chopped parsley. Serve hot.

MOROCCAN CHICKEN OVER COUSCOUS

PREPARATION TIME: 15 minutes   COOKING TIME: 20 minutes   SERVES 6

Moderate GI

Per serving: Cal 360 ■ Carb 43 g ■ Fat 9 g ■ Fiber 4 g

2 teaspoons ground cumin
2 teaspoons ground coriander
1 teaspoon ground fennel
1 15-oz. can chickpeas, drained and patted dry
1 tablespoon olive oil, plus a little extra
2 cloves garlic, finely chopped
2 small hot red peppers, finely chopped
1 lb. skinless chicken breast cutlets
½ bunch flat-leaf parsley, coarsely chopped
1 lemon, thinly sliced
½ cup dry white wine
1 cup couscous, uncooked
½ cup raisins
juice of 1 lemon
salt and freshly ground black pepper

1. Combine the cumin, coriander, and fennel in a mixing bowl, and toss the chickpeas in the spices.

2. Heat 1 tablespoon of olive oil in a large wok or frying pan. Add the garlic and hot peppers and cook, stirring, for 1 minute.

3. Toss the chickpeas into the pan and cook until the aroma of the spices comes through—about 2 minutes. Place the chickpeas in a large bowl and set aside.

4. Add a little extra olive oil to the pan and cook the chicken for approximately 4 minutes or until just cooked through. Add to the chickpeas, and stir in the chopped parsley and lemon slices.

5. To make a sauce, deglaze the pan with the wine, simmering for 2 minutes.

6. Pour over the chicken mixture and keep warm.

7. Place the couscous in a large mixing bowl and pour 1 cup of boiling water over the top. As the couscous plumps up, gently mix in the raisins, lemon juice, and salt and pepper, and serve with the chicken.

SPICY BEEF RAGOUT

Here's a warm comfort food, full of flavor and packed with nutrients.

PREPARATION TIME: 25 minutes   COOKING TIME: 1 hour 40 minutes
SERVES 8

Low GI

Per serving: Cal 320 ■ Carb 40 g ■ Fat 7 g ■ Fiber 8 g

1 lb. rump steak, diced
⅓ cup white flour
salt and freshly ground black pepper
1 tablespoon olive oil
2 medium onions, finely diced
3 cloves garlic, coarsely chopped
1 red hot pepper, coarsely chopped
3 large (3½ lbs.) sweet potatoes, peeled and coarsely diced
1½ quarts beef stock
2 tablespoons tomato paste
1 tablespoon grainy mustard
2 stalks celery, sliced
2 large red peppers, halved, seeded, and coarsely diced
1 cup corn kernels
1 28-oz. can peeled chopped tomatoes, undrained
1 15-oz. can pinto beans, drained
1 cup spiral noodles, cooked
½ cup kalamata olives
½ bunch parsley, coarsely chopped

1. Toss the steak in flour seasoned with salt and black pepper in a large mixing bowl.

2. Heat the oil in a large 6-quart casserole dish or metal pan and gently cook the onions, garlic, and red hot pepper for 1 minute. Add the steak and brown on all sides.

3. Add the sweet potato, beef stock, tomato paste, mustard, celery, peppers, corn kernels, and tomatoes. Season with salt and pepper. Simmer gently, with lid on, for 1½ hours, stirring occasionally.

4. Remove the lid and add the pinto beans, cooked noodles, and olives. Simmer for 5 minutes, stir in the parsley, and serve immediately.

STEAMED MUSSELS OVER RATATOUILLE AND BASMATI RICE

The ratatouille flavor improves with time, so make it the day before and reheat gently.

PREPARATION TIME: 45 minutes   COOKING TIME: 1 hour   SERVES 4

Moderate GI

Per serving: Cal 390 ■ Carb 56 g ■ Fat 7 g ■ Fiber 6 g

1 large eggplant, cut into small cubes	3 cups water
1 tablespoon canola oil	4 bay leaves
1 large red pepper, halved, seeded and diced (½-inch pieces)	2 sprigs fresh thyme
	salt and freshly ground black pepper
4 zucchini, sliced into 1-inch rings	8 fresh basil leaves, roughly chopped
1 large onion, roughly chopped	1 cup basmati rice
3 cloves garlic, roughly chopped	1 lb. mussels (approximately 20)
1 15-oz. can chopped tomatoes, undrained	1 cup dry white wine
	10 black peppercorns

1. Place the eggplant in a colander, sprinkle with salt, and leave for 30 minutes. Wash under cold water, drain, and pat dry with a paper towel.

2. Heat the oil in a large saucepan and add the eggplant, pepper, zucchini, onion, and garlic. Toss in the hot oil for 2 minutes, then add the tomatoes, 2 cups of the water, 2 bay leaves, and the thyme. Season with salt and pepper. Reduce the heat and simmer for 45 minutes, stirring occasionally.

3. Remove the bay leaves and thyme sprigs. Stir in the basil.

4. Meanwhile, bring 2 quarts of water to a boil and cook the rice for 11 minutes. Immediately drain and keep warm.

5. Prepare the mussels by discarding any broken shells and soaking in cold water. Pull the "beard" from the side of the shell with a sharp tug toward the pointed end of the mussel.

6. Bring the wine, the remaining water and bay leaves, and the peppercorns to a boil, reduce the heat, and add the mussels. Cover the saucepan and simmer for approximately 2 minutes, removing each mussel as it fully opens. Discard any unopened shells.

7. To serve, arrange half a cup of rice in the middle of the plate, top with spoonfuls of ratatouille, and arrange the cooked mussel shells over the top.

FISH FILLETS OVER SWEET POTATO WEDGES WITH OVEN-ROASTED TOMATOES

Everyone will love the delicate combination of flavors in this dish.

PREPARATION TIME: 20 minutes   COOKING TIME: 45 minutes   SERVES 6

Moderate GI

Per serving: Cal 310 ■ Carb 26 g ■ Fat 11 g ■ Fiber 4 g

6 large ripe Roma tomatoes, halved lengthwise
1 teaspoon olive oil
2 cloves garlic, finely chopped
6 basil leaves, finely sliced
salt and freshly ground pepper
6 small (about 1½ lbs.) fish fillets, such as catfish, flounder, or halibut
⅓ cup white flour, seasoned with salt and freshly ground black pepper
2 omega-3–enriched eggs, lightly whisked
3 large (about 1¾ lbs.) sweet potatoes (orange flesh), peeled and thinly sliced
2 tablespoons olive oil
3 cups baby spinach leaves
1 tablespoon toasted sesame seeds
6 lemon wedges

1. Preheat the oven to 350°F.

2. Place the tomatoes, cut side up, on a lightly oiled baking tray. Top the tomatoes with a little olive oil, half the garlic, the basil leaves, and seasonings. Place in the oven and bake for 30 minutes.

3. Dip the fish fillets in the seasoned flour and eggs. Cover and set aside in the refrigerator.

4. Heat 1½ tablespoons olive oil in a heavy-based frying pan and spread the sweet potato slices over it, seasoning the layers with salt and pepper and the remaining garlic. Cook until the underside turns golden and slightly crisp, then turn once and cook the other side. Keep warm.

5. Heat ½ tablespoon olive oil in a heavy-based frying pan and cook the fish fillets for approximately 4 minutes, turning once only, until golden brown and flaky.

6. Serve the fish atop the sweet potato chips on a bed of baby spinach. Sprinkle with toasted sesame seeds and serve with lemon wedges and oven-roasted tomatoes.

PORK AND NOODLE STIR-FRY WITH CASHEWS

A classic, flavorful dish that is easy to prepare.

PREPARATION TIME: 20 minutes   COOKING TIME: 25 minutes   SERVES 4

Low GI

Per serving: Cal 580 ■ Carb 56 g ■ Fat 19 g ■ Fiber 8 g

1 tablespoon oil
1 lb. pork strips
10 oz. plain Chinese noodles
1 medium red pepper, sliced into thin strips
8 oz. broccoli, chopped into small florets
1 clove garlic, crushed
2 teaspoons finely grated fresh ginger
5 oz. snow peas, ends cut off and sliced diagonally into thirds
8 oz. button mushrooms, thinly sliced
1 baby bok choy, washed, trimmed, and cut lengthways into 8 pieces
6 green onions, chopped diagonally
1 tablespoon reduced-salt soy sauce
1 tablespoon hoisin sauce
1 tablespoon honey
½ cup roasted cashew nuts

1. Heat a large frying pan or wok over high heat. Add half the oil and when the oil is hot, add one-third of the pork strips and stir-fry for 1–2 minutes until just cooked. Repeat with the remaining 2 batches of pork, transferring to a plate covered loosely with foil to keep warm.

2. Prepare the noodles according to package directions and drain.

3. Add the remaining oil to the pan over high heat. Add the pepper, broccoli, garlic, and ginger and stir-fry for about 1 minute. Add the remaining vegetables and stir-fry 1–2 minutes until the vegetables are tender-crisp, sprinkling in a little water if necessary.

4. Combine the sauces and honey together in a bowl.

5. Return the pork to the pan with the noodles and sauces. Toss until well combined and heated through. Put into bowls to serve, and sprinkle with the cashew nuts.

GLAZED CHICKEN WITH MASHED SWEET POTATO AND STIR-FRIED GREENS

Here's a yummy stir-fry that's ready in no time.

PREPARATION TIME: 20 minutes   COOKING TIME: 35 minutes   SERVES 2

Moderate GI

Per serving: Cal 530 ■ Carb 49 g ■ Fat 15 g ■ Fiber 9 g

Mashed Sweet Potato
1 medium (1 lb.) sweet potato (orange flesh), peeled and cut into chunks
⅓ cup low-fat milk
1 tablespoon sweet chili sauce

Glazed Chicken
2 12-oz. chicken breasts, sliced into strips across the grain
1 teaspoon oil
1 cup chicken stock
2 teaspoons reduced-salt soy sauce
1 tablespoon sweet chili or duck sauce
1 tablespoon cornstarch
2 teaspoons grated fresh ginger
few sprigs of fresh coriander leaves

Stir-fried Greens
1 teaspoon oil
large handful of snow peas, trimmed and chopped
bunch of Chinese greens, such as baby bok choy, chopped
2 medium zucchini, sliced

1. Boil or microwave the sweet potato until tender. When cooked, drain and mash with milk and sweet chili sauce. Keep warm.
2. Heat a wok or large frying pan with the oil and stir-fry the chicken until browned.
3. Remove from pan and set aside. Keep warm.
4. Heat another teaspoon of oil in the wok or frying pan. When hot, add the green vegetables. Stir-fry until lightly cooked.
5. Combine remaining ingredients in a separate bowl and add to the pan with the cooked chicken and stir until thickened slightly.
6. Serve the chicken and greens over the mashed sweet potato.

WARM LAMB AND CHICKPEA SALAD

A delicious new way to prepare lamb.

PREPARATION TIME: 20 minutes   COOKING TIME: 20 minutes   SERVES 4

Low GI

Per serving: Cal 430 ■ Carbs 23 g ■ Fat 25 g ■ Fiber 9 g

1 lb. lamb cutlets
1 tablespoon olive oil
1 onion, finely chopped
3 garlic cloves, crushed
½ teaspoon ground cumin
½ teaspoon ground coriander
½ teaspoon ground ginger
½ teaspoon paprika
2 15-oz. cans chickpeas, drained and rinsed
salt and black pepper to taste
1 tomato, diced
1 cup cilantro, finely chopped
1 cup flat-leaf parsley, finely chopped
1 cup mint, finely chopped
3 tablespoons extra-virgin olive oil
juice of 1 lemon
baby spinach leaves, washed, to serve

1. Cook the lamb cutlets in a lightly oiled frying pan, over medium heat, about 3 minutes on each side. Transfer to a plate and cover with foil to keep warm. Set aside.

2. Heat the tablespoon of olive oil in the frying pan and cook the onion for 5 minutes or until soft. Add the garlic and spices and cook for 5 minutes over low heat, stirring occasionally. Add the chickpeas and heat through, stirring until warm and well coated with the spice mixture. Remove from the heat and add the salt and pepper, tomato, chopped herbs, extra oil, and lemon juice.

3. Cut the lamb cutlets into thick slices, diagonally. Toss in the chickpea-herb mixture.

4. Arrange the baby spinach leaves on plates and top with the chickpeas and lamb. Serve immediately.

SPICY PILAF WITH CHICKPEAS

A meatless rice dish that serves three to four people for a light meal.

Garam masala, the key spice here, is a blend of Indian spices (peppercorns, cardamom, cinnamon, cloves, coriander, nutmeg, turmeric, and/or fennel seeds) found in Indian specialty shops, markets, or international sections of large supermarkets. Slivered almonds can be toasted easily by placing in a dry pan over medium heat. Once the pan gets hot, toss the almonds around to toast them. This will take no more than a minute. Don't leave unattended, as the almonds toast rapidly.

PREPARATION TIME: 15 minutes COOKING TIME: 20 minutes SERVES 3 to 4

Low GI

Per serving: Cal 230 ■ Carb 32 g ■ Fat 8 g ■ Fiber 4 g

1 teaspoon poly- or monounsaturated margarine
2 teaspoons olive oil
1 medium onion, peeled and finely diced
6 oz. button mushrooms, quartered or halved
1 clove garlic, crushed
⅔ cup basmati rice
1 teaspoon garam masala
½ cup canned chickpeas
1 bay leaf
1½ cups chicken stock
1 tablespoon slivered almonds, toasted

1. Heat margarine and oil in a medium-sized frying pan over medium heat. Add the onion, cover, and cook 3 minutes, stirring occasionally. Add mushrooms and garlic and cook, uncovered, another 5 minutes, stirring occasionally.

2. Add the rice and spice, stirring to combine until aromatic. Add the chickpeas and bay leaf and pour the stock over. Bring to a boil. Reduce the heat to very low. Cover with a tight-fitting lid and simmer (without lifting the lid) for at least 12 minutes or until rice is tender and all liquid has been absorbed.

3. Sprinkle with toasted almonds and serve with a salad.

MOROCCAN KEBABS

These North African flavors are delicious and quick to make.

Moroccan seasoning is available in jars in the spice section of the super-market. Alternatively, flavor the patties with 1 clove of crushed garlic and ½ teaspoon each of ground coriander, cumin, paprika, black pepper, and dried rosemary. The optional hummus can be purchased in the refrig-erated section of the supermarket or in delicatessens.

PREPARATION TIME: 15 minutes   COOKING TIME: 20 minutes   SERVES 4

Low GI

Per serving: Cal 470 ■ Carb 65 g ■ Fat 9 g ■ Fiber 11 g

4 large pieces of pita bread
12 oz. lean ground beef
½ cup cracked wheat (bulgur)
2 teaspoons Moroccan seasoning
1 medium white onion, very finely chopped
1 egg, lightly beaten
3 medium tomatoes, diced
1 tablespoon mint, roughly chopped
2 teaspoons olive oil
2 teaspoons red wine vinegar
lettuce leaves
hummus (optional)

1. Wrap the pita bread in foil and heat in the oven for 15 minutes.

2. Meanwhile, combine the beef, cracked wheat, seasoning, onion, and egg in a bowl. Shape the mixture into 8 patties.

3. Heat a nonstick frying pan with cooking spray over medium heat and cook the patties about 4 to 5 minutes on each side.

4. Combine the tomato and mint with the olive oil and vinegar in a bowl and serve with the patties and lettuce on the pita bread spread with hummus (if you are using).

WINTER VEGETARIAN STEW

A hearty vegetarian meal that can be prepared in around 30 minutes.

PREPARATION TIME: 15 minutes   COOKING TIME: 30 minutes   SERVES 4 to 6

Low GI

Per serving: Cal 260 ■ Carb 47 g ■ Fat 1.5 g ■ Fiber 12 g

1 teaspoon oil
1 onion, finely chopped
2 cloves garlic, crushed, or 2 teaspoons minced garlic
2 sticks celery, sliced
2 squash or 2 small zucchini, sliced
8 oz. button mushrooms
1 15-oz. can kidney beans, rinsed and drained
1 28-oz. can tomatoes, undrained and chopped
1 teaspoon minced hot pepper
2 tablespoons tomato paste
1½ cups prepared vegetable stock
1¼ cups small macaroni pasta
freshly ground black pepper
chopped fresh parsley, to serve

1. Heat the oil in a nonstick frying pan, add the onion and garlic and cook for about 5 minutes or until soft.

2. Add the celery, squash or zucchini, and mushrooms, and cook, stirring, for 5 minutes.

3. Stir in the beans, tomatoes, chili pepper, tomato paste, and stock, and bring to a boil.

4. Add the pasta, reduce the heat, and simmer for about 20 minutes or until the pasta is tender.

5. Add pepper to taste and serve sprinkled with parsley.

EASY TUNA BAKE

PREPARATION TIME: 25 minutes   COOKING TIME: 55 minutes   SERVES 4

Low GI

Per serving: Cal 567 ■ Carb 49 g ■ Fat 22 g ■ Fiber 6.5 g

olive oil spray
1 cup pasta spirals (or small shapes
   like macaroni)
15 oz. can tuna in oil, drained, flaked
1 small red pepper, diced
3 green onions, sliced
⅓ cup cornstarch
2 cups reduced-fat milk
⅓ cup finely grated Parmesan cheese
3 tablespoons finely chopped parsley

freshly ground black pepper
2 cups frozen corn and pea mix
1 tablespoon Dijon mustard

Topping
⅔ cup fresh low GI bread crumbs
½ teaspoon paprika
1½ tablespoons reduced-fat
   margarine

1. Preheat the oven to 350°F. Spray an 8 x 8 x 2 inch square baking dish with olive oil spray.

2. Cook the pasta according to the directions on the packet until only just al dente (remember you are going to be baking it as well), drain, cover, and set aside.

3. In a large bowl, combine the tuna, pepper, and green onions.

4. Stir the cornstarch with a little of the milk in a small cup until it dissolves. Heat the remaining milk in a large saucepan and bring just to a boil. Add the cornstarch mix and stir until the mixture boils, then reduce the heat to low and simmer for 1 minute while continuing to stir. Turn off the heat and stir in the cheese, parsley, and freshly ground black pepper.

5. Add tuna mix to the mixture in the saucepan along with the corn and pea mix, mustard, and the pasta and combine well. Spoon the mixture into the prepared baking dish and smooth the top.

6. For the topping, combine bread crumbs and paprika and rub in margarine. Sprinkle this evenly over the tuna mixture. Bake in the oven for 40 minutes or until the top is golden and crunchy. Serve with a garden salad.

LAMB CURRY WITH SPINACH RICE PILAF

PREPARATION TIME: 25 minutes COOKING TIME: 35 minutes SERVES 4

Low GI

Per serving: Cal 452 ■ Carb 38 g ■ Fat 17 g ■ Fiber 9 g

1½ tablespoons curry powder
14 oz. lamb cutlets, diced into
   1–1¼ inch pieces
1 tablespoon canola oil
1 onion, chopped
2 cloves garlic, crushed
1 teaspoon grated ginger
2 carrots, chopped into 1-inch chunks
1 15-oz. can chopped tomatoes
2 cups cauliflower florets
¾ cup reduced-salt chicken stock
1 cup frozen green peas

Spinach Rice Pilaf
1 tablespoon canola oil
1 onion, chopped
½ cup basmati rice
1 cup gluten-free reduced-salt chicken
   stock
1 bay leaf
1 15-oz. can lentils, drained and
   rinsed
1½ cups baby spinach leaves

1. Sprinkle 2 teaspoons of the curry powder over the lamb to coat lightly. Heat 2 teaspoons of the oil in a large, heavy-based saucepan, add the lamb and brown for 2–3 minutes in 2 batches. Spoon the browned meat into a dish, cover, and set aside, keeping warm.

2. Heat the remaining oil in the pan. Add the onion and cook for 3–4 minutes until soft and golden. Add the garlic, ginger, remaining curry powder, and carrots, and cook, stirring, for 1 minute. Return the meat to the pan with the tomatoes, cauli-flower, and stock. Bring to a boil, then reduce the heat to low, cover, and simmer gently for 20 minutes. Add the peas and cook for another 2 minutes.

3. Meanwhile, to make the rice pilaf, heat the oil in a medium-sized saucepan. Add the onion and cook for 3–4 minutes until soft and golden. Add the rice and cook, stirring, for 1 more minute. Add the stock and bay leaf and bring to a boil. Reduce the heat to low, cover, and simmer very gently for 15 minutes.

4. Stir in the lentils, heat through, and then stir through the spin-ach. Serve topped with the curry.

Desserts and Sweet Treats

■

Cinnamon Muesli Cookies

Granola Bars

Oat Munchies

Mixed Berry and Cinnamon Compote

Bread and Hazelnut Chocolate Pudding

Apple Cranberry Crisp

Cinnamon Raisin Bread and Butter Pudding

Creamy Rice with Sliced Pears

Apricot, Honey, and Coconut Crunch

Fresh Fruit Cheesecake

Winter Fruit Salad

Yogurt Berry Jello

CINNAMON MUESLI COOKIES

Delicious, good-for-you cookie treats.

PREPARATION TIME: 10 minutes   COOKING TIME: 25 minutes
MAKES APPROXIMATELY 10 cookies

Moderate GI

Per serving: Cal 30 ■ Carb 21 g ■ Fat 4 g ■ Fiber 2 g

2 tablespoons canola oil
3 tablespoons maple syrup
⅓ cup orange juice
1 cup unsweetened rolled-oat muesli
1 cup unbleached all-purpose flour
1 tablespoon cinnamon
powdered sugar

1. Preheat the oven to 350°F.
2. Line a baking tray with parchment paper.
3. Measure the oil and maple syrup into a large mixing bowl. Add the orange juice and mix.
4. Add the muesli, flour, and cinnamon and mix to a soft dough.
5. Place spoonfuls of the mixture onto the prepared tray, leaving about 1 inch between each cookie.
6. Bake immediately for 15–20 minutes, until just golden brown. Cool on a wire rack and sprinkle with a little powdered sugar.

GRANOLA BARS

These bars have a wholesome texture and make a very sustaining snack.

PREPARATION TIME: 20 minutes   COOKING TIME: 20 minutes   MAKES 12 bars

Low GI

Per serving: Cal 140 ■ Carb 15 g ■ Fat 8 g ■ Fiber 3 g

½ cup whole-wheat flour
½ cup unbleached all-purpose flour
1¾ teaspoons baking powder
½ teaspoon mixed spice
½ teaspoon ground cinnamon
1½ cups rolled oats
1 cup dried-fruit medley or dried fruit of choice, chopped
¼ cup sunflower seed kernels
½ cup apple juice
¼ cup oil
1 egg, lightly beaten
2 egg whites, lightly beaten

1. Preheat oven to 400°F. Line an 8 x 12 inch baking pan with parchment paper.

2. Sift the flours, baking powder, and spices into a large bowl. Stir in the oats, fruit, and seeds and stir to combine.

3. Add the apple juice, oil, and whole egg; mix well. Gently mix in the egg whites until combined.

4. Press the mixture evenly into the prepared pan and press firmly with the back of a spoon. Mark the surface into 12 bars using a sharp knife.

5. Bake in hot oven for about 15 to 20 minutes or until lightly browned. Cool and cut into bars.

OAT MUNCHIES

Crunchy cookies that make handy, low GI snacks.

PREPARATION TIME: 15 minutes   COOKING TIME: 10 minutes
MAKES 16 cookies

Low GI

Per serving: Cal 140 ■ Carb 17 g ■ Fat 6 g ■ Fiber 3 g

6½ tablespoons poly- or monounsaturated margarine
¼ cup honey
1 egg
½ teaspoon vanilla extract
2½ cups rolled oats
2 tablespoons sunflower seed kernels
¼ cup self-rising flour, sifted

1. Preheat oven to 375°F. Melt the margarine and honey in a small saucepan.
2. Whisk the egg and vanilla extract together in a large bowl.
3. Add the margarine mixture, muesli, sunflower seed kernels, and flour to the egg mixture; stir until combined.
4. Place small spoonfuls of the mixture onto a lightly greased baking tray, spacing evenly.
5. Bake in hot oven for about 10 minutes or until golden brown. Let stand on tray until firm, then loosen and place on a wire rack to cool.

MIXED BERRY AND CINNAMON COMPOTE

Fifteen minutes is all it takes for this scrumptious dessert, which is delicious as a topping on your favorite pudding; it pairs beautifully with Cinnamon Raisin Bread and Butter Pudding (page 293).

A COOK'S NOTE: Before you squeeze the oranges for juice, zest the skin using a zester or vegetable peeler.

PREPARATION TIME: 10 minutes   COOKING TIME: 15 minutes   SERVES 6 to 8

Low GI

Per serving: Cal 145 ■ Carb 36 g ■ Fat negligible ■ Fiber 2 g

¾ cup freshly squeezed orange juice
1 cup sugar
2 cinnamon sticks
zest of 1 orange, finely sliced
4 cups mixed berries (raspberries, blackberries, blueberries, strawberries)

1. Place the orange juice, sugar, cinnamon sticks, and orange zest in a large stainless-steel saucepan, and slowly bring to a boil.

2. Add the mixed berries and simmer gently for 2 minutes, just until the berries warm through and swell.

3. Serve warm or as a topping on your favorite pudding.

BREAD AND HAZELNUT CHOCOLATE PUDDING

A healthy dessert that includes Nutella in a costarring role.

PREPARATION TIME: 25 minutes   COOKING TIME: 55 minutes   SERVES 4
Low GI
Per serving: Cal 340 ■ Carb 55 g ■ Fat 7 g ■ Fiber 2 g

1 tablespoon raisins
1 tablespoon rum (optional)
4 slices sourdough bread
2 tablespoons Nutella or other chocolate hazelnut spread
2 eggs, lightly beaten
½ teaspoon ground cinnamon
½ cup superfine sugar
1 cup low-fat milk
1 tablespoon pudding mix

1. Preheat oven to 400°F. If you want to plump the raisins with rum, place them in a small bowl with the alcohol, and heat in the microwave for 20 seconds or until the fruit is swollen.

2. Spread the Nutella thickly over 2 slices of the bread. Dot with the raisins and make a sandwich with the remaining 2 slices of bread. Cut each sandwich into 4 triangular quarters and stand upright in a 1-quart baking dish, squashing together to fit.

3. Combine the beaten eggs with the remaining ingredients by whisking together in a deep bowl. Pour the egg mixture over the sandwiches in the baking dish and let stand for 10 minutes while the bread absorbs the pudding.

4. Stand the baking dish in another ovenproof dish and add hot water to the larger dish to come halfway up the sides (hot-water-bath style). Bake for 40 minutes in preheated oven until the custard around the bread is set and golden in color.

APPLE CRANBERRY CRISP

This is a version of Jane Brody's recipe in her now-classic Jane Brody's Good Food Cookbook—*and a delicious late autumn or early winter, low GI dessert. Tart cranberries and sweet apples virtually melt together beneath the crumb topping.*

PREPARATION TIME: 15 minutes   COOKING TIME: 40 minutes   SERVES 8

Low GI

Per serving: Cal 267 ■ Carb 43 g ■ Fat 10 g ■ Fiber 5 g

3 cups cranberries (1 12-oz. package)
2 large apples, peeled, cored, and chopped into cranberry-size pieces
½ cup sugar
2 teaspoons cinnamon
¼ cup all-purpose flour, divided
3 tablespoons packed brown sugar
¾ cup rolled oats
½ cup chopped walnuts (optional)
3 tablespoons mono- or polyunsaturated margarine, melted

1. Preheat the oven to 375°F. Combine the cranberries, apples, sugar, cinnamon, and 1 tablespoon of flour in a mixing bowl. Transfer the mixture to a 6-cup shallow baking dish sprayed with cooking spray.

2. Combine the remaining flour, brown sugar, oats, and nuts (if desired) in the same mixing bowl (it need not be washed). Stir in the melted butter or margarine, and mix the ingredients well—the mixture will be crumbly. Sprinkle the oat mixture over the fruit mixture.

3. Bake the crisp in a hot oven for 40 minutes or until the crisp is lightly browned. Let the crisp stand for 10 minutes before serving.

CINNAMON RAISIN BREAD AND BUTTER PUDDING

Served with the Mixed Berry and Cinnamon Compote, this is an ideal early-autumn dessert.

PREPARATION TIME: 20 minutes   COOKING TIME: 1 hour   SERVES 6 to 8
Low GI
Per serving: Cal 175 ■ Carb 25 g ■ Fat 4 g ■ Fiber 1 g

2½ cups low-fat milk
3 omega-3–enriched eggs
2 tablespoons sugar
1 teaspoon vanilla extract
4 slices cinnamon raisin bread
1 tablespoon margarine
½ cup raisins, soaked in 2 tablespoons brandy
1 teaspoon ground cinnamon

1. Preheat the oven to 325°F. Lightly grease a 1½-quart ovenproof dish. Boil 4–6 cups of water.
2. Whisk the milk, eggs, sugar, and vanilla extract in a large mixing bowl.
3. Remove the crusts from the bread and spread generously with the margarine, cutting each slice in half diagonally. Stack the triangles of bread upright across the prepared dish. Scatter the cut slices with the presoaked raisins, and pour the custard mixture over. Gently push the slices down to soak up the custard. Sprinkle with cinnamon.
4. Place the bread-and-butter pudding dish in the center of a large, deep, baking dish. Pour boiling water slowly into the outer dish to come at least three-quarters of the way up the sides of the pudding dish (hot-water-bath style).
5. Bake for approximately 1 hour or until the custard is set, puffy, and a light golden brown.
6. Serve with the Mixed Berry and Cinnamon Compote (page 290).

CREAMY RICE WITH SLICED PEARS

A rice pudding with a healthy twist.

PREPARATION TIME: 10 minutes   COOKING TIME: 30 minutes   SERVES 4

Low GI

Per serving: Cal 295 ■ Carb 65 g ■ Fat negligible ■ Fiber 3 g

2 cups water
1 cup Uncle Ben's converted or basmati rice
¾ cup canned evaporated skim milk
¼ cup firmly packed brown sugar
1 teaspoon vanilla extract
1 16-oz. can pear slices (in natural juice), drained

1. Bring the water to a boil in a saucepan, add the rice and boil for 15 minutes; drain.

2. Return the rice to the saucepan with the milk. Stir over a low heat until all the milk is absorbed. Stir in the sugar and vanilla extract; cool.

3. Using an ice cream scoop, serve scoops of rice with the pear slices fanned out next to it.

APRICOT, HONEY, AND COCONUT CRUNCH

Apricots, honey, and yogurt on a coconut-cookie base.
To toast coconut, cook in a nonstick frying pan over low heat, stirring for 2 minutes or until just golden. Remove from the pan to cool.

PREPARATION TIME: 20 minutes   COOKING TIME: 45 minutes   SERVES 8

Low GI

Per serving: Cal 255 ■ Carb 32 g ■ Fat 12 g ■ Fiber 2 g

Base
¼ cup dried, shredded coconut, toasted
16 oatmeal cookies, finely crushed
4 tablespoons poly- or monounsaturated margarine, melted

Topping
1 cup dried apricots
½ cup boiling water
2 8-oz. containers low-fat apricot yogurt
¼ cup honey
2 eggs

1. Line a 6½ x 10½ inch rectangular pan with foil.
2. For the base, combine the ingredients in a bowl and mix well. Press the mixture evenly over the bottom of the prepared pan.
3. Bake in a 350°F oven for about 10 minutes or until browned. Remove from the oven and allow to cool.
4. For the topping, cover the apricots with the boiling water and let stand for 30 minutes or until soft. Process in a blender or food processor until smooth. Add the yogurt, honey, and eggs and blend until smooth.
5. Spread the topping mixture over the prepared base. Bake in a 350°F oven for about 30 to 35 minutes or until set.
6. Cool, then refrigerate several hours before serving.

FRESH FRUIT CHEESECAKE

A delicious lower-fat cheesecake that leaves you feeling good after you eat it, not weighed down with fat.

Avoid using pineapple or kiwi for the chopped fresh fruit in the filling, because these tend to prevent the gelatin from setting.

PREPARATION TIME: 20 minutes   COOKING TIME: 15 minutes
CHILLING TIME: 1 hour   SERVES 8

Low GI

Per serving: Cal 335 ■ Carb 35 g ■ Fat 14 g ■ Fiber 1 g

Crust
32 oatmeal cookies, crushed
6½ tablespoons poly- or monounsaturated margarine, melted

Filling
2 teaspoons gelatin
2 tablespoons boiling water
1 8-oz. container low-fat fruit yogurt
1 8-oz. container low-fat pineapple cottage cheese
¼ cup honey
½ teaspoon vanilla extract
1 cup chopped fresh fruit (e.g., apple, orange, cantaloupe, strawberries, pear, grapes)

1. For the crust, combine the cookie crumbs and margarine in a bowl. Press evenly into a 9-inch pie dish. Bake in a 350°F oven for 10 minutes. Cool.

2. For the filling, sprinkle the gelatin over the boiling water in a cup, stand the cup in a small pan of simmering water, and stir until dissolved; cool slightly.

3. Process the cooled gelatin with the yogurt, cottage cheese, honey, and vanilla extract in a blender or food processor until smooth.

4. Arrange the chopped fruit over the prepared crust and pour the yogurt mixture over.

5. Refrigerate for about 1 hour or until set.

WINTER FRUIT SALAD

Oranges, apples, and bananas tend to be available year-round, and this combination is ideal when other fruits are out of season.

PREPARATION TIME: 10 minutes   COOKING TIME: none
CHILLING TIME: 1 hour   SERVES 2

Low GI

Per serving: Cal 150 ■ Carb 33 g ■ Fat 1 g ■ Fiber 5 g

1 orange, peeled and separated into segments
1 medium red apple, cut into bite-sized cubes
2 teaspoons sugar
1 teaspoon fresh lemon juice
1 small banana
1 tablespoon shredded coconut

1. Cut the orange segments in half. Place the apple and orange chunks in a bowl. Sprinkle with the sugar and lemon juice and mix thoroughly. Cover and refrigerate for at least 1 hour.

2. Just before serving, stir in the sliced banana. Sprinkle with coconut to serve.

YOGURT BERRY JELLO

An easy dessert. You can make it with low-calorie or sugar-free jello if you want to reduce the calories.

PREPARATION TIME: 10 minutes   COOKING TIME: 5 minutes   CHILLING TIME: 40 minutes   SERVES 4

Low GI

Per serving: Cal 85 ■ Carb 16 g ■ Fat negligible ■ Fiber 1 g

1 3-oz. package berry-flavored gelatin powder
1 cup boiling water
1 cup strawberries or frozen raspberries
1½ cups low-fat berry yogurt

1. Stir the boiling water into the gelatin in a bowl until completely dissolved; cool, but do not allow to set.
2. Roughly chop the strawberries (frozen raspberries will tend to break up on stirring).
3. Fold the yogurt and berries into the gelatin; mix well. Pour into serving bowls, cover, and refrigerate until set.

The Authoritative Tables of GI Values

23

An Introduction and How to Use the Tables

THIS ALL-NEW EDITION of our authoritative table of GI values presents the completely updated tables, organized alphabetically by category.

These tables will help you put those low GI food choices into your shopping cart and onto your plate.

Each entry lists an individual food and its GI value. We also list the nominal serving size, the amount of carbohydrate per serving, the GL, and whether the food's GI is low, medium, or high.

High, Medium, or Low GI . . .

- A high GI value is 70 or more.
- A medium/moderate GI value is 56–69 inclusive.
- A low GI value is 55 or less.

Where Did the GI Cut-offs Come From?

The GI cut-offs have been commonly used for some time, but we are often asked for their scientific basis. During the 1980s when the GI of few foods was known, we developed diets broadly categorized as high and low GI, based on the knowledge that most breads, rices, and potatoes had a GI of around 70 or above, while pasta, legumes, dairy products, and many fruits had GI values in the 30s to 50s. In the absence of formal guidelines, our research dietitians conducting studies gave practical instructions to choose carbohydrate foods of 55 or less for those following a low GI diet, and 70 or more for those following the conventional diet.

In clinical trials, the low GI diets, so defined, were associated with lower glycated hemoglobin levels (HbA1c) and improved carbohydrate tolerance. These informal cut-offs were therefore validated and henceforth recommended in lay publications and adopted by dietitians.

Nonetheless, there is a need to recognize the difference between a low GI diet and a low GI food. Because a low GI food is defined as 55 or less, it is sometimes assumed that a diet that averages less than 55 represents a low GI eating pattern. In fact, population studies show that the median GI of a Western diet already hovers around 56–58. The lowest risk of chronic disease, however, is associated with an average GI of around 45. Since this represents a self-selected diet and is sustainable in "real life," it becomes a logical basis for defining a low GI diet (i.e., 45 or less).

You can use the table to:

- Find the GI of your favorite foods.
- Compare carb-rich foods within a category (two types of bread or breakfast cereal, for example).
- Identify the best carbohydrate choices.
- Improve your diet by finding a low GI substitute for high GI foods.
- Put together a low GI meal.
- Find foods with a high GI but low GL.

Each food appears alphabetically within a food category, such as "Bread" or "Fruit." This makes it easy to compare the kinds of foods you eat every day and helps you see which high GI foods you can replace with low GI versions.

The food categories are listed alphabetically, but if you need to find one quickly, check the category index below. For instance, if you wanted to find the GI value of an apple, you would look under the food category "Fruit."

The food categories used in the tables and the pages on which they begin, are:

- **Beans, peas, and legumes**, including baked beans, chickpeas, lentils, and split peas—page 305
- **Beverages**, including fruit and vegetable juices, soft drinks, flavored milk, and sports drinks—page 306
- **Bread**, including sliced white and whole grain breads, fruit breads, flat breads, and crispbreads—page 309
- **Breakfast cereals**, including processed cereals, muesli, oats, and oatmeal—page 311
- **Cakes and muffins**, including other baked goods—page 313
- **Cereal grains**, including couscous, bulgur, and barley—page 315
- **Cookies and crackers**—page 315
- **Dairy products**, including milk, yogurt, ice cream, and dairy desserts—page 317
- **Fruit**, including fresh, canned, and dried fruit—page 320
- **Gluten-free products**—page 322
- **Meals, prepared and convenience**—page 323
- **Meat, seafood, eggs, and protein**—page 325
- **Nutritional supplements**—page 327
- **Nuts and seeds**—page 328
- **Oils and dressings**—page 329
- **Pasta and noodles**—page 329
- **Rice**—page 332
- **Snack foods**, including chocolate, fruit bars, muesli bars, nuts, and seeds—page 334
- **Soups**—page 339
- **Soy products**, including soy milk and soy yogurt—page 341
- **Spreads and sweeteners**, including sugars, honey, and jam—page 341
- **Vegetables**, including green vegetables, salad vegetables, and root vegetables—page 343

In the table, you will sometimes see these symbols:

★ indicates that a food contains little or no carbohydrate. We have included these foods—such as vegetables and protein-rich foods—because so many people ask us for their GI.

ⓖ indicates that a food is part of the GI symbol program. Foods with the GI symbol have had their GI tested properly and are a healthy choice for their food category.

To make a fair comparison, all foods have been tested using an internationally standardized method. Gram for gram of carbohydrates, the higher the GI, the higher the blood glucose levels after consumption. If you can't find the GI value in these tables for a food you eat regularly, check our Website (www.glycemicindex.com), where we maintain an international database of published GI values that have been tested by a reliable laboratory. Alternatively, please write to the manufacturer and encourage it to have the food tested by an accredited laboratory. In the meantime, choose a similar food from the table as a substitute.

The GI values in this book are correct at the time of publication. However, the formulation of commercial foods can change, and the GI may change as well. You can rely on foods showing the GI symbol. Although some manufacturers include the GI on the nutritional label, you would need to know that the testing was carried out independently by an accredited laboratory.

24
The Authoritative Tables of GI Values

Beans & Legumes

Food	GI Value	Nominal Serving Size	Available Carbs	GL Value	GI Level
Baked beans, canned in tomato sauce, Heinz	49	5 oz	18	9	low
Black beans, boiled	30	2¼ oz	15	5	low
Black-eyed beans, soaked, boiled	42	4¼ oz	17	7	low
Broad beans, frozen, reheated	63	3 oz	7	4	med
Butter beans, canned, drained	36	6 oz	17	6	low
Butter beans, dried, boiled	31	5¼ oz	17	5	low
Butter beans, soaked overnight, boiled 50 mins	26	5¼ oz	17	4	low
Cannellini beans, canned, drained	31	5 oz	14	4	low
Chickpeas, canned, drained	38	5 oz	25	10	low
Chickpeas, canned in brine	40	4 oz	16	6	low
Chickpeas, dried, boiled	28	3 oz	14	4	low
Cranberry beans, canned, drained	41	2¼ oz	17	7	low
Four bean mix, canned, drained	37	3½ oz	14	5	low
Green beans, cooked, canned	38	2¼ oz	13	5	low
Green beans, dried, boiled	33	4 oz	15	5	low
Kidney beans, dark red, canned, drained	43	3½ oz	14	6	low
Kidney beans, red, canned, drained	36	6½ oz	19	7	low
Kidney beans, red, dried, boiled	28	3 oz	13	4	low
Kidney beans, red, soaked overnight, boiled 60 mins	51	3 oz	13	7	low

★ little or no carbs   ⓖ program participant

305

Beans & Legumes

Food	GI Value	Nominal Serving Size	Available Carbs	GL Value	GI Level
Lentils, brown, canned, drained	42	5¼ oz	21	9	low
Lentils, green, canned	48	4¾ oz	13	6	low
Lentils, green, dried, boiled	30	4½ oz	12	4	low
Lentils, red, dried, boiled	26	4½ oz	12	3	low
Lentils, red, split, boiled 25 mins	21	4½ oz	12	3	low
Lima beans, baby, frozen, reheated	32	4 oz	15	5	low
Mung beans, boiled	39	5 oz	16	6	low
Peas, dried, boiled	22	6¼ oz	13	3	low
Peas, green, frozen, boiled	48	5½ oz	13	6	low
Pinto beans, canned, drained	45	4 oz	18	8	low
President's Choice Blue Menu low fat 4-bean salad	13	3 oz	9	1	low
Refried pinto beans, canned, Casa Fiesta	38	4 oz	20	8	low
Romano beans	46	5 oz	9	4	low
Soy beans, canned, drained	14	6 oz	5	1	low
Soy beans, dried, boiled	18	6 oz	2	0	low
Split peas, yellow, boiled 20 mins	32	6¼ oz	13	4	low
Split peas, yellow, dried, soaked overnight, boiled 55 mins	25	6¼ oz	13	3	low

Beverages

Food	GI Value	Nominal Serving Size	Available Carbs	GL Value	GI Level
All Sport Body Quencher	53	8 fl oz	16	8	low
Apple and Cherry juice, pure	43	8 fl oz	33	14	low
Apple and Mango juice, pure	47	8 fl oz	33	16	low
Apple and Pineapple juice	48	8 fl oz	34	16	low
Apple juice, filtered, pure	44	8 fl oz	30	13	low
Apple juice, Granny Smith, unsweetened	44	8 fl oz	30	13	low
Apple juice, no added sugar	40	8 fl oz	28	11	low
Apple juice with fiber	37	8 fl oz	28	10	low
Beer (4.6% alcohol)	66	25 fl oz	15	10	med
Campbell's, 100% vegetable juice	43	6 fl oz	6	3	low
Campbell's, tomato juice	33	12 fl oz	11	4	low
Campbell's V8 Splash, tropical blend fruit drink	47	8 fl oz	27	13	low
Carrot juice, freshly made	43	8 fl oz	14	6	low

★ little or no carbs Ⓖ program participant

Beverages

Food	GI Value	Nominal Serving Size	Available Carbs	GL Value	GI Level
Chocolate Daydream shake, fructose, Revival Soy	33	8 fl oz	36	12	low
Chocolate Daydream shake, sucralose, Revival Soy	25	8 fl oz	7	2	low
Chocolate-flavored milk	37	8 fl oz	24	9	low
Chocolate milkshake, commercial	21	16 fl oz	68	14	low
Cinch Chocolate weight management powder, prepared with skim milk, Shaklee Corporation	16	8 fl oz	31	5	low
Cinch Vanilla weight management powder, prepared with skim milk, Shaklee Corporation	22	8 fl oz	29	6	low
Coca-Cola	53	12 fl oz	41	22	low
Cocoa with water	★	8 fl oz	0	0	
Coffee, black	★	8 fl oz	0	0	
Coffee, cappuccino	★	8 fl oz	4	0	
Coffee, milk	★	8 fl oz	2	0	
Cola, artificially sweetened	★	8 fl oz	0	0	
Cranberry juice cocktail	52	8 fl oz	34	18	low
Diet Coke	★	8 fl oz	0	0	
Diet dry ginger ale	★	8 fl oz	0	0	
Diet ginger beer	★	8 fl oz	0	0	
Diet lemonade	★	8 fl oz	0	0	
Diet orange fruit drink	★	12 fl oz	3	0	
Fanta orange lite	★	8 fl oz	1	0	
Fanta orange soft drink	68	8 fl oz	30	20	med
Fruit punch	67	8 fl oz	29	19	med
Gatorade	78	8 fl oz	15	12	high
Grapefruit juice, unsweetened	48	8 fl oz	18	9	low
Hot chocolate mix made with hot water	51	6 fl oz	23	12	low
Lemonade	54	8 fl oz	28	15	low
Lemonade, artificially sweetened	★	8 fl oz	0	0	
Ⓖ Lo-Gly Acai Blue	31	8 fl oz	34	11	low
Ⓖ Lo-Gly Mango Mojito	24	8 fl oz	35	8	low
Ⓖ Lo-Gly Pomegranate	28	8 fl oz	35	10	low
Ⓖ Lo-Gly Pomegranate Mojito	32	8 fl oz	31	10	low
Mango smoothie	32	8 fl oz	30	10	low
Malted powder in full fat milk	33	8 fl oz	30	10	low
Malted powder in reduced fat milk	36	8 fl oz	30	11	low
Malted powder in skim milk	39	8 fl oz	30	12	low
Mineral water	★	8 fl oz	0	0	

★ little or no carbs   Ⓖ program participant

Beverages

Food	GI Value	Nominal Serving Size	Available Carbs	GL Value	GI Level
MonaVie E^{MV}	52	8 fl oz	40	21	low
Nesquik powder, Chocolate, in 2% fat milk	41	8 fl oz	26	11	low
Nesquik powder, Strawberry, in 2% fat milk	35	8 fl oz	26	9	low
Orange juice, unsweetened, fresh	50	8 fl oz	19	10	low
Orange juice, unsweetened, from concentrate	53	8 fl oz	19	10	low
Pepsi Max	★	8 fl oz	0	0	
Pineapple juice, unsweetened	46	8 fl oz	24	11	low
President's Choice Blue Menu Oh Mega j orange juice	48	8 fl oz	30	14	low
President's Choice Blue Menu Orange Delight Cocktail with pulp	44	8 fl oz	16	7	low
President's Choice Blue Menu Soy Beverage, Chocolate flavored	40	8 fl oz	28	11	low
President's Choice Blue Menu Soy Beverage, Original flavored	15	8 fl oz	9	1	low
President's Choice Blue Menu Soy Beverage, Vanilla flavored	28	8 fl oz	16	4	low
President's Choice Blue Menu Tomato juice, low sodium	23	8 fl oz	7	2	low
Prune juice	43	8 fl oz	36	11	low
Rice milk, low fat	86	8 fl oz	27	23	high
Slim Fast French Vanilla ready-to-drink shake	37	11 fl oz	35	13	low
Smoothie, banana	30	8 fl oz	26	8	low
Smoothie, banana and strawberry, V8 Splash	44	8 fl oz	20	9	low
Smoothie, fruit	35	8 fl oz	28	10	low
Smoothie, mango	32	8 fl oz	26	8	low
Soda water	★	8 fl oz	0	0	
Sprite Zero lemonade	★	8 fl oz	0	0	
Strawberry-flavored milk	37	8 fl oz	22	8	low
Tea, black	★	8 fl oz	0	0	
Tea, white	★	8 fl oz	1	0	
Tomato juice, no added sugar	38	8 fl oz	11	4	low
Tonic water, artificially sweetened	★	8 fl oz	0	0	
Tropical blend fruit drink	47	8 fl oz	20	9	low

★ little or no carbs Ⓖ program participant

Bread

Food	GI Value	Nominal Serving Size	Available Carbs	GL Value	GI Level
3 Grain bread, sprouted grains	55	1 oz	17	9	low
9 Grain muffin	43	1 oz	11	5	low
9 Grain, multigrain bread	43	1¼ oz	13	6	low
100% whole grain bread	51	1 oz	11	6	low
Apricot fruit bread	56	1½ oz	24	13	med
Bagel, white	72	1 oz	16	12	high
Baguette, traditional French bread	77	2 oz	31	24	high
Black rye bread	76	1½ oz	18	14	high
Bread roll, white	71	1 oz	17	12	high
Bread roll, whole wheat	70	1¼ oz	17	11	high
COBS Bread Higher-Fibre Low GI White Roll	50	2¼ oz	37	19	low
Continental fruit loaf	47	¾ oz	12	6	low
Corn tortilla	53	1 oz	14	7	low
Country grain bread	61	2½ oz	28	17	med
Croissant, plain	67	1 oz	13	9	med
Crumpet	69	1¼ oz	16	11	med
Flaxseed and soy bread	55	3 oz	26	14	low
Fruit and spice loaf	54	2 oz	29	16	low
Gluten-free buckwheat bread	72	1 oz	11	8	high
Hamburger bun, white	61	1 oz	18	11	med
Homemade white bread	70	1¼ oz	18	13	high
Hot dog roll, white	68	1½ oz	22	15	med
Italian bread	73	1¼ oz	18	13	high
Kaiser roll, white	73	1 oz	15	11	high
Lebanese bread, white	75	1 oz	19	14	high
Light rye bread	68	1 oz	14	10	med
Melba toast, plain	70	½ oz	11	8	high
Multigrain sandwich bread	65	1 oz	14	9	med
Natural Ovens English Muffin bread	77	1 oz	15	12	high
Natural Ovens Happiness, cinnamon, raisin, pecan bread	63	1 oz	12	8	med
Natural Ovens Hunger Filler, whole grain bread	59	1 oz	11	6	med
Organic stoneground whole wheat sourdough bread	59	1¼ oz	17	10	med
Pita bread, white	63	1¼ oz	17	11	med
Pita bread, white, mini	68	1 oz	16	11	med
President's Choice Blue Menu 100% Whole Wheat Gigantico Burger Buns	62	2¾ oz	31	19	med

★ little or no carbs   Ⓖ program participant

Bread

Food	GI Value	Nominal Serving Size	Available Carbs	GL Value	GI Level
President's Choice Blue Menu 100% Whole Wheat Gigantico Hot Dog Rolls	62	3¼ oz	36	22	**med**
President's Choice Blue Menu Multi-grain Flax Loaf	51	3 oz	32	16	**low**
President's Choice Blue Menu Oatmeal Loaf	63	3¼ oz	43	27	**med**
President's Choice Blue Menu tortillas, flax	53	2 oz	29	15	**low**
President's Choice Blue Menu tortillas, whole wheat	59	2 oz	27	16	**med**
President's Choice Blue Menu Whole Grain Baguette	73	1¾ oz	21	15	**high**
President's Choice Blue Menu Whole Grain Chipotle Red Pepper Tortilla	35	2¼ oz	32	11	**low**
President's Choice Blue Menu Whole Grain Cinnamon Raisin Bagel	52	2 oz	31	16	**low**
President's Choice Blue Menu Whole Grain English muffins	51	2 oz	20	10	**low**
President's Choice Blue Menu Whole Grain Multi-Grain English Muffin	45	2 oz	20	9	**low**
President's Choice Blue Menu Whole Grain Multi-Grain Flax Bagel	58	2 oz	28	16	**med**
President's Choice Blue Menu Whole Grain Jalapeno Corn Tortilla	55	2¼ oz	32	18	**low**
President's Choice Blue Menu Whole Grain Oatmeal Bagel	63	2 oz	30	19	**med**
President's Choice Blue Menu Whole Wheat Soy Loaf	45	3 oz	27	12	**low**
Pumpernickel bread	50	1 oz	14	7	**low**
Raisin toast	63	1 oz	17	11	**med**
Rye bread, whole grain	58	1 oz	12	7	**med**
Schinkenbrot, dark rye bread	86	1¼ oz	18	15	**high**
Sourdough rye bread	48	1¼ oz	18	9	**low**
Sourdough wheat bread	54	1 oz	11	6	**low**
Spelt multigrain bread	54	1¼ oz	14	8	**low**
Stuffing, bread	74	2¾ oz	17	13	**high**
Traditional sourdough bread	58	3 oz	42	24	**med**

★ little or no carbs   Ⓖ program participant

Bread

Food	GI Value	Nominal Serving Size	Available Carbs	GL Value	GI Level
Tortilla, reduced carbohydrate	51	1 oz	7	4	low
Turkish bread, white	87	3 oz	40	35	high
White bread, high fiber, low GI	52	1¼ oz	15	8	low
White bread, regular, sliced	71	1 oz	13	9	high
White Vienna bread	66	1½ oz	23	15	med
Whole grain rye bread	58	1 oz	15	9	med
Whole wheat country grain bread	53	2½ oz	28	15	low
Whole wheat sandwich bread	71	1 oz	12	9	high
Wonder White	80	1 oz	12	10	high
Ⓖ Wonder White Low GI sandwich bread	54	1 oz	13	7	low

Breakfast Cereals

Food	GI Value	Nominal Serving Size	Available Carbs	GL Value	GI Level
All-Bran, Kellogg's	49	1 oz	23	11	low
All-Bran Complete Wheat Flakes, Kellogg's	60	1 oz	21	13	med
All-Bran Bran Buds, Kellogg's	58	1 oz	24	14	med
Bran Chex, Nabisco	58	1 oz	39	23	med
Bran Flakes, Kellogg's	74	¾ oz	14	10	high
Cheerios, General Mills	74	1 oz	21	16	high
Coco Pops, Kellogg's	80	1 oz	26	21	high
Corn Flakes, Kellogg's	86	1 oz	24	21	high
Corn Pops, Kellogg's	80	1 oz	26	21	high
Cream of Wheat	66	6 oz	29	19	med
Cream of Wheat, Instant	74	6 oz	33	24	high
Crispix, Kellogg's	87	1 oz	25	22	high
Froot Loops, Kellogg's	69	¾ oz	17	12	med
Frosted Flakes, Kellogg's	55	¾ oz	17	9	low
Gluten-free muesli	39	1½ oz	13	5	low
Golden Grahams, General Mills	71	1 oz	25	18	high
Grape-nuts, Post	71	8 oz	48	34	high
Grape-nuts Flakes, Post	80	1.1 oz	24	19	high
Hi-Bran Weet-Bix, regular	61	1 oz	17	10	med
Honey Smacks, Kellogg's	71	1 oz	23	16	high
Just Right, Kellogg's	60	1½ oz	32	19	med
Kashi 7 Whole Grain Puffs	65	0.7 oz	14	9	med
Life, Quaker Oats	66	1 oz	24	16	med

★ little or no carbs   Ⓖ program participant

Breakfast Cereals

Food	GI Value	Nominal Serving Size	Available Carbs	GL Value	GI Level
Muesli, gluten and wheat free with psyllium	50	1½ oz	13	7	low
Muesli, mixed berry & apple	64	1½ oz	30	19	med
Muesli, Natural	40	1 oz	16	6	low
Muesli, Swiss Formula	56	1 oz	18	10	med
Muesli, yeast and wheat free	44	1½ oz	13	6	low
Nutri-Grain, Kellogg's	66	¾ oz	14	9	med
Oat bran, raw, unprocessed	59	1 oz	17	10	med
Oatmeal, instant, made with water	82	6 oz	18	15	high
Oatmeal, made from steel-cut oats with water	52	6 oz	18	9	low
Oatmeal, multigrain, made with water	55	1 oz	17	9	low
Oatmeal, regular, made from oats with water	58	6 oz	18	10	med
Oats, rolled, raw	55	1 oz	15	8	low
President's Choice Blue Menu Bran Flakes	65	1 oz	24	16	med
President's Choice Blue Menu Fiber-First, multi-bran cereal	55	1 oz	23	13	low
President's Choice Blue Menu Granola Clusters, original, low-fat	63	2 oz	40	25	med
President's Choice Blue Menu Granola Clusters, Raisin Almond, low-fat	70	2 oz	40	28	high
President's Choice Blue Menu Multi-Grain Instant Oatmeal–Regular and Cinnamon & Spice	55	1½ oz	26	14	low
President's Choice Blue Menu Omega-3 Granola Cereal	43	2 oz	32	14	low
President's Choice Blue Menu Soy Crunch Multi-Grain Cereal	47	2 oz	36	17	low
President's Choice Blue Menu Steel-Cut Oats	51	1¼ oz	29	15	low
Puffed buckwheat	65	¾ oz	15	10	med
Puffed Wheat, Quaker Oats	67	1 oz	21	14	med
Quick oats	65	6 oz	19	12	med
Quick oats porridge	80	¾ oz	15	12	high
Raisin Bran, Kellogg's	61	1 oz	23	14	med
Rice Krispies, Kellogg's	82	1.2 oz	29	24	high
Semolina, cooked	87	¾ oz	17	15	high

★ little or no carbs Ⓖ program participant

Breakfast Cereals

Food	GI Value	Nominal Serving Size	Available Carbs	GL Value	GI Level
Shredded Wheat, Post	83	1.6 oz	37	31	high
Special K, Kellogg's	69	1.1 oz	22	15	med
Total, General Mills	76	1 oz	23	17	high
Weetabix	74	1 oz	28	21	high

Cakes & Muffins

Food	GI Value	Nominal Serving Size	Available Carbs	GL Value	GI Level
9 grain muffin	43	1 oz	11	5	low
Angel food cake	67	1 oz	15	10	med
Apple, oat, raisin muffin	54	1½ oz	36	19	low
Apple berry crumble, commercially made	41	3½ oz	40	16	low
Apple muffin, homemade	46	1½ oz	17	8	low
Apricot, coconut and honey muffin	60	1½ oz	34	20	med
Banana, oat and honey muffin	65	1½ oz	17	11	med
Banana cake, homemade	51	1½ oz	17	9	low
Blueberry muffin	59	1½ oz	22	13	med
Blueberry muffin, commercially made	59	1½ oz	17	10	med
Bran muffin, commercially made	60	1½ oz	16	10	med
Carrot cake	36	1 oz	12	4	low
Carrot muffin, commercially made	62	1½ oz	17	11	med
Chocolate butterscotch muffin	53	1½ oz	31	16	low
Chocolate cake, made from packet mix with frosting, Betty Crocker	38	1 oz	14	5	low
Chocolate muffin	53	1½ oz	18	10	low
Croissant, plain	67	1 oz	13	9	med
Crumpet, white	69	1½ oz	18	12	med
Cupcake, strawberry-iced	73	1 oz	15	11	high
Double chocolate muffin	46	1½ oz	24	11	low
Doughnut, cinnamon sugar	76	1½ oz	18	14	high
Doughnut, commercially made	75	1½ oz	22	17	high
Egg custard	35	4 oz	15	5	low
Macaroons, coconut	32	1 oz	22	7	low
NutriSystem Apple Strudel Scone	43		26	11	low
NutriSystem Blueberry Bran Muffin	28	2 oz	11	3	low
NutriSystem Cranberry Orange Pastry	28	1.8 oz	19	5	low

★ little or no carbs ⓖ program participant

Cakes & Muffins

Food	GI Value	Nominal Serving Size	Available Carbs	GL Value	GI Level
Oatmeal muffin, made from mix	69	1½ oz	17	12	med
Pancakes, buckwheat, gluten-free, packet mix	102	¾ oz	15	15	high
Pancakes, homemade	66	3 oz	20	13	med
Pancakes, prepared from mix (6-inch diameter)	67	2 oz	18	12	med
Pastry, puff	59	1 oz	15	9	med
Pound cake, Sara Lee	54	1 oz	14	8	low
President's Choice Blue Menu Cranberry & Orange Soy Muffin	48	2½ oz	29	14	low
President's Choice Blue Menu Doughnut, cake type	76	1½ oz	23	17	high
President's Choice Blue Menu Raisin Bran Flax Muffin	51	2½ oz	33	17	low
President's Choice Blue Menu Raspberry & Pomegranate Whole Grain Muffin	58	2½ oz	33	19	med
President's Choice Blue Menu Raspberry Coffee Cake	50	1¾ oz	22	11	low
President's Choice Blue Menu Whole Grain Banana & Prune Muffin	39	2½ oz	39	15	low
President's Choice Blue Menu Whole Grain Carrots, Dates, Pineapples & Walnuts Muffin	53	2½ oz	34	18	low
President's Choice Blue Menu Wild Blueberry 10-Grain Muffins	57	2½ oz	39	22	med
Scones, plain, made from packet mix	92	1 oz	17	16	high
Sponge cake, plain, unfilled	46	1 oz	14	6	low
Vanilla cake, made from packet mix with vanilla frosting, Betty Crocker	42	1½ oz	19	8	low
Waffle, plain	76	1¼ oz	16	12	high
Waffle, toasted	76	1¼ oz	16	12	high

★ little or no carbs   Ⓖ program participant

Cereal Grains

Food	GI Value	Nominal Serving Size	Available Carbs	GL Value	GI Level
Barley, pearled, boiled	25	2 oz	14	4	low
Buckwheat, boiled	54	3 oz	17	9	low
Bulgur, cracked wheat	48	3 oz	15	7	low
Millet, boiled	71	2½ oz	16	11	high
Polenta (cornmeal), boiled	68	6¾ oz	16	11	med
Quinoa, boiled	53	3½ oz	15	8	low
Rye, whole kernels	34	1 oz	14	5	low
Semolina, cooked	55	6 oz	13	7	low
Whole-wheat kernels, boiled	41	4 oz	16	7	low

Cookies & Crackers

Food	GI Value	Nominal Serving Size	Available Carbs	GL Value	GI Level
Apricot fruit cookies (97% fat free)	47	1 oz	16	8	low
Arrowroot, McCormicks's	63	¾ oz	16	10	med
Arrowroot plus, McCormicks's	62	¾ oz	16	10	med
Blueberry fruit cookies (97% fat free)	47	1 oz	16	8	low
Breton wheat crackers	67	1 oz	14	9	med
Chocolate chip cookies	43	1 oz	18	8	low
Corn Thins, puffed corn cakes, gluten-free	87	1 oz	16	14	high
Digestives, plain	62	¾ oz	15	9	med
Highland Oatcakes, Walker's	57	1 oz	13	7	med
Kavli Norwegian crispbread	71	¾ oz	14	10	high
Macaroons, coconut	32	1 oz	22	7	low
Milk Arrowroot	69	¾ oz	13	9	med
Oatmeal cookies	54	¾ oz	14	8	low
Premium Soda Crackers	74	1 oz	21	16	high
President's Choice Blue Menu Ancient Grains Snack Crackers	65	¾ oz	12	8	med
President's Choice Blue Menu Cranberry Orange Cookies	60	¾ oz	15	9	med
President's Choice Blue Menu Fat-free Fruit Bar, Apple	90	1½ oz	30	27	high
President's Choice Blue Menu Fat-free Fruit Bar, Raspberry	74	1½ oz	31	23	high
President's Choice Blue Menu Fruit Bar, Fig	70	1½ oz	30	21	high
President's Choice Blue Menu Fruit & Nut Whole Grain Soft Cookie	51	1¼ oz	24	12	low

★ little or no carbs ⓖ program participant

Cookies & Crackers

Food	GI Value	Nominal Serving Size	Available Carbs	GL Value	GI Level
President's Choice Blue Menu Ginger and Lemon Cookies	64	¾ oz	15	10	med
President's Choice Blue Menu Oatmeal Double Chocolate Soft Cookie	49	1¼ oz	18	9	low
President's Choice Blue Menu Oatmeal Raisin Whole Grain Soft Cookie	56	1¼ oz	24	13	med
President's Choice Blue Menu Wheat and Onion Snack Crackers	60	¾ oz	14	8	med
President's Choice Blue Menu Wheat and Sesame Snack Crackers	56	¾ oz	14	8	med
President's Choice Blue Menu Wheat Snack Crackers	65	¾ oz	14	9	med
President's Choice Blue Menu Whole Wheat Fig Bar, 60%	72	1½ oz	29	21	high
Puffed crispbread	81	1 oz	18	15	high
Puffed Rice Cakes, white	82	¾ oz	15	12	high
Rice cracker, plain	91	½ oz	11	10	high
Rich tea biscuits	55	¾ oz	18	10	low
Rye crispbread	63	1 oz	28	18	med
Ryvita Fruit Crunch crispbread	66	½ oz	8	5	med
Ryvita Original Rye crispbread	69	¾ oz	10	7	med
ⒼRyvita Pumpkin Seeds and Oats crispbread	48	1 oz	10	5	low
Ryvita Sesame Rye crispbread	64	¾ oz	9	8	med
ⒼRyvita Sunflower Seeds and Oats crispbread	48	1 oz	9	4	low
Shortbread biscuits, plain	64	1 oz	15	10	med
Shredded Wheat cookies	62	¾ oz	15	9	med
Spicy Apple fruit cookies (97% fat free)	47	1 oz	16	8	low
Sticky Date fruit cookies (97% fat free)	47	1 oz	16	8	low
Stoned Wheat Thins	67	1 oz	19	13	med
Vanilla wafer cookies, plain	77	1 oz	16	12	high
Water cracker	63	1 oz	15	9	med
Wheat cracker, plain	70	1 oz	18	13	high
Zesty Ginger fruit cookies (97% fat free)	47	1 oz	16	8	low

★ little or no carbs.   Ⓖ program participant

Dairy Products: Cheeses

Food	GI Value	Nominal Serving Size	Available Carbs	GL Value	GI Level
Brie	★	1 oz	0	0	
Camembert	★	1 oz	0	0	
Cheddar	★	1 oz	0	0	
Cheddar, 25% reduced fat	★	1 oz	0	0	
Cheddar, 50% reduced fat	★	1 oz	0	0	
Cheddar, low fat	★	1 oz	0	0	
Cheddar, reduced salt	★	1 oz	0	0	
Cheese spread, cheddar	★	1 oz	1	0	
Cheese spread, cheddar, reduced fat	★	1 oz	2	0	
Cottage cheese	★	1 oz	1	0	
Cottage cheese, low fat	★	1 oz	1	0	
Cream cheese	★	1 oz	1	0	
Cream cheese dip	★	1 oz	3	0	
Cream cheese, reduced fat	★	1 oz	1	0	
Feta	★	1 oz	0	0	
Feta, low salt	★	1 oz	0	0	
Feta, reduced fat	★	1 oz	0	0	
Mozzarella	★	1 oz	0	0	
Mozzarella, reduced fat	★	1 oz	0	0	
Parmesan	★	1 oz	0	0	
Ricotta	★	1 oz	0	0	
Ricotta, reduced fat	★	1 oz	0	0	
Soy cheese	★	1 oz	0	0	

★ little or no carbs   Ⓖ program participant

Dairy Products: Ice Cream, Custards, Puddings & Desserts

Food	GI Value	Nominal Serving Size	Available Carbs	GL Value	GI Level
Chocolate pudding, instant, made from packet with full fat milk	47	4½ oz	20	9	low
Chocolate shake, low fat chocolate soft serve with skim milk and malted milk powder	21	10 fl oz	38	8	low
Custard, homemade from milk, wheat starch and sugar	43	2 oz	14	6	low
Custard, low fat	38	4 fl oz	18	7	low
Gelato, sucrose-free, chocolate	37	2 oz	14	5	low
Gelato, sucrose-free, vanilla	39	2 oz	14	5	low
Ice cream, light creamy low fat, chocolate	27	2½ fl oz	16	4	low
Ice cream, light creamy low fat, English toffee	27	2½ fl oz	14	4	low
Ice cream, light creamy low fat, mango	30	2½ fl oz	13	4	low
Ice cream, light creamy low fat, vanilla	36	2½ fl oz	17	6	low
Ice cream, low carbohydrate, chocolate	32	3½ fl oz	5	2	low
Ice cream, regular, full fat, average	47	2½ fl oz	15	7	low
Low fat chocolate soft serve ice cream	24	2 oz	9	2	low
Low fat chocolate soft serve eaten with a plain cone	44	4 oz	20	9	low
Low fat chocolate soft serve eaten with a waffle cone	55	4 oz	28	15	low
President's Choice Blue Menu Frozen yogurt, Mochaccino	51	4 fl oz	21	11	low
President's Choice Blue Menu Frozen yogurt, Strawberry Banana	55	4 fl oz	20	11	low
President's Choice Blue Menu Frozen yogurt, Vanilla	46	4 fl oz	21	10	low
Tapioca pudding, boiled, with milk	81	4 oz	18	15	high
Vanilla frozen yogurt	46	2½ oz	17	8	low
Vanilla pudding, instant, made from packet mix with full fat milk	40	3 oz	15	6	low
Wild Berry, non-dairy, frozen fruit dessert	59	1¾ fl oz	12	7	med

★ little or no carbs　Ⓖ program participant

Dairy Products: Milk & Alternatives

Food	GI Value	Nominal Serving Size	Available Carbs	GL Value	GI Level
Blue Diamond Unsweetened Chocolate Breeze (almond beverage)	23	8 fl oz	3	1	low
Blue Diamond Unsweetened Original Breeze (almond beverage)	23	8 fl oz	2	0	low
Blue Diamond Unsweetened Vanilla Breeze (almond beverage)	23	8 fl oz	2	0	low
Chocolate-flavored, low fat milk	27	8½ fl oz	25	7	low
Chocolate-flavored milk	37	5¼ fl oz	15	6	low
Condensed milk, sweetened, full fat	61	1 oz	14	9	med
Milk, calcium-enriched, low fat (1%)	34	8 fl oz	17	6	low
Milk, low fat (1%)	32	8 fl oz	12	4	low
Milk, reduced fat (2%)	30	8 fl oz	12	4	low
Milk, whole (3.25%)	27	8 fl oz	12	3	low
Milk, with omega-3	27	8½ fl oz	16	4	low
Mocha-flavored, low fat milk	27	8½ fl oz	17	5	low
Mocha-flavored milk	32	8½ fl oz	24	8	low
Probiotic fermented milk drink with *Lactobacillus casei*	46	2¼ fl oz	12	6	low
Strawberry-flavored milk	37	6 fl oz	15	6	low
Vitasoy Light Original, soy milk	45	8 fl oz	8	4	low
Vitasoy Organic soy milk	43	8 fl oz	16	7	low
Yakult, fermented milk drink with *Lactobacillus casei*	46	2.2 fl oz	12	6	low
Yakult Light, fermented milk drink with *Lactobacillus casei*	36	2.2 fl oz	9	3	low

★ little or no carbs   Ⓖ program participant

Dairy Products: Yogurt

Food	GI Value	Nominal Serving Size	Available Carbs	GL Value	GI Level
Yogurt, low fat, natural	35	7 oz	15	5	low
Yogurt, low fat, no added sugar, vanilla or fruit	20	7 oz	17	3	low
Yoplait Original Mixed Berry yogurt	25	3½ oz	17	4	low
Yoplait Original French Vanilla yogurt	27	3½ oz	17	5	low
Yoplait Original Mango yogurt	37	3½ oz	17	6	low
Yoplait Original Strawberry yogurt	25	3½ oz	17	4	low
Yoplait Light Apple Turnover yogurt	18	7 oz	19	3	low
Yoplait Light Apricot Mango yogurt	20	7 oz	19	4	low
Yoplait Light Banana Cream Pie yogurt	18	7 oz	20	4	low
Yoplait Light Berries 'N Cream yogurt	16	7 oz	19	3	low
Yoplait Light Red Raspberry yogurt	16	7 oz	19	3	low
Yoplait Light Strawberry yogurt	16	7 oz	19	3	low

Fruit

Food	GI Value	Nominal Serving Size	Available Carbs	GL Value	GI Level
Apple	38	4 oz	13	5	low
Apple, canned, solid pack without juice	42	4½ oz	10	4	low
Apple, dried	29	1 oz	16	5	low
Apricots	57	6 oz	13	7	med
Apricots, canned, in light syrup	64	4½ oz	16	10	med
Apricots, dried	30	1 oz	16	5	low
Apricot halves, canned in fruit juice	51	4½ oz	12	6	low
Avocado	★	2¾ oz	0	0	
Banana	52	3 oz	16	8	low
Blueberries, wild	53	3½ oz	9	5	low
Breadfruit	62	2 oz	26	16	med
Cantaloupe	65	12 oz	16	10	med
Cherimoya	54	3 oz	13	7	low
Cherries, dark	63	4½ oz	15	9	med
Cherries, dried, tart	58	1½ oz	30	17	med
Cherries, frozen, tart	54	3½ oz	6	3	low
Cherries, raw, sour	22	5 oz	22	5	low
Cherries, sour, pitted, canned	41	4 oz	21	9	low
Cranberries, dried, sweetened	64	¾ oz	17	11	med

★ little or no carbs   Ⓖ program participant

Fruit

Food	GI Value	Nominal Serving Size	Available Carbs	GL Value	GI Level
Dates, medjool, vacuum-packed	39	2 oz	18	7	low
Dates, pitted	45	1 oz	17	8	low
Figs	★	2 oz	8	0	
Figs, dried, tenderized	61	1 oz	16	10	med
Fruit and nut mix	15	1¼ oz	17	3	low
Fruit cocktail, canned	55	5 oz	16	9	low
Fruit salad, canned in fruit juice	54	4½ oz	15	8	low
Grapefruit	25	11 oz	15	4	low
Grapefruit, ruby red segments in juice	47	4½ oz	20	9	low
Grapes	53	3½ oz	15	8	low
Kiwi	53	6¾ oz	19	10	low
Kumquats	★	¾ oz	2	0	
Lemon	★	½ oz	0	0	
Lime	★	½ oz	0	0	
Loganberries	★	2½ oz	4	0	
Lychees, canned, in syrup, drained	79	3 oz	15	12	high
Lychees, fresh	57	2 oz	7	4	med
Mandarin segments in juice	47	4½ oz	12	6	low
Mango	51	3½ oz	13	7	low
Mixed fruit, dried	60	1 oz	18	11	med
Mixed nuts and raisins	21	1 oz	17	4	low
Mulberries	★	2½ oz	3	0	
Nectarine, fresh	43	4 oz	10	4	low
Orange	42	7 oz	15	6	low
Orange & grapefruit segments in juice	53	4½ oz	19	10	low
Papaya	56	5 oz	12	7	med
Peach	42	7 oz	13	5	low
Peach and pineapple in fruit juice	45	4½ oz	13	6	low
Peaches, canned, in heavy syrup	58	5 oz	14	8	med
Peaches, canned, in light syrup	57	4½ oz	17	10	med
Peaches, canned, in natural juice	45	5½ oz	15	7	low
Peaches, dried	35	1 oz	16	6	low
Peaches and grapes, canned in fruit juice	46	4½ oz	13	6	low
Pear	38	4 oz	16	6	low
Pear, canned, in fruit juice	43	4½ oz	14	6	low
Pear, canned, in natural juice	44	5 oz	15	7	low
Pear, dried	43	1 oz	16	7	low
Pear halves, canned, in reduced-sugar syrup, lite	25	3½ oz	15	4	low
Pineapple	59	6 oz	13	8	med

★ little or no carbs   Ⓖ program participant

Fruit

Food	GI Value	Nominal Serving Size	Available Carbs	GL Value	GI Level
Pineapple & papaya pieces, canned in juice	48	4½ oz	18	9	low
Pineapple pieces, canned in fruit juice	49	4½ oz	19	9	low
Plum	39	9 oz	19	7	low
Prunes, pitted, Sunsweet	40	1½ oz	22	9	low
Raisins	64	¾ oz	14	9	med
Raspberries	★	2 oz	3	0	
Rhubarb, stewed, unsweetened	★	3½ oz	1	0	
Strawberries	40	17 oz	13	5	low
Tropical fruit and nut mix	49	1 oz	17	8	low
Watermelon	76	10 oz	14	11	high

Gluten-free Products

Food	GI Value	Nominal Serving Size	Available Carbs	GL Value	GI Level
Apricot and Apple Fruit Strips	29	¾ oz	16	5	low
Apricot spread, no added sugar	29	1 oz	13	4	low
Buckwheat pancakes, gluten-free, packet mix	102	¾ oz	15	15	high
Cookie, chocolate-coated	35	1½ oz	18	6	low
Corn pasta	78	2 oz	15	12	high
Corn Thins, puffed corn cakes, gluten-free	87	¾ oz	16	14	high
Marmalade spread, no added sugar	27	1 oz	14	4	low
Muesli Breakfast Bar, gluten-free	50	¾ oz	13	7	low
Multigrain bread	79	1 oz	15	12	high
Pancakes, gluten-free, made from packet mix	61	3 oz	53	32	med
Pasta, rice and corn, dry	76	1 oz	19	14	high
Peach and Pear Fruit Strips	29	¾ oz	15	4	low
Plum and Apple Fruit Strips	29	1 oz	16	5	low
Raspberry spread, no added sugar	26	1 oz	14	4	low
Rice pasta, enriched (Gluten, Maize, Wheat, and Soya free)	51	¾ oz	18	9	low
Spaghetti, enriched (Gluten, Wheat, and Soya free)	51	¾ oz	19	10	low
Strawberry spread, no added sugar	29	1 oz	14	4	low

★ little or no carbs Ⓖ program participant

Meals, Prepared & Convenience

Food	GI Value	Nominal Serving Size	Available Carbs	GL Value	GI Level
Baked potato with baked beans	62	7 oz	26	16	low
Beef and ale casserole, prepared convenience meal	53	10½ oz	17	9	low
Burrito, made with corn tortilla, refried beans and tomato salsa	39	3½ oz	19	7	low
Cannelloni, spinach and ricotta, prepared convenience meal	15	8 oz	30	5	low
Chicken curry and rice, prepared convenience meal	45	10½ oz	20	9	low
Chicken fajitas	42	3 oz	6	3	low
Chicken nuggets, frozen, reheated in microwave 5 mins	46	4 oz	16	7	low
Chicken tandoori curry with rice, prepared meal	45	10 oz	53	24	low
Chow mein, chicken, prepared convenience meal	51	10½ oz	18	9	low
Creamy carbonara whole grain pasta & sauce meal	39	5 oz	21	8	low
Fish fingers	38	2½ oz	13	5	low
French fries, frozen, reheated in microwave	75	5 oz	19	14	high
French-style chicken with rice, prepared convenience meal	36	7 oz	32	12	low
Grape leaves, stuffed with rice and lamb, served with tomato sauce	30	4 oz	15	5	low
Hamburger, commercially prepared	66	3 oz	28	18	med
Lamb moussaka, prepared convenience meal	35	10½ oz	20	7	low
Lasagna, beef, commercially made	47	5 oz	17	8	low
Mashed potato, instant	85	4 oz	14	12	high
McDonald's Chicken McNuggets consumed with Sweet 'N Sour Sauce	55	4½ oz	26	14	low
McDonald's Fillet-O-Fish Burger	66	4½ oz	30	20	med
McDonald's Hamburger	66	3½ oz	25	17	med
McDonald's McChicken Burger	66	6½ oz	40	26	med
NutriSystem, Beef Stroganoff with Noodles	41	9 oz	21	9	low
NutriSystem, Cheese Tortellini	41	8 oz	25	10	low
NutriSystem, Chicken Cacciatore Parmesan	27	8 oz	16	4	low
NutriSystem, Chicken Pasta	41	9 oz	20	8	low
NutriSystem, Hearty Beef Stew	26	8 oz	16	4	low

★ little or no carbs Ⓖ program participant

Meals, Prepared & Convenience

Food	GI Value	Nominal Serving Size	Available Carbs	GL Value	GI Level
NutriSystem, Lasagna with Meat Sauce	26	8 oz	26	7	low
NutriSystem, Rotini with Meatballs	29	9 oz	25	7	low
Pizza, cheese	60	5 oz	52	31	med
Pizza, Super Supreme, pan, Pizza Hut	36	1¾ oz	14	2	low
Pizza, Super Supreme, Thin 'n Crispy, Pizza Hut	30	2½ oz	18	5	low
Pizza, Veggie Lovers, Thin 'n Crispy, Pizza Hut	49	1¾ oz	15	7	low
President's Choice Blue Menu 3-Rice Bayou Blend Rice & Beans Sidedish	44	2 oz	34	15	low
President's Choice Blue Menu 4-Rice Pilaf Rice & Beans Sidedish	46	2 oz	36	17	low
President's Choice Blue Menu 9-Vegetable Vegetarian Patty (frozen)	54	4 oz	25	14	low
President's Choice Blue Menu Barley Risotto with Herbed Chicken	38	10 oz	37	14	low
President's Choice Blue Menu Cauliflower Topped Shepherd's Pie	21	8 oz	13	3	low
President's Choice Blue Menu Deluxe Cheddar Macaroni & Cheese Dinner	34	2 oz	39	13	low
President's Choice Blue Menu Ginger Glazed Salmon	40	11 oz	45	18	low
President's Choice Blue Menu Lentil and Bean Vegetarian Patty	55	4 oz	27	15	low
President's Choice Blue Menu Linguine with Shrimp Marinara	40	11 oz	28	11	low
President's Choice Blue Menu Pasta Sauce, Tomato and Basil	33	4 oz	8	3	low
President's Choice Blue Menu Penne with Roasted Vegetable Entrée	39	11 oz	43	17	low
President's Choice Blue Menu Rice & Lentils Espana Sidedish	49	2 oz	36	18	low

★ little or no carbs   Ⓖ program participant

Meals, Prepared & Convenience

Food	GI Value	Nominal Serving Size	Available Carbs	GL Value	GI Level
President's Choice Blue Menu Tricolour Linguini Sun-Dried Tomato, Basil and Original Nest	42	4 oz	57	24	low
President's Choice Blue Menu Vegetarian Chili	39	8 oz	29	11	low
President's Choice Blue Menu Whole Grain Pizza Kit	59	3¼ oz	28	17	med
Sausages	28	4 oz	9	3	low
Sausages and mashed potato, prepared convenience meal	61	10 oz	27	16	med
Shepherds' pie	66	10½ oz	22	15	med
Sirloin steak with mixed vegetables and mashed potato, homemade	66	10½ oz	25	17	med
Spaghetti bolognese, homemade	52	10½ oz	65	34	low
Stir-fried vegetables with chicken and boiled white rice, homemade	73	10½ oz	62	45	high
Sushi, salmon	48	2¾ oz	19	9	low
Taco shells, cornmeal-based, baked	68	1 oz	16	11	med

Meat, Seafood, Eggs & Protein

Food	GI Value	Nominal Serving Size	Available Carbs	GL Value	GI Level
Bacon, fried	★	1 oz	1	0	
Bacon, grilled	★	1 oz	1	0	
Beef, corned silverside	★	¾ oz	0	0	
Beef, corned silverside, canned	★	1¾ oz	0	0	
Beef, roast	★	1 oz	0	0	
Beef steak, fat trimmed	★	6 oz	0	0	
Brains, cooked	★	2 oz	0	0	
Burger, fried	★	1¾ oz	3	0	
Calamari, fried	★	2 oz	0	0	
Calamari rings, squid, not battered or crumbed	★	3 oz	2	0	
Chicken breast, baked without skin	★	3 oz	0	0	
Chicken breast, grilled without skin	★	3 oz	0	0	
Chicken chopped, cooked	★	3½ oz	0	0	
Chicken drumstick, grilled without skin	★	1½ oz	0	0	
Chicken loaf	★	¾ oz	2	0	

★ little or no carbs Ⓖ program participant

Meat, Seafood, Eggs & Protein

Food	GI Value	Nominal Serving Size	Available Carbs	GL Value	GI Level
Chicken roll	★	¾ oz	1	0	
Chicken thigh fillet grilled, without skin	★	1¾ oz	0	0	
Chicken wing grilled, without skin	★	¾ oz	0	0	
Cod, fried	★	4 oz	3	0	
Crab, cooked	★	2 oz	1	0	
Duck, roasted, without skin	★	2 oz	0	0	
Egg, whole, raw	★	2 fl oz	0	0	
Egg white, raw	★	1 fl oz	0	0	
Egg yolk, raw	★	½ fl oz	0	0	
Flounder, fried	★	4 oz	3	0	
Frankfurter	★	2 oz	1	0	
Ham, canned leg	★	1½ oz	0	0	
Hamburger patty	★	2¾ oz	0	0	
Kingfish (Mackerel), fried	★	4 oz	4	0	
Lamb, ground, cooked	★	3½ oz	0	0	
Lamb, grilled chop, fat trimmed	★	1¾ oz	0	0	
Lamb, roasted loin, fat trimmed	★	2 oz	0	0	
Ling (Lingcod), fried	★	4 oz	3	0	
Liver, cooked	★	2 oz	2	0	
Liverwurst	★	1 oz	0	0	
Lobster, cooked	★	2 oz	0	0	
Mullet, fried	★	4 oz	4	0	
Mussels, cooked	★	2 oz	4	0	
Nutolene	★	3 oz	4	0	
Ocean perch, fried	★	4 oz	4	0	
Octopus, cooked	★	2 oz	1	0	
Oysters, natural, plain	★	3 oz	3	0	
Pancetta	★	¾ oz	0	0	
Pepperoni	★	¾ oz	1	0	
Pork, grilled chops, fat trimmed	★	3 oz	0	0	
Prosciutto	★	1½ oz	0	0	
Quail	★	2¾ oz	0	0	
Salami	★	¾ oz	0	0	
Salmon, pink, no added salt, drained	★	2 oz	0	0	
Salmon, red, no added salt, drained	★	2 oz	0	0	
Sardines, canned in oil, drained	★	2 oz	0	0	
Sausages, fried	★	2 oz	4	0	
Scallops, cooked	★	2 oz	0	0	
Seafood marinara, canned	★	2 oz	3	0	
Shark, fried	★	4 oz	3	0	
Shrimp	★	1 oz	0	0	

★ little or no carbs   Ⓖ program participant

Meat, Seafood, Eggs & Protein

Food	GI Value	Nominal Serving Size	Available Carbs	GL Value	GI Level
Shrimp, cooked	★	2 oz	0	0	
Snapper, fried	★	4 oz	4	0	
Sole, fried	★	4 oz	3	0	
Spam, lite	★	2 oz	2	0	
Spam, regular	★	1½ oz	1	0	
Speck	★	3½ oz	0	0	
Steak, lean	★	7 oz	0	0	
Tofu, cooked	★	4½ oz	1	0	
Tofu, plain, unsweetened	★	3½ oz	0	0	
Trout, cooked	★	4 oz	0	0	
Trout, fresh or frozen	★	5¾ oz	0	0	
Trout, fried	★	4 oz	4	0	
Tuna, cooked	★	4 oz	0	0	
Tuna in brine, drained	★	2 oz	0	0	
Tuna in oil	★	2 oz	0	0	
Turkey breast, deli-sliced	★	¾ oz	0	0	
Turkey breast, rolled roast	★	3 oz	0	0	
Turkey breast, smoked, without skin	★	3 oz	0	0	
Turkey leg, roasted without skin	★	3 oz	0	0	
Turkey, roasted breast without skin	★	2¾ oz	0	0	
Veal, roasted, fat trimmed	★	3 oz	0	0	
Vegetarian sausages	★	3 oz	3	0	

Nutritional Supplements

Food	GI Value	Nominal Serving Size	Available Carbs	GL Value	GI Level
Ensure, vanilla drink	48	8 fl oz	38	18	low
Ensure Plus, vanilla	40	8 fl oz	47	19	low
Jevity, 1 cal, unflavored	48	8 fl oz	33	16	low
Jevity, 1.2 cal, unflavored	59	8 fl oz	36	21	med
Nutrimeal meal replacement drink, Usana	20	8 fl oz	17	3	low
Promote with Fiber nutritional supplement	49	8 fl oz	30	15	low
Prosure, ready-to-drink nutritional supplement, vanilla flavor	55	8 fl oz	41	23	low
TwoCal HN, high nitrogen nutritional supplement, vanilla flavor	55	8 fl oz	51	28	low

★ little or no carbs   Ⓖ program participant

Nuts & Seeds

Food	GI Value	Nominal Serving Size	Available Carbs	GL Value	GI Level
Almonds, raw	★	½ oz	1	0	
Almonds, roasted	★	½ oz	1	0	
Blue Diamond Whole Natural Almonds	25	1 oz	6	2	low
Brazil nuts	★	½ oz	0	0	
Cashew nuts, raw	22	½ oz	2	0	low
Cashew nuts, roasted and salted	22	½ oz	3	1	low
Coconut, fresh	★	½ oz	1	0	
Coconut cream	★	4 fl oz	5	0	
Coconut milk, canned	★	4 fl oz	5	0	
Coconut milk, fresh	★	4 fl oz	4	0	
Flaxseeds	★	½ oz	2	0	
Hazelnuts	★	½ oz	1	0	
Macadamia nuts, raw	★	½ oz	1	0	
Macadamia nuts, roasted	★	½ oz	1	0	
Mixed nuts, fruit, seeds	21	½ oz	4	1	low
Mixed nuts, raw	★	½ oz	1	0	
Mixed nuts, roasted, salted	24	½ oz	4	1	low
Mixed nuts, roasted, unsalted	★	½ oz	1	0	
Nut & raisin mix	★	½ oz	5	0	
Nut & seed mix	★	½ oz	1	0	
Peanut butter	★	½ oz	2	0	
Peanut butter, no added sugar	★	½ oz	1	0	
Peanuts, raw	23	1 oz	3	1	low
Peanuts, roasted	23	½ oz	3	1	low
Pecans, raw	★	½ oz	2	0	
Pine nuts	★	½ oz	1	0	
Pistachio nuts, raw	★	½ oz	2	0	
Pistachio nuts, roasted	★	½ oz	2	0	
Poppy seeds	★	¼ oz	0	0	
Pumpkin seeds, raw	★	½ oz	2	0	
Sesame seeds	★	⅓ oz	1	0	
Sunflower seeds, raw	★	½ oz	0	0	
Sunflower seeds, roasted	★	½ oz	0	0	
Walnuts	★	½ oz	0	0	

★ little or no carbs   Ⓖ program participant

Oils & Dressings

Food	GI Value	Nominal Serving Size	Available Carbs	GL Value	GI Level
Caesar salad dressing	★	1 fl oz	0	0	
Canola oil	★	⅓ fl oz	0	0	
Cream, pure, >35% fat	★	1 fl oz	1	0	
Cream, sour, >35% fat	★	1 oz	1	0	
Cream, thickened, >35% fat	★	¾ fl oz	1	0	
Dripping, pork	★	⅓ fl oz	0	0	
French dressing	★	1 fl oz	4	0	
French dressing, fat free, artificially sweetened	★	1 fl oz	0	0	
Ghee	★	⅓ oz	0	0	
Italian dressing	★	1 fl oz	2	0	
Italian dressing, fat free, artificially sweetened	★	1 fl oz	0	0	
Lard	★	⅓ oz	0	0	
Margarine, cooking	★	⅓ oz	0	0	
Mayonnaise	★	½ fl oz	3	0	
Mayonnaise, creamy, 97% fat free	★	¾ fl oz	5	0	
Salad dressing, homemade oil & vinegar	★	1 fl oz	0	0	
Safflower oil	★	⅓ fl oz	0	0	
Sesame oil	★	⅓ fl oz	0	0	
Soybean oil	★	⅓ fl oz	0	0	
Suet	★	⅓ oz	1	0	
Sunflower oil	★	⅓ fl oz	0	0	
Tartar sauce	★	1 fl oz	2	0	
Thousand Island dressing	★	¾ fl oz	4	0	
Vinegar	★	½ fl oz	0	0	

Pasta & Noodles

Food	GI Value	Nominal Serving Size	Available Carbs	GL Value	GI Level
Beef ravioli, fresh, commercially made	43	5 oz	40	17	low
Beef & vegetable ravioli, fresh, commercially made	47	5 oz	45	21	low
Cannelloni, spinach and ricotta, prepared convenience meal	15	8 oz	30	5	low
Capellini pasta, white, boiled	45	2 oz	15	7	low

★ little or no carbs   Ⓖ program participant

Pasta & Noodles

Food	GI Value	Nominal Serving Size	Available Carbs	GL Value	GI Level
Cheese & vegetable ravioli, fresh, commercially made	51	5 oz	46	23	low
Cheese tortellini, cooked	50	1¾ oz	15	8	low
Chicken & garlic ravioli, fresh, commercially made	44	5 oz	38	17	low
Corn pasta, gluten-free, boiled	78	1¾ oz	13	10	high
Couscous, boiled 5 mins	65	5½ oz	15	10	med
Creamy carbonara whole grain pasta & sauce meal	39	5 oz	21	8	low
Creamy sun-dried tomato pasta sauce	19	6 oz	15	3	low
Fettuccine, egg, fresh	54	5 oz	36	19	low
Fusilli twists, tricolor, boiled	51	2½ oz	19	10	low
Gnocchi, cooked	68	1¾ oz	15	10	med
Ⓖ Israeli Couscous, Osem brand, boiled	52	2.2 oz	20	10	low
Italian tomato & garlic pasta sauce	40	6 oz	12	5	low
Lasagna, beef, commercially made	47	5 oz	17	8	low
Lasagna sheets, fresh	49	2½ oz	22	11	low
Linguine, thick, durum wheat, boiled	46	2 oz	15	7	low
Linguine, thin, durum wheat, boiled	52	2 oz	15	8	low
Macaroni, white, durum wheat, boiled	47	2 oz	15	7	low
Macaroni and cheese, from packet mix, Kraft	64	2½ oz	19	12	med
Meat pasta sauce	24	6 oz	13	3	low
Mung bean noodles, dried, boiled	33	1¾ oz	13	4	low
Noodles, dried rice, boiled	61	2½ oz	16	10	med
Noodles, fresh rice, boiled	40	2½ oz	17	7	low
President's Choice Blue Menu 100% Whole Wheat Lasagna pasta	46	3 oz	56	26	low
President's Choice Blue Menu 100% Whole Wheat Penne Rigate pasta	51	3¼ oz	56	29	low
President's Choice Blue Menu 100% Whole Wheat Spaghetti pasta	45	3¼ oz	56	25	low
President's Choice Blue Menu 100% Whole Wheat Spaghettini	56	3¼ oz	56	31	med

★ little or no carbs   Ⓖ program participant

Pasta & Noodles

Food	GI Value	Nominal Serving Size	Available Carbs	GL Value	GI Level
President's Choice Blue Menu Fettuccini	55	4 oz	56	31	low
President's Choice Blue Menu Whole Grain Lasagna Sheets	52	2¼ oz	34	18	low
President's Choice Blue Menu Whole Wheat Rotini	57	3 oz	56	32	med
Ravioli, meat-filled, durum wheat flour, boiled	39	2 oz	13	5	low
Rice and corn pasta, gluten-free	76	2½ oz	16	12	high
Rice pasta, brown, boiled	92	5 oz	41	38	high
Rice vermicelli noodles, dried, boiled, Chinese	58	2 oz	16	9	med
Ricotta & spinach agnolotti, fresh, commercially made	47	5 oz	41	19	low
Soba noodles/buckwheat noodles	59	4 oz	24	14	med
Soba noodles, instant, served in soup	46	1¾ oz	14	6	low
Spaghetti, gluten-free, canned in tomato sauce	68	4 oz	14	10	med
Spaghetti, protein-enriched, boiled	27	1¾ oz	15	4	low
Spaghetti, white, durum wheat, boiled 10–15 mins	44	2 oz	15	7	low
Spaghetti, whole wheat, boiled	42	2 oz	15	6	low
Spaghetti with meat sauce, homemade	52	5 oz	23	12	low
Spicy tomato & bacon pasta sauce	24	6 oz	13	3	low
Spirali, white, durum wheat, boiled	43	2 oz	15	6	low
Toasted pasta, Osem brand, boiled	52	2.2 oz	20	10	low
Udon noodles, plain, boiled	62	2 oz	13	8	med
Veal tortellini, fresh, commercially made	48	5 oz	37	18	low
Vermicelli pasta, white, durum wheat, boiled	35	2 oz	15	5	low
Whole grain ricotta & spinach ravioli, fresh, commercially made	39	5 oz	37	14	low

★ little or no carbs   Ⓖ program participant

Rice

Food	GI Value	Nominal Serving Size	Available Carbs	GL Value	GI Level
Arborio risotto rice, white, boiled, SunRice	69	6.5 oz	53	37	med
Basmati rice, white, boiled	58	5.5 oz	45	26	med
Broken rice, Thai, white, cooked in rice cooker	86	6.5 oz	52	45	high
Brown Pelde rice, boiled	76	6.75 oz	46	35	high
Calrose rice, brown, medium-grain, boiled	87	6.75 oz	46	40	high
Calrose rice, white, medium-grain, boiled	83	6.5 oz	53	44	high
Doongara Clever rice, SunRice	54	5.5 oz	45	24	low
Doongara rice, brown, SunRice	66	6.75 oz	46	30	med
Glutinous rice, white, cooked in rice cooker	98	6 oz	37	36	high
Instant rice, white, cooked 6 mins with water	87	6 oz	43	37	high
Jasmine fragrant rice, SunRice	89	6 oz	48	43	high
Jasmine rice, white, long-grain, cooked in rice cooker	109	6 oz	48	52	high
Long-grain rice, white, Mahatma, boiled 15 mins	50	5.5 oz	45	23	low
Moolgiri rice	54	5.5 oz	45	24	low
Pelde parboiled rice, Sungold	87	6 oz	48	42	high
Sunbrown Quick rice, Ricegrowers, boiled	80	6.5 oz	57	46	high
SunRice Japanese-Style Sushi Rice, white	85	6 oz	47	40	high
SunRice Koshihikari rice, Ricegrowers	73	6 oz	48	35	high
SunRice Long Grain White Rice in 90 seconds, microwaved	76	4½ oz	49	37	high
SunRice Medium Grain brown rice	59	6.75 oz	46	27	med
SunRice Medium Grain Brown Rice in 90 seconds, microwaved	59	4½ oz	43	25	med
SunRice Medium Grain white rice, boiled	75	6 oz	49	37	high
SunRice Premium White Long Grain rice	59	5.5 oz	45	27	med
Uncle Ben's Converted, white, long grain, boiled 20–30 mins	50	5.5 oz	44	22	low
Uncle Ben's Original Converted, white	45	5.5 oz	44	20	low

★ little or no carbs　Ⓖ program participant

Rice

Food	GI Value	Nominal Serving Size	Available Carbs	GL Value	GI Level
Uncle Ben's Ready Rice Long Grain & Wild (pouch)	52	5 oz	41	21	**low**
Uncle Ben's Ready Rice Original Long Grain (pouch)	48	5 oz	39	19	**low**
Uncle Ben's Ready Rice Roasted Chicken Flavored (pouch)	51	5 oz	39	20	**low**
Uncle Ben's Ready Rice Whole Grain Brown Rice (pouch)	48	5 oz	37	18	**low**
Uncle Ben's Ready Rice Whole Grain Chicken Flavored Brown Rice (pouch)	46	5¼ oz	38	17	**low**
Uncle Ben's Santa Fe, Ready Whole Grain Medley (pouch)	48	5.5 oz	37	18	**low**
Uncle Ben's Spanish Style, Ready Rice (pouch)	51	5 oz	38	19	**low**
Uncle Ben's Vegetable Harvest, Ready Whole Grain Medley (pouch)	48	5 oz	39	19	**low**
Wild rice, boiled	57	5.5 oz	35	20	**med**

★ little or no carbs   Ⓖ program participant

Snack Foods

Food	GI Value	Nominal Serving Size	Available Carbs	GL Value	GI Level
Apricot-filled fruit bar, wholemeal pastry	50	1 oz	12	6	low
Cadbury's milk chocolate, plain	49	1 oz	16	8	low
Cashew nuts, salted	22	1¾ oz	13	3	low
Chickpea chips	44	2 oz	25	11	low
Chocolate #9 (gourmet chocolate sauce, sweetened with agave)	46	1 oz	15	7	low
Chocolate, dark, Dove	23	1 oz	23	5	low
Chocolate, dark, plain, regular	41	1 oz	15	6	low
Chocolate, milk, plain, Nestlé	42	1 oz	17	7	low
Chocolate, milk, plain, reduced sugar	35	1 oz	17	6	low
Chocolate, milk, plain, regular	41	1 oz	17	7	low
Chocolate, milk, plain, with fructose instead of regular sugar	20	1 oz	17	3	low
Chocolate brownies	42	2 oz	36	15	low
Chocolate candy, sugar free, Dove	23	1.2 oz	14	3	low
Chocolate Raspberry Zing bar, Revival Soy	47	1 bar	10	5	low
Cinch Chocolate weight management bar, Shaklee Corporation	29	1 oz	15	4	low
Cinch Lemon Cranberry weight management bar, Shaklee Corporation	23	1 oz	15	3	low
Cinch Peanut Butter weight management bar, Shaklee Corporation	22	1 oz	15	3	low
Clif bar, Chocolate Brownie Energy bar	57	2¼ oz	45	26	med
Clif Bar, Cookies 'n Cream	101	2¼ oz	42	42	high
Combos Snacks Cheddar Cheese Crackers	54	1¾ oz	30	16	low
Combos Snacks Cheddar Cheese Pretzels	52	1¾ oz	33	17	low
Corn chips	74	1 oz	17	13	high
Corn chips, plain, salted	42	1 oz	17	7	low
Dove milk chocolate	45	1 oz	17	8	low
ExtendBar Apple Cinnamon Delight Bar	33	1.35 oz	21	7	low
ExtendBar Chocolate Delight Bar	41	1.35 oz	21	9	low
ExtendBar Peanut Delight Bar	32	1.35 oz	21	7	low
Fruit and nut mix	32	2 oz	25	8	low

★ little or no carbs   Ⓖ program participant

Snack Foods

Food	GI Value	Nominal Serving Size	Available Carbs	GL Value	GI Level
Gummi confectionary, based on glucose syrup	94	¾ oz	15	14	high
Ironman PR bar, chocolate	39	1½ oz	19	7	low
Jell-O, Raspberry flavor	53	4 oz	18	10	low
Jelly beans	78	¾ oz	15	12	high
Kudos Milk Chocolate Granola Bars, Peanut Butter Flavor	45	1 oz	17	8	low
Kudos Milk Chocolate Granola Bars, with M&M's	52	¾ oz	16	8	low
Licorice, soft	78	1 oz	14	11	high
Life Savers, peppermint	70	½ oz	16	11	high
Luna Cookie Dough Bar	18	1½ oz	21	4	low
Luna Protein Chocolate Peanut Butter Bar	28	1½ oz	19	5	low
Mars Bar, regular	62	1 oz	18	11	med
Marshmallows, plain, pink and white	62	½ oz	15	9	med
Milky Bar, white, Nestlé	44	1 oz	17	7	low
Milky Way Bar	62	2 oz	40	25	med
M&M's, peanut	33	1 oz	17	6	low
Muesli bar, chewy, with choc chips or fruit	54	1 oz	15	8	low
Muesli bar, crunchy, with dried fruit	61	¾ oz	14	9	med
Munch Peanut Butter bar, M&M/Mars	27	1.35 oz	22	6	low
NutriSystem, Apple Cinnamon Soy Chips	36	1 oz	10	4	low
NutriSystem Apple Granola bar	52	1.4 oz	28	15	low
NutriSystem, Blueberry Dessert Bar	36	1½ oz	21	8	low
NutriSystem, Chocolate Crunch Bar	41	1 oz	15	6	low
NutriSystem, Chocolate	48	1½ oz	18	9	low
NutriSystem Cinnamon Swirl Granola bar	47	1.4 oz	27	13	low
NutriSystem Cranberry Granola bar	50	1.4 oz	27	14	low
NutriSystem Fudge Brownie	41	1.2 oz	22	9	low
NutriSystem Honey Mustard Pretzels	32	1 oz	7	2	low
NutriSystem Peanut Butter Granola bar	32	1.4 oz	18	6	low
Nuts, mixed, roasted and salted	24	½ oz	4	1	low

★ little or no carbs   ⓖ program participant

Snack Foods

Food	GI Value	Nominal Serving Size	Available Carbs	GL Value	GI Level
Peanut Butter Chocolate Buddy bar, Revival Soy	52	1 bar	30	16	low
Peanuts, roasted, salted	14	5½ oz	14	2	low
Pecan nuts, raw	★	½ oz	2	0	
Performance Chocolate energy bar, Power Bar	53	2.2 oz	44	23	low
Pirate's Booty, Aged White Cheddar snack	70	1 oz	19	13	high
Pop-Tarts, double chocolate	70	1 oz	19	13	high
Popcorn, plain, cooked in microwave	72	1 oz	14	10	high
Potato chips, plain, salted	51	1¾ oz	27	14	low
PowerBar, Chocolate	53	2 oz	40	21	low
President's Choice Blue Menu 60% Whole Wheat Fig Fruit bar	72	1.35 oz	31	22	high
President's Choice Blue Menu Apple Fruit Bar, Fat-Free	90	1.35 oz	30	27	high
President's Choice Blue Menu Chewy Chocolate Chip & Marshmallow Granola Bar	78	0.9 oz	21	16	high
President's Choice Blue Menu Chewy Cranberry Apple Granola Bar	58	0.9 oz	21	12	med
President's Choice Blue Menu Fig Fruit Bar	70	1.35 oz	31	22	high
President's Choice Blue Menu Flaxseed Tortilla Chips, Sea Salt	64	1¾ oz	20	13	med
President's Choice Blue Menu Flaxseed Tortilla Chips, Spicy	64	1¾ oz	20	13	med
President's Choice Blue Menu Fruit & Nut Bar, Apple & Almonds	65	1 oz	20	13	med
President's Choice Blue Menu Fruit & Nut Mixed Berries & Almonds Chewy Multi-Grain Bars	63	1¼ oz	26	16	med
President's Choice Blue Menu Fruit & Yogurt Apple Cinnamon Chewy Bars (Soy)	34	1½ oz	21	7	low
President's Choice Blue Menu Fruit & Yogurt Cranberry Blueberry Bars (Soy)	33	1½ oz	21	7	low

★ little or no carbs   Ⓖ program participant

Snack Foods

Food	GI Value	Nominal Serving Size	Available Carbs	GL Value	GI Level
President's Choice Blue Menu Japanese Wasabi & Honey Rice & Corn Crisps	82	1¾ oz	40	33	high
President's Choice Blue Menu Microwave Popping Corn, butter flavor	72	1½ oz	31	22	high
President's Choice Blue Menu Microwave Popping Corn, natural flavor	58	1½ oz	31	18	med
President's Choice Blue Menu Original & Tomato Basil Vegetable Sticks	65	1¾ oz	38	25	med
President's Choice Blue Menu Raspberry Fruit bar, fat-free	74	1.35 oz	32	24	high
President's Choice Blue Menu Rice & Corn Chips, Japanese Tamari	91	1¾ oz	38	35	high
President's Choice Blue Menu Rice & Corn Chips, Thai Curry	84	1¾ oz	39	33	high
Pretzels, oven-baked, traditional wheat flavor	83	¾ oz	13	11	high
Rice Krispie Treat bar, Kellogg's	63	¾ oz	17	11	med
Roll-Ups, processed fruit snack	99	¾ oz	14	14	high
Skittles	70	¾ oz	18	13	high
SlimFast Meal Options bar, rich chocolate brownie flavor	64	2 oz	34	22	med
SmartZone Crunchy Chocolate Brownie Flavor Nutrition Bar	23	1.7 oz	18	4	low
SmartZone Crunchy Chocolate Caramel Flavor Nutrition Bar	16	1.7 oz	21	3	low
SmartZone Crunchy Chocolate Peanut Butter Flavor Nutrition Bar	14	1.7 oz	18	3	low
Snickers Bar	43	2 oz	34	15	low
Snickers Marathon Nutrition Bar, Dark Chocolate Crunch flavor	49	1.4 oz	15	7	low
Snickers Marathon Nutrition Bar, Honey & Toasted Almond flavor	41	1.4 oz	15	6	low
Snickers Marathon Protein Performance Bar, Caramel Nut Rush Flavor	26	2¾ oz	30	8	low

★ little or no carbs Ⓖ program participant

Snack Foods

Food	GI Value	Nominal Serving Size	Available Carbs	GL Value	GI Level
Snickers Marathon Protein Performance Bar, Chocolate Nut Burst Flavor	32	2¾ oz	26	8	low
SoLo GI Nutrition Bar, Berry Bliss	28	1¾ oz	22	6	low
SoLo GI Nutrition Bar, Chocolate Charger	28	1¾ oz	22	6	low
SoLo GI Nutrition Bar, Lemon Lift	28	1¾ oz	22	6	low
SoLo GI Nutrition Bar, Mint Mania	23	1¾ oz	22	5	low
SoLo GI Nutrition Bar, Peanut Power	27	1¾ oz	20	5	low
SoLo GI Snack Bar, Berry Bliss	28	1 oz	11	3	low
SoLo GI Snack Bar, Chocolate Charger	28	1 oz	10	3	low
SoLo GI Snack Bar, Lemon Lift	28	1 oz	11	3	low
SoLo GI Snack Bar, Mint Mania	23	1 oz	10	2	low
SoLo GI Snack Bar, Peanut Power	27	1 oz	10	3	low
Stretch Island Fruit Co Summer Strawberry fruit leather	29	½ oz	11	3	low
Twisties, cheese-flavored snack	74	1 oz	15	11	high
Twix bar	44	½ oz	12	5	low
VO2 Max Chocolate Energy Bar, M&M/Mars	49	2.2 oz	45	22	low
ZonePerfect nutrition bar, double chocolate flavor	44	1.7 oz	20	9	low

★ little or no carbs   Ⓖ program participant

Soups

Food	GI Value	Nominal Serving Size	Available Carbs	GL Value	GI Level
Black bean, canned	64	8 oz	18	12	med
Campbell's Minestrone, condensed, prepared with water	48	8 oz	28	13	low
Chicken and mushroom soup	58	8 oz	18	10	med
Clear consommé, chicken or vegetable	★	8 fl oz	2	0	
Green pea, canned	66	9 oz	19	13	med
Lentil, canned	44	9 oz	13	6	low
Minestrone, traditional	39	9 oz	13	5	low
President's Choice Blue Menu Barley Vegetable Low Fat Instant Soup	41	9 oz	28	11	low
President's Choice Blue Menu Chicken & Rotini Soup	38	9 oz	11	4	low
President's Choice Blue Menu Indian Lentil Low Fat Instant Soup	55	9 oz	20	11	low
President's Choice Blue Menu Lentil Soup	56	9 oz	19	11	med
President's Choice Blue Menu Minestrone & Pasta Instant soup, low-fat	54	9 oz	46	25	low
President's Choice Blue Menu Mushroom Barley, Ready-to-Serve	45	9 oz	9	4	low
President's Choice Blue Menu Pasta e Fagioli Soup, Ready-to-Serve	52	9 oz	22	11	low
President's Choice Blue Menu Soupreme, Carrot Soup	35	9 oz	13	5	low
President's Choice Blue Menu Soupreme, Tomato and Herb Soup	47	9 oz	14	7	low
President's Choice Blue Menu Soupreme, Winter Squash Soup	41	9 oz	10	4	low
President's Choice Blue Menu Spicy Black Bean Low Fat Instant Soup	57	9 oz	32	18	med
President's Choice Blue Menu Spicy Black Bean with Vegetables Soup	46	9 oz	34	16	low

★ little or no carbs   Ⓖ program participant

Soups

Food	GI Value	Nominal Serving Size	Available Carbs	GL Value	GI Level
President's Choice Blue Menu Spicy Thai Instant Noodles with Vegetables Low Fat Instant Soup	56	9 oz	31	17	med
President's Choice Blue Menu Vegetable CousCous Low Fat Instant Soup Cup	57	9 oz	33	19	med
President's Choice Blue Menu Vegetarian Chili, Ready-to-Serve	39	9 oz	29	11	low
President's Choice Blue Menu Vegetarian Chili Low Fat Instant Cup	36	9 oz	29	10	low
Pumpkin, Creamy, Heinz	76	7 oz	16	12	high
Split pea, canned	60	8 oz	27	16	med
Tomato, canned	45	9 oz	14	6	low
Tomato soup, condensed, prepared with water, Campbell's	52	8 oz	40	21	low
Vegetable soup	60	8 oz	18	11	med

★ little or no carbs Ⓖ program participant

Soy Products

Food	GI Value	Nominal Serving Size	Available Carbs	GL Value	GI Level
Flaxseed and soy bread	55	3 oz	26	14	low
NutriSystem, Apple Cinnamon Soy Chips	36	1 oz	10	4	low
NutriSystem, Sour Cream and Onion Soy Chips	41	1 oz	10	4	low
President's Choice Blue Menu Soy Beverage, Chocolate flavored	40	8 fl oz	28	11	low
President's Choice Blue Menu Soy Beverage, Original flavored	15	8 fl oz	9	1	low
President's Choice Blue Menu Soy Beverage, Vanilla flavored	28	8 fl oz	16	4	low
Soy beans, canned, drained	14	6 oz	5	1	low
Soy beans, dried, boiled	18	6 oz	2	0	low
Soy yogurt, Peach and Mango, 2% fat, with sugar	50	3½ oz	8	4	low
Vitasoy Light Original, soy milk	45	12 fl oz	15	7	low
Vitasoy Organic soy milk	43	8 fl oz	16	7	low

Spreads & Sweeteners

Food	GI Value	Nominal Serving Size	Available Carbs	GL Value	GI Level
Anchovy fish paste	★	¾ oz	1	0	
Apricot 100% Pure Fruit spread, no added sugar	43	½ oz	9	4	low
Apricot fruit spread, reduced sugar	55	½ oz	6	3	low
Butter	★	⅓ oz	0	0	
Cashew spread	★	⅓ oz	3	0	
Cottee's 100% Fruit Jam Apricot	50	1 oz	15	8	low
Cottee's 100% Fruit Jam Blackberry	46	1 oz	15	7	low
Cottee's 100% Fruit Jam Breakfast Marmalade	55	1 oz	17	9	low
Cottee's 100% Fruit Jam Raspberry	46	1 oz	15	7	low
Cottee's 100% Fruit Jam Strawberry	46	1 oz	15	7	low
Dairy blend, with canola oil	★	⅓ oz	0	0	
Extra virgin olive oil spread	★	¼ oz	0	0	
Fructose, pure	19	½ oz	15	3	low

★ little or no carbs   Ⓖ program participant

Spreads & Sweeteners

Food	GI Value	Nominal Serving Size	Available Carbs	GL Value	GI Level
Ginger Marmalade, original	50	¾ oz	14	7	low
Glucose Syrup	100	¾ oz	16	16	high
Glucose tablets or powder	100	½ oz	15	15	high
Golden syrup	63	¾ oz	15	9	med
Honey, Capilano, blended	64	¾ oz	18	12	med
Honey, general	52	¾ oz	18	9	low
Honey, Ironbark	48	¾ oz	18	9	low
Honey, Red Gum	53	¾ oz	18	10	low
Honey, Salvation Jane	64	¾ oz	18	12	med
Honey, Stringybark	44	¾ oz	18	8	low
Honey, Yapunya	52	¾ oz	18	9	low
Honey, Yellow-box	35	¾ oz	18	6	low
Hummus (chickpea dip)	22	1 oz	6	1	low
Jam, sweetened with aspartame	★	⅓ oz	0	0	
Jam, sweetened with sucralose	★	⅓ oz	0	0	
Jelly, grape	52	½ oz	10	5	low
Lemon butter, homemade	★	⅓ oz	3	0	
Maple syrup, pure, Canadian	54	¾ oz	13	7	low
Margarine, canola	★	⅓ oz	0	0	
Marmalade, orange	48	½ oz	13	6	low
Marmalade, sweetened with aspartame	★	⅓ oz	0	0	
Marmalade, sweetened with sucralose	★	⅓ oz	0	0	
Nutella, hazelnut spread	33	1 oz	17	6	low
Ⓖ Premium Agave Nectar, Sweet Cactus Farms	19	¾ oz	16	3	low
President's Choice Blue Menu Twice the Fruit Apricot spread	49	½ oz	6	3	low
President's Choice Blue Menu Twice the Fruit Spread– Strawberry & Rhubarb	69	½ oz	6	4	med
Raspberry 100% Pure Fruit spread, no added sugar	26	½ oz	9	2	low
Strawberry jam, regular	51	¾ oz	13	7	low
Sugar, brown	61	½ oz	17	10	med
Sugar, white	65	½ oz	17	11	med
Tahini	★	¾ oz	0	0	

★ little or no carbs   Ⓖ program participant

Vegetables

Food	GI Value	Nominal Serving Size	Available Carbs	GL Value	GI Level
Alfalfa sprouts	★	½ oz	0	0	
Artichoke, globe	★	4 oz	2	0	
Artichoke hearts, whole, canned	★	1½ oz	1	0	
Artichokes in brine	★	1½ oz	2	0	
Artichoke hearts in brine, drained	★	3 oz	1	0	
Arugula	★	¾ oz	1	0	
Asparagus	★	3 oz	1	0	
Asparagus, canned, drained	★	3 oz	1	0	
Asparagus green/white spears, canned	★	2 oz	1	0	
Asparagus in springwater	★	2 oz	1	0	
Baby corn, cut, canned	★	1¾ oz	2	0	
Baby corn spears, whole, canned	★	1¾ oz	2	0	
Bamboo shoots, canned	★	1 oz	0	0	
Bean sprouts, cooked	★	2 oz	1	0	
Bean sprouts, raw	★	1 oz	0	0	
Beans, green	★	1¾ oz	1	0	
Beans, Chinese long	★	2½ oz	1	0	
Beets, canned	64	6 oz	16	10	med
Bok choy	★	3 oz	1	0	
Broccoflower	★	1½ oz	1	0	
Broccoli	★	3½ oz	1	0	
Brussels sprouts	★	2¾ oz	2	0	
Cabbage, Chinese	★	3 oz	1	0	
Cabbage, green, cooked	★	3 oz	2	0	
Cabbage, green, raw	★	3 oz	2	0	
Cabbage, red, cooked	★	3 oz	3	0	
Cabbage, red, raw	★	3 oz	3	0	
Carrots, peeled, boiled	39	3 oz	6	2	low
Cauliflower	★	3 oz	2	0	
Celery, cooked	★	2½ oz	2	0	
Celery, raw	★	1 oz	1	0	
Chili, banana, cooked	★	1¾ oz	1	0	
Chili, banana, raw	★	2 oz	1	0	
Chili, hot thin, cooked	★	¾ oz	1	0	
Chili, hot thin, raw	★	1 oz	1	0	
Chives	★	¼ oz	0	0	
Chayote	★	1½ oz	2	0	
Cucumber	★	1 oz	0	0	
Cucumber, Persian	★	1 oz	1	0	
Eggplant, cooked	★	1¾ oz	1	0	
Eggplant, raw	★	1½ oz	1	0	

★ little or no carbs   Ⓖ program participant

Vegetables

Food	GI Value	Nominal Serving Size	Available Carbs	GL Value	GI Level
Endive	★	3 oz	0	0	
Fennel, cooked	★	2½ oz	3	0	
Fennel, raw	★	1¾ oz	2	0	
Garlic	★	¼ oz	0	0	
Ginger	★	⅒ oz	0	0	
Green beans, sliced, canned	★	3 oz	5	0	
Green plantain, peeled, boiled, 10 mins	39	4 oz	37	14	low
Green plantain, peeled, fried in vegetable oil	40	4 oz	37	15	low
Hash browns	75	2 oz	15	11	high
Herbs, fresh or dried	★	⅒ oz	0	0	
Horseradish	★	¼ oz	1	0	
Kohlrabi	★	3 oz	4	0	
Leeks, cooked	★	3 oz	3	0	
Leeks, raw	★	3 oz	3	0	
Lettuce, Boston, Bibb	★	¾ oz	0	0	
Lettuce, cos	★	¾ oz	0	0	
Lettuce, iceberg	★	¾ oz	0	0	
Mashed potato, made with milk	85	4 oz	15	13	high
Mashed potato, made with milk and margarine	71	4.2 oz	20	14	high
Mixed vegetables, Chinese, canned	★	3 oz	5	0	
Mushrooms	★	1¼ oz	1	0	
Mushrooms, canned	★	1 oz	1	0	
Mushrooms, shiitake, canned	★	1 oz	1	0	
Okra	★	3 oz	1	0	
Onion	★	1 oz	2	0	
Onions, canned, sautéed and diced	★	1¾ oz	3	0	
Onions, sautèed and diced	★	½ oz	1	0	
Parsley, cooked	★	1½ oz	0	0	
Parsley, raw	★	¼ oz	0	0	
Parsnips, boiled	52	2¾ oz	8	4	low
Peas, green	45	7 oz	15	7	low
Pepper, green, canned	★	1½ oz	1	0	
Pepper, green, raw	★	1½ oz	1	0	
Pepper, red, canned	★	1½ oz	2	0	
Pepper, red, cooked	★	1½ oz	2	0	
Potato, baked, without skin	85	3½ oz	14	12	high
Potato, wedge, with skin	75	1¼ oz	17	13	high
Potato salad, canned	63	4 oz	16	10	med
Potato chips, deep fried	75	1½ oz	14	11	high

★ little or no carbs   Ⓖ program participant

Vegetables

Food	GI Value	Nominal Serving Size	Available Carbs	GL Value	GI Level
Potatoes, baked, Russet Burbank potatoes, baked, without fat	76	5.75 oz	41	31	high
Potatoes, boiled	59	5.75 oz	36	21	med
Potatoes, Désirée, red-skinned type, peeled, boiled 35 mins	101	4 oz	16	16	high
Potatoes, instant, mashed, Idahoan	88	4 oz	16	14	high
Potatoes, new, canned, microwaved 3 mins	65	5 oz	16	10	med
Potatoes, new, unpeeled, boiled 20 mins	78	5 oz	16	12	high
Potatoes, Ontario, white, baked in skin	60	5.75 oz	41	25	med
Potatoes, Pontiac, peeled, boiled 15 mins, mashed	91	4 oz	14	13	high
Potatoes, Pontiac, peeled, boiled whole 30–35 mins	72	4 oz	16	12	high
Potatoes, Pontiac, peeled, microwaved 7 mins	79	4 oz	16	13	high
Potatoes, red, boiled with skin on in salted water 12 mins	89	5.75 oz	37	33	high
Potatoes, red, cubed, boiled in salted water 12 mins, stored overnight in refrigerator, consumed cold	56	5.75 oz	37	21	med
Potatoes, Sebago, white, peeled, boiled 35 mins	87	4 oz	16	14	high
Pumpkin, boiled	66	7½ oz	15	10	med
Radishes, red	★	2 oz	1	0	
Rutabaga	72	5.75 oz	18	13	high
Sauerkraut, canned	★	2½ oz	1	0	
Seaweed	★	1½ oz	0	0	
Shallots, cooked	★	1 oz	1	0	
Shallots, raw	★	½ oz	1	0	
Snowpeas, cooked	★	2¾ oz	4	0	
Snowpeas, raw	★	1 oz	2	0	
Spinach, cooked	★	3 oz	1	0	
Spinach, raw	★	1 oz	0	0	
Spring onions	★	½ oz	1	0	
Squash	★	2½ oz	2	0	
Squash, butternut, boiled	51	2¾ oz	6	3	low
Sweet corn, Honey 'n Pearl variety, boiled	37	2¾ oz	15	6	low

★ little or no carbs   ⓖ program participant

Vegetables

Food	GI Value	Nominal Serving Size	Available Carbs	GL Value	GI Level
Sweet corn, on the cob, boiled	48	2¾ oz	15	7	low
Sweet corn, whole kernel, canned, drained	46	3 oz	16	7	low
Sweet potato, baked	46	3 oz	16	7	low
Sweet potato, peeled, cubed, boiled in salted water 15 mins	59	5 oz	31	18	med
Swiss chard	★	4 oz	2	0	
Taro, boiled	54	1½ oz	15	8	low
Tomato, onion, pepper, celery	★	3 oz	3	0	
Tomato puree	★	2 oz	3	0	
Tomatoes	★	1¾ oz	1	0	
Tomatoes, in tomato juice	★	3 oz	3	0	
Tomatoes, Italian diced	★	4½ oz	5	0	
Tomatoes, Italian whole peeled Roma	★	4½ oz	5	0	
Tomatoes, whole peeled, no added salt	★	4½ oz	4	0	
Turnips	★	1¾ oz	2	0	
Water chestnuts, drained	★	¾ oz	2	0	
Watercress	★	¼ oz	0	0	
Yam, peeled, boiled	54	2½ oz	16	9	low
Zucchini, cooked	★	3 oz	2	0	
Zucchini, raw	★	2 oz	1	0	

★ little or no carbs   Ⓖ program participant

Glossary
An A to Z of Key Terms Used Throughout This Book

A1c See **HbA1c**.

Alternative sweeteners include nutritive sweeteners (which add calories to the diet) and nonnutritive sweeteners, which are calorie-free. *Nutritive sweeteners,* including sugars, sugar-alcohols, and oligosaccharides (medium-sized chains of glucose), are simply different types of carbohydrate with varying levels of sweetness. The sugar alcohols sorbitol, mannitol, and maltitol are generally not as sweet as table sugar, provide fewer calories, and have less of an impact on blood glucose levels. *Nonnutritive sweeteners* (such as Equal, Splenda, Stevia, NutraSweet, or saccharin, for example) are all much sweeter than table sugar and have essentially no effect on your blood glucose levels because most are used in such small quantities and are not absorbed into or metabolized by the body. Because they are used in only minute amounts, the number of calories they provide is insignificant. Nonnutritive sweeteners made of protein molecules often break down when heated for long periods and lose their sweetness.

Area under the curve refers, in the context of the GI testing of food, to the mathematical space under blood glucose response to any food. It is calculated using a computer program.

Atherosclerosis, or hardening of the arteries, is a slow, progressive disease that produces problems such as angina, heart attack, or stroke.

347

Most heart disease is caused by atherosclerosis clogging on the inside wall of the coronary arteries through the slow build-up of fatty deposits (called plaque) that narrow the arteries and reduce the blood flow. If the plaque ruptures, clots form, causing a more acute, total blockage. If the blood vessel is providing blood to the heart, the result is a heart attack. Atherosclerosis can affect the arteries to the heart and in the brain, kidneys, and the arms and legs.

Autoimmune disease is a disorder in which the body's immune system mistakenly attacks and destroys body tissue or organs that it believes to be foreign; type 1 diabetes (see below) is an autoimmune condition.

Beta cells produce the hormone insulin. They are found grouped together in "islands" (the Islets of Langerhans) in the pancreas.

Blood glucose (blood sugar or **glucose**) is the most common kind of sugar found in the blood and is a major source of energy for most of the body's organs and tissues and the only source of fuel for the brain. When the body's digestive organs process carbohydrates, they end up mostly as glucose, which passes through the walls of the intestine into the bloodstream to the liver and eventually into general circulation. From here, glucose enters individual cells or tissues throughout the body to be used for fuel and energy.

Blood glucose level (BGL) is the amount of glucose in the bloodstream. If you haven't eaten in the past few hours (and you don't have diabetes), your blood glucose level will normally fall within the range of 70–130 mg/dL (4–6 mmol/L). If you eat, this will rise, but rarely above 180 mg/dL (10 mmol/L), unless you have diabetes. The extent of the increase will vary depending on your glucose tolerance (your own physiological response) and the type of food you have just eaten.

Blood pressure is the pressure of the blood on the inside walls of your blood vessels caused by the beating of the heart. It is expressed as a ratio such as "120/80." The first number is the *systolic* pressure, or the pressure when the heart pushes the blood out into the arteries. The second number is the *diastolic* pressure, or the pressure when the heart rests between beats. High blood pressure (or hypertension), above 140/90, is the most common cardiovascular risk factor. High blood pressure is more prevalent in people with diabetes and increases the risk of stroke, heart attack, and diseases of the kidney and eye. Your blood pressure should be measured when you visit your doctor for checkups or at least twice a year, with a goal of 130/80 mm Hg or lower.

Blood sugar. See **blood glucose**.

BMI (Body Mass Index) is a measure that evaluates body weight relative to height to find out if an individual is underweight, in the healthy weight range, overweight, or obese. It has limitations: it can overestimate body fat in athletes and others who have a muscular build, such as body builders, and in pregnant women, and it can underestimate body fat in older people or people with a disability who have lost muscle mass. It's not appropriate for children and young people under eighteen. For an easy online calculator, go to www.nhlbisupport.com/bmi/

BMI categories:

Less than 18.5	Underweight
18.5–24.9	Healthy weight range
25–29.9	Overweight
Over 30	Obese

For Maori and Pacific Island people: BMI is 20–26 for the healthy weight range, 27–31 for overweight, and over 32 for obese.

Calorie (or kilocalorie, to be technically correct) is the old unit that measures the energy you get from the food you eat (your energy intake). The term is used in the United States, while the rest of the world uses kilojoules (although calories is still used and understood), the metric equivalent. You can convert calories to kilojoules by multiplying by 4.2; you can convert kilojoules to calories by dividing by 4.2.

Carbohydrate is one of the three main macronutrients in food; protein and fat are the other two. Carbohydrate is the starchy part of foods like rice, bread, legumes, potatoes, and pasta and the sugars in foods like fruit, milk, and honey, and most types of fiber. Some foods contain a large amount of carbohydrate (cereals, potatoes, sweet potatoes, yams, taro, and legumes), while other foods, such as carrots, broccoli, and salad vegetables, are very dilute sources. *See also* **fiber**, **starches**, and **sugars**.

Carbohydrate counting is a method of meal planning for people with diabetes based on counting the grams of carbohydrate in food. It ignores the type of carbohydrate and its GI.

Carbohydrate exchange is an amount of food typically containing an average of fifteen grams of carbohydrate. It is one of several approaches to meal planning for people with diabetes. Lists set out the serving sizes of different carb foods. A dietitian assigns a certain number of exchanges to each meal over the course of the day. The system is intended to promote consistency in the amount of carbohydrate eaten from day to day. It was developed long before research on the glycemic index was published, and thus the emphasis is on carbohydrate quantity rather than carbohydrate quality.

Cardiovascular disease, or CVD, refers to the diseases that involve the heart and/or blood vessels (arteries and veins), particularly those related to atherosclerosis in the heart, brain, and lower limbs.

Cardiovascular system is the heart and blood vessels. It is the means by which blood is pumped from the heart and circulated through the body. As the blood circulates, it carries nourishment and oxygen to all the body's tissues. It also removes waste products.

Celiac disease is a condition in which the lining of the small intestine is damaged due to an immune reaction from the body to gluten, a small protein. Gluten is found in certain grain foods, such as wheat, rye, triticale (a hybrid of wheat and rye), and barley, and in much smaller amounts in oats (as a contaminant). The only treatment for celiac disease at present is a gluten-free diet.

Central obesity, or a high waist measurement, is often a better predictor of your health risks than BMI. Abdominal fat increases your risk of heart disease, high blood pressure, and diabetes. The cutoff waist measurements are:

For people of Caucasian (European) origin:

Men	37 inches (94 cm.)
Women	31.5 inches (80 cm.)

For people from South Asia, China, and Japan:

Men	35.5 inches (90 cm.)
Women	31.5 inches (80 cm.)

Until more specific data are available:

Ethnic South and Central Americans should use South Asian data. Sub-Saharan Africans should use European data. Eastern Mediterranean and Middle East (Arab) populations should use European data.

Cholesterol is a soft waxy substance found in the blood and in all the body's cells. It is an important part of a healthy body because it is part of the membrane around all the body's cells and is a major component of many of the hormones the body produces. All of the cholesterol the body needs can be manufactured by the liver. It is found in animal foods (eggs, milk, cheese, liver, meat, and poultry), but not plants. High levels of cholesterol in the blood are related to excessive intake of saturated fat, rather than dietary cholesterol. A high level can lead to blocked arteries, heart attack, and stroke. Cholesterol and other fats can't dissolve in the blood. They have to be transported to and from the cells by special carriers called *lipoproteins*. The most common ones are low-density lipoprotein (LDL) cholesterol and high-density lipoprotein (HDL) cholesterol.

HDL cholesterol is known as "good" cholesterol because higher levels of HDL protect against heart attack and stroke. HDL tends to sweep excess cholesterol from the blood back to the liver, where it is eliminated from the body. *LDL cholesterol* is the main form of cholesterol in the blood and does most of the damage to blood vessels; it's a red flag for cardiovascular disease. If there is too much LDL cholesterol in the blood, it can slowly build up in the walls of the blood vessels that feed the heart, brain, and other important organs, causing a heart attack or stroke. Recommended ranges for people with diabetes:

Total cholesterol	<200 mg/dL (<5.1 mmol/L)
Triglycerides	<150 mg/dL (<1.7 mmol/L)
HDL cholesterol	
men:	>40 mg/dL (>1.0 mmol/L)
women:	>50 mg/dL (>1.3 mmol/L)
LDL cholesterol	<100 mg/dL (<2.5 mmol/L)

Total cholesterol/HDL ratio men: <5.0; women: <4.0

Complications are the harmful effects of diabetes, including damage to the blood vessels, heart, nervous system, eyes, feet, kidneys, teeth, and gums. Studies show that keeping blood glucose, blood pressure, and cholesterol levels within the recommended ranges can help to prevent or delay these problems.

Diabetes *Type 1 diabetes* is characterized by high blood glucose levels due to the body's complete inability to produce insulin. It occurs when the body's immune system attacks the insulin-producing beta cells in the pancreas and destroys them. The pancreas then produces very little or no insulin. Type 1 diabetes occurs most often in young people but can develop in adults.

Type 2 diabetes is characterized by high blood glucose levels caused by an insufficiency of insulin and the body's inability to use insulin efficiently. It occurs when the body becomes excessively **insulin resistant**. The pancreas compensates initially by producing more insulin, then eventually becomes "exhausted" and fails to produce enough insulin. Type 2 diabetes occurs most often in middle-aged and older people but is being seen increasingly in younger people at the time of puberty. *See also* **gestational diabetes**.

Energy The foods we eat provide energy (fuel for the body), which is measured in kilojoules or calories. Just how much energy a food provides depends on the amount of carbohydrate, protein, and fat it contains. The technical term for this used to be "calorie," but "kilojoule" tends now to be accepted internationally. The terms *kilojoule* and *calorie* allow us to talk about how much energy a food contains and how much energy is burned up during exercise.

Energy density The number of kilojoules in a food, per gram or per serving size.

Fasting blood glucose is a blood test in which a sample of your blood is drawn after an overnight fast (eight–twelve hours) to measure the amount of glucose in your blood. The test is used to diagnose diabetes and prediabetes and to monitor people who already have type 2 diabetes.

Fat is one of the three main nutrients in food and provides 9 calories or 37 kilojoules per gram. Today's health message is to focus on the good fats (mono- and omega-3 polyunsaturated fats) and avoid the bad fats (saturated fats and trans fats). All fats are actually mixtures of saturated and unsaturated fats.

Saturated fats are solid or semisolid at room temperature. They are found in both plant and animal foods. Saturated fats raise blood cholesterol levels by increasing the amount of cholesterol produced by the liver, causing it to build up in the bloodstream and become part of the plaque that forms on the walls of the blood vessels.

Monounsaturated fat is a type of unsaturated fat that can be found in both animal and plant foods. It's considered to be healthy fat; in fact, studies show that it can boost levels of good HDL cholesterol and that a diet rich in monounsaturated fats may reduce the risk of heart disease. Rich sources include olive oil, canola oil, and nuts.

Polyunsaturated fat is a type of unsaturated fat that also comes from both animal and plant foods. It's healthier than saturated fat, but some forms lower levels of both bad LDL cholesterol *and* good HDL cholesterol. Sources include safflower, sunflower, soybean, corn, and cottonseed oils. Salmon, tuna, and other fish contain large amounts of omega-3 polyunsaturated fats, which are the healthiest of all.

Transfatty acids or *trans fats* occur naturally in small amounts in the fat of dairy products and meat. They are also formed by hydrogenation—a chemical process that changes a liquid oil into a solid fat. The United States now requires that food manufacturers list the amount of trans fat in the Nutrition Facts panel on the label. Trans fats can raise cholesterol levels and are linked with an increased risk of cardiovascular disease.

Fatty liver disease is the build-up of excessive amounts of triglycerides and other fats inside liver cells; also known as nonalcoholic fatty liver (NAFL) or *steatohepatitis* or *NASH* (nonalcoholic steatohepatitis).

Fiber Dietary fibers are mainly carbohydrate molecules made up of many different sorts of *monosaccharides*. They are different from starches and sugars in that they are not broken down by human digestive enzymes, and they reach the large intestine largely unchanged. Once there, bacteria begin to ferment and break down the fibers. Dietary fiber comes mainly from the outer bran layers of grains (corn, oats, wheat, and rice and in foods containing these grains), fruits and vegetables, and nuts and legumes (dried beans, peas, and lentils). There are three main types of fiber—soluble, insoluble, and resistant starch.

Soluble fibers can be dissolved in water—the gel, gum, and often jellylike components of apples, oats, and legumes. Some soluble fibers are very viscous when in solution. By slowing down the time it takes for food to pass through the stomach and small intestine, soluble fiber can lower the glycemic response to a food. Good sources include oatmeal, oat bran, nuts, and seeds, legumes (beans, peas, and lentils), apples, pears, strawberries, and blueberries.

Insoluble fibers such as cellulose, are insoluble, meaning they are not soluble in water and don't reduce blood glucose directly. Indirectly, they improve insulin sensitivity and glucose tolerance. They are dry and branlike and are commonly called roughage. All cereal grains and products that retain the outer coat of the grain they are made from are sources of insoluble fiber, e.g., whole-wheat bread and All-Bran, but not all foods containing insoluble fiber are low GI. Insoluble fibers will only lower the GI of a food when they exist in their original, intact form, for example, in whole grains of wheat. Here they act as a physical barrier, delaying access of digestive enzymes and water to the starch within the cereal grain. Good sources include whole grains, whole-wheat breads, barley, couscous, brown rice, bulgur, wheat bran, seeds, and most vegetables.

Resistant starch. See page 363.

Fructose. See **sugars**.

Fuel hierarchy The body runs on fuel the way a car runs on gasoline. The fuels the body burns are derived from a mixture of the protein, fat, carbohydrate, and alcohol you consume. The fuel hierarchy describes the priority for burning the fuels in food. Alcohol is burned first, because the body has no place to store unused alcohol and it is potentially toxic to many of the body's organs and tissues. Excess protein comes second, followed by carbohydrate, while fat is last in line. In practice, the fuel mix is usually a combination of carbohydrate and fat in varying proportions—after meals, the mix is mainly carbohydrate; before meals, it is mainly fat.

Gestational diabetes can develop during pregnancy but usually goes away following the birth of the baby. Type 2 diabetes often develops later in life. Hormones released by the placenta during pregnancy reduce the effectiveness of the mother's insulin. This insulin resistance of pregnancy is normal, but in some women, it is more than the beta-cells can deal with. It is usually managed successfully with healthy eating and regular physical activity. Some women may require insulin as well.

Glucose is a simple form of sugar (a *monosaccharide*) that is created when the body's digestive processes break down the carbohydrate foods you eat, such as bread, cereals, and fruit. It is this glucose that is absorbed from the intestine and becomes the fuel that circulates in the bloodstream.

Glucose tolerance test (GTT) a test used in the diagnosis of diabetes and prediabetes. Glucose in the blood is measured at regular intervals for a couple of hours before and after a person has drunk 75 grams of pure glucose, after an overnight fast.

Glycemia is the concentration of glucose in the blood. Hence the adjective **glycemic**.

Glycemic index (GI) Ranks carbohydrate foods according to their glycemic potency. Some carbs break down quickly during digestion and release glucose rapidly into the bloodstream; others break down gradually and slowly trickle glucose into the blood stream. The glycemic index, or GI, is a numerical ranking on a scale of 0 to 100 that describes this difference. It is a measure of carbohydrate quality. After testing hundreds of carbohydrate foods around the world, scientists have found that foods with a low GI will have less effect on your blood glucose than foods with a high GI. High-GI foods tend to cause spikes in your glucose levels, whereas low GI foods tend to cause gentle increases. All foods are compared with a reference food and tested using an internationally standardized method.

Glycemic Index Symbol Program is a program that helps consumers make nutritious carbohydrate choices, whatever the GI. Manufacturers must have their carbohydrate foods GI-tested at an accredited laboratory and show the value on the food's packaging. Foods that are part of the GISP must meet strict nutrition criteria to ensure that they are healthy foods. They are easily identified by the program's distinct symbol ⓖ. More details can be found at the program's Website, www.gisymbol.com.au.

Glycemic load (GL) is a number that depends on both the quality of the carbohydrate (its GI) and the quantity of carbohydrate in the meal. You can think of the GL as the *amount* of carbohydrate adjusted for its glycemic impact. It is calculated by multiplying the GI of a food by the available carbohydrate content (carbohydrate minus fiber) in the serving (expressed in grams), divided by 100 (GL = GI ÷ 100 × available carbs per serving).

Glycemic response or **glycemic impact** describes the actual change or pattern of change in blood glucose after you have consumed a food or a meal. Glucose response can be fast or slow, short or prolonged. It varies from person to person, from day to day, and with the amount of carbohydrate and the kind of carbohydrate in the meal.

Glycosylated hemoglobin. See **HbA1c**.

Gram is a unit of weight in the metric system. One ounce equals twenty-eight grams (often rounded up to thirty). One typical slice of bread is thirty grams.

Glycogen is the name given to the glucose stores in the body. It can be readily broken down into glucose to maintain normal blood glucose levels. Approximately 60 percent of the body's glycogen is found in the muscles and 40 percent in the liver. The total stores of glycogen in the body are relatively small, however, and will be exhausted in about twenty-four hours during fasting or starvation.

HbA1c (also called **A1c**, **hemoglobin A1c**, or **glycosylated** or **glycolated hemoglobin**) a blood test that measures your average blood glucose level over the previous two to three months. It indicates the percentage of hemoglobin (the part of the red blood cell that carries oxygen) that has become "glycated." *Glycated* means it has a glucose molecule riding on its back. This is always proportional to the amount of glucose in the blood. The higher the level of HbA1c, the greater the risk of developing diabetic complications. If you have diabetes, it should be measured two to four times a year, depending on your type, and you should aim to keep it under 7 percent.

HDL cholesterol. *See* **cholesterol**.

High blood glucose. *See* **hyperglycemia**.

Hormones are "chemical messengers" made in one part of the body and released into the bloodstream to trigger or regulate particular functions of another part of the body. For example, insulin is a hormone made in the pancreas that plays a master role in growth and metabolism.

Hyperglycemia is a condition that occurs when there are excessively high levels of glucose in the blood. The symptoms usually occur when blood glucose levels go above 270 mg/dL (15 mmol/L), and include extreme thirst, frequent urination and large volumes of urine, weakness, and weight loss. If left untreated, it can lead to the *ketoacidosis* and eventually unconsciousness, coma, and death.

Hyperinsulinemia is a condition when the level of insulin in the blood is higher than normal. It is caused by excessive secretion of insulin by the pancreas and is related to **insulin resistance**.

Hypertension. See **blood pressure**.

Hypoglycemia (also called an insulin reaction) occurs when a person's blood glucose falls below normal levels—usually less than 70 mg/dL (3.5 mmol/L). It is treated by consuming a carb-rich food, such as a glucose tablet or juice. It may also be treated with an injection of *glucagon* if the person is unconscious or unable to swallow. See also **reactive hypoglycemia**.

Immune system is the body's defense system, which protects itself from viruses, bacteria, and any "foreign" substances.

Impaired fasting glucose is a condition in which the fasting blood glucose level is 100–125mg/dL (5.6 and 6.9mmol/L) after an overnight fast but is not high enough to be classified as diabetes. It is sometimes called **prediabetes**.

Impaired glucose tolerance is a condition in which the blood glucose level is elevated (140–199 mg/dL; >7.8mmol/L) after a two-hour oral glucose tolerance test, but is not high enough to be classified as diabetes. It is now called prediabetes. People with impaired glucose tolerance are at increased risk of developing diabetes, heart disease, and stroke.

Insulin is a hormone produced by the pancreas that facilitates the passage of glucose into muscle cells, where it is used to create energy for the body. The pancreas should automatically produce the right amount of insulin to move glucose into the cells. When the body cannot make enough insulin, it has to be taken by injection or through use of an insulin pump. It can't be taken by mouth, because it will be broken down by the body's digestive juices. Insulin is not only involved in regulating blood glucose levels, but also plays a key part in determining whether we burn fat or carbohydrate to meet our energy needs; it switches muscle cells from fat burning to carb burning. For this reason, lowering insulin levels is one of the secrets to weight control.

Insulinemia simply means the presence of insulin in the blood; hyperinsulinemia is excessive amounts of insulin in the blood.

Insulin resistance means that your muscle and liver cells are resisting glucose uptake. Chances are you'll have very high insulin levels even long after a meal, as the body tries to metabolize the carbohydrate in the meal. When insulin levels in the body are chronically raised, the cells that usually respond to insulin become resistant to its signals. The body then responds by secreting more and more insulin, a never-ending vicious cycle that spells trouble on many fronts. Insulin resistance is at the root of prediabetes and type 2 diabetes, many forms of heart disease, and polycystic ovarian syndrome (PCOS).

Insulin resistance syndrome. See **metabolic syndrome.**

Insulin sensitivity If you are insulin sensitive, your muscle and liver cells take up glucose rapidly without the need for a lot of insulin. Exercise keeps you insulin sensitive; so does a moderately high carbohydrate intake.

Ketones are the breakdown products of fat, which can be used as a source of fuel if required. They occur in higher concentrations when the body is unable to use glucose as a fuel source. Ketones are strong acids, and when they are produced in large quantities, they can upset the body's delicate acid-base balance. They are normally released into the urine, but if levels are very high or if the person is dehydrated, they may begin to build up in the blood. High blood levels of ketones may cause bad breath; loss of appetite; nausea or vomiting; fast, deep breathing (to blow off the acid in the form of carbon dioxide); and excessive urination (to eliminate the extra acid). In severe cases, it may lead to coma and death. In a pregnant woman, even a moderate amount of ketones in the blood may harm the baby and impair brain development. The excessive formation of ketones in the blood is called *ketosis*. Large amounts of ketones in the urine may signal *diabetic ketoacidosis,* a dangerous condition that is caused by very high blood glucose levels.

Ketosis is the metabolic state in which the body is burning only fat for fuel. Normally, carbohydrates are the main source of fuel for your brain and nervous system, kidneys, and many other organs.

Kilojoule (kJ) is the metric system for measuring the amount of energy produced when food is completely metabolized in the body. You can convert kilojoules to calories by dividing by 4.2; you can convert calories to kilojoules by multiplying by 4.2.

LDL cholesterol. *See* **cholesterol.**

Lipid profile is a blood test that measures total cholesterol, triglycerides, and HDL cholesterol. LDL cholesterol is then usually calculated from the results, though it can sometimes be measured separately. Your lipid profile is one measure of your risk of cardiovascular disease.

Lipids is a term for fat in the body and in food. The most common lipids are cholesterol and triglycerides (sometimes called triacylglycerols).

Macronutrients are the three main components in foods: carbohydrate, protein, and fat.

Metabolic syndrome is a cluster of risk factors for heart disease and diabetes. A person with metabolic syndrome will have central or abdominal obesity plus two of the following risk factors: high triglycerides, low HDL cholesterol, raised blood pressure, raised blood glucose. Tests on patients with the metabolic syndrome show that insulin resistance is very common.

Metabolism is the term used to describe how the cells of the body chemically change the food you consume and make the protein, fats, and carbohydrates into forms of energy or use them for growth and repair.

mg/dL stands for milligrams per deciliter—a unit of measure that shows the concentration of a substance in a specific amount of fluid. In the United States, blood glucose test results are reported as mg/dL. Medical journals and other countries, including Canada, use millimoles per liter (mmol/L). To convert blood glucose levels to mg/dL from mmol/L, multiply mmol/L by 18. Example: 10 mmol/L × 18 = 180 mg/dL.

mmol/L stands for millimoles per liter—a unit of measure that shows the concentration of a substance in a specific amount of fluid. In most of the world, including Canada, blood glucose test results are reported as mmol/L. In the United States, milligrams per deciliter (mg/dL) is used. To convert blood glucose results to mmol/L from mg/dL, divide mg/dL by 18. Example: 180 mg/dL ÷ 18 = 10 mmol/L.

Monounsaturated fat. *See* **fat.**

Nurses' Health Study Established in 1976 by Dr. Frank Speiser at Harvard's Channing Laboratory, one of the largest ongoing studies of the risk factors in women for developing major chronic diseases. The study follows registered nurses, because, due to their medical background, they can easily and accurately answer specific, health-related questions. Every two years, more than 100,000 nurses provide personal information about diseases and health, including diet and nutrition, smoking, hormones, and general quality of life. The study is now conducted under the aegis of the Harvard School of Public Health.

Obesity is defined as when a person's BMI is >30 kg/m². The risk of developing prediabetes, type 2 diabetes, heart disease, stroke, and arthritis is very high when a person is obese.

Overweight is defined as when a person's BMI is between 25 and 29.9 kg/m². The healthy weight range is 18.5–24.9 kg/m². The risk of developing prediabetes, type 2 diabetes, heart disease, and stroke starts to increase when a person is overweight.

Pancreas is a vital organ near the stomach that secretes the digestive juices that help break down food during digestion and produces the hormones insulin and glucagon.

PCOS (polycystic ovarian syndrome) can have a number of different causes. Elements of PCOS are thought to affect one in four women in developed countries. At the root of PCOS is insulin resistance. The signs of PCOS range from subtle symptoms such as faint facial hair to a "full house" syndrome—lack of periods, infertility, heavy body-hair growth, acne or skin pigmentation, obstinate body fat, diabetes, and cardiovascular disease.

Postprandial glucose The increase in blood glucose that occurs immediately after a meal that contains appreciable (>10 grams per serving) amounts of carbohydrate.

Prediabetes is a condition in which blood glucose levels are higher than normal but not high enough for a diagnosis of diabetes. People with prediabetes may have impaired fasting glucose or impaired glucose tolerance. Some people have both. Studies show that most people with prediabetes will develop type 2 diabetes within ten years if they don't make lifestyle changes such as losing weight, eating a healthy diet, and exercising more. They are also at increased risk of having a heart attack or stroke.

Protein is one of the three main macronutrients from food along with fat and carbohydrate. The body uses protein to build and repair body tissue—muscles, bones, skin, hair, and virtually every other body part are made of protein. The best sources are meat, egg, fish, seafood, poultry, and dairy foods. Other sources are plant proteins—legumes (beans, chickpeas, and lentils), tofu, cereal grains (especially whole grains), and nuts and seeds. Because our bodies can't stockpile amino acids (the building blocks of protein) from one day to the next as it does fat or carbs, we need a daily supply. Women on average need about forty-five grams of protein a day (more if they are pregnant or breast-feeding) and men about fifty-five grams. Active people may need more, as do growing children and teenagers. In practice, we eat much more protein than we actually need and break down the excess as a source of energy.

Polyunsaturated fat. *See* **fat**.

Reactive hypoglycemia is a lay term to describe blood glucose levels rising too quickly after you have eaten, causing the release of too much insulin. This then draws too much glucose out of the blood, your blood glucose levels fall below normal, and you suffer a variety of unpleasant symptoms, including sweating, tremor, anxiety, palpitations, weakness, restlessness, irritability, poor concentration, lethargy, and drowsiness. Most doctors believe it is in people's imaginations, but it's not.

Resistant starch is the starch that completely resists digestion in the small intestine. It cannot contribute to glycemia because it is not absorbed, but passes through to the large intestine, where it acts just like dietary fiber to improve bowel health. Sources of resistant starch are foods such as unprocessed cereals and whole grains, firm (unripe) bananas, legumes, and especially starchy foods that have been cooked and then cooled (such as cold potatoes). Resistant starch is also added to some refined cereal products, including breads and breakfast cereals, to increase their fiber content.

Retinopathy is damage to the retina of the eye caused by high blood glucose and blood pressure. It is a major cause of blindness in people with diabetes. Modern laser therapy may be used to treat people with this condition.

Risk factor is anything that increases your chances of developing a disease.

Satiety is the feeling of fullness and satisfaction we experience after eating. Carbohydrate-rich foods and protein provide the best satiety.

Saturated fats. *See* **fat**.

Starches are long chains of sugar molecules. They are called *poly-saccharides* (*poly* meaning *many*). They are not sweet-tasting. There are two sorts—amylose and amylopectin. *Amylose* is a straight-chain molecule, like a string of beads. These tend to line up in rows and form tight, compact clumps that are harder to gelatinize and therefore digest. *Amylopectin* is a string of glucose molecules with lots of branching points, such as you see in some types of seaweed. Amylopectin molecules are larger and more open, and the starch is easier to gelatinize and digest. *See also* **resistant starch**.

Starch gelatinization occurs when starch granules have swollen and burst during cooking—the starch is said to be fully gelatinized. The starch in raw food is stored in hard, compact granules that make it difficult to digest. Most starchy foods need to be cooked for this reason. During cooking, water and heat expand the starch granules to different degrees; some granules actually burst and free the individual starch molecules. The swollen granules and free starch molecules are very easy to digest, because the starch-digesting enzymes in the small intestine have a greater surface area to attack. A food containing starch that is fully gelatinized will therefore have a high GI value.

Sugars are a type of carbohydrate. The simplest is a single-sugar molecule called a *monosaccharide* (*mono* meaning *one, saccharide* meaning *sweet*). Glucose is a monosaccharide that occurs in food (as glucose itself and as the building block of starch). If two mono-saccharides are joined together, the result is a *disaccharide* (*di* meaning *two*). *Sucrose,* or common table sugar, is a disaccharide, as is *lactose,* the sugar in milk. As the number of monosaccharides in the chain increases, the carbohydrate becomes less sweet. Maltodextrins are *oligosaccharides* (*oligo* meaning a *few*) that are five or six glucose residues long and commonly used as a food ingredient. They taste only faintly sweet.

Syndrome X. Now known as metabolic syndrome. *See* **metabolic syndrome**.

Trans fats. *See* **fat**.

Triglycerides, also known as **triacylglycerols** or **blood fats**, are another type of fat linked to increased risk of heart disease. Having too much triglyceride often goes hand in hand with having too little HDL cholesterol. Having high levels of triglycerides can be inherited, but it's most often associated with being overweight or obese. People with diabetes should aim to keep their triglyceride levels under 150 mg/dL (1.7 mmol/L), as they are at greater risk of cardiovascular disease.

Type 1 diabetes. *See* diabetes.

Type 2 diabetes. *See* diabetes.

Unsaturated fat. *See* **fat**.

Vasodilation is the normal increase in the diameter of blood vessels that occurs after a meal.

Further Reading
Sources and References

Amano, Kawakubo, and Lee, "Correlation between dietary glycemic index and cardiovascular disease risk factors among Japanese women," *European Journal of Clinical Nutrition*, 58(11), 1472–8, 2004.

Bahadori, Yazdani-Biuki, Krippl et al., "Low-fat, high-carbohydrate (low-glycaemic index) diet induces weight loss and preserves lean body mass in obese healthy subjects: results of a 24-week study," *Diabetes, Obesity and Metabolism*, 7(3), 290–3, 2005.

Barclay, Flood, Rochtchina et al., "Glycemic Index, dietary fibre and risk of type 2 diabetes in a cohort of older Australians," *Diabetes Care*, 30, 2811–13, 2007.

Benton and Nabb, "Carbohydrate, memory, and mood," *Nutrition Reviews*, 61(5), S61–7, 2003.

Benton, "Carbohydrate ingestion, blood glucose and mood," *Neuroscience and Biobehavioral Reviews*, 26(3), 293–308, 2002.

Benton, Ruffin, Lassel et al., "The delivery rate of dietary carbohydrates affects cognitive performance in both rats and humans," *Psychopharmacology*, 166(1), 86–90, 2003.

Beulens, de Bruijne, Stolk et al., "High dietary glycemic load and glycemic index increase risk of cardiovascular disease among middle-aged women: a population-based follow-up study," *Journal of the American College of Cardiology*, 50(1), 14–21, 2007.

Brand-Miller, Hayne, Petocz et al., "Low-glycemic index diets in the management of diabetes: a meta-analysis of randomized controlled trials," *Diabetes Care*, 26(8), 2261–7, 2003.

Chiu, Hubbard, Armstrong et al., "Dietary glycemic index and carbohydrate in relation to early age-related macular degeneration," *American Journal of Clinical Nutrition,* 83(4), 880–6, 2006.

Davis, Miller, Mitchell et al., "More favorable dietary patterns are associated with lower glycemic load in older adults," *Journal of the American Dietetic Association,* 104(12), 1828–35, 2004.

DeMarco, Sucher, Cisar et al., "Pre-exercise carbohydrate meals: application of glycemic index," *Medicine and Science in Sports and Exercise,* 31(1), 164–70, 1999.

Ebbeling, Leidig, Sinclair et al., "A reduced-glycemic load diet in the treatment of adolescent obesity," *Archives of Pediatric and Adolescent Medicine,* 157(8), 773–9, 2003.

FAO/WHO, Expert consultation, Carbohydrates in human nutrition, FAO Food and Nutrition Paper, 66, 1997.

Foster-Powell, Holt, Brand-Miller et al., "International table of glycemic index and glycemic load values: 2002," *American Journal of Clinical Nutrition,* 76(1), 5–56, 2002.

Frost, Wilding, and Beecham, "Dietary advice based on the glycaemic index improves dietary profile and metabolic control in type 2 diabetic patients," *Diabetic Medicine,* 11(4), 397–401, 1994.

Galgani, Aguirre, Díaz et al., "Acute effect of meal glycemic index and glycemic load on blood glucose and insulin responses in humans," *Nutrition Journal,* 5(5), 22, 2006.

Gilbertson, Brand-Miller, Thorburn et al., "The effect of flexible low glycemic index dietary advice versus measured carbohydrate exchange diets on glycemic control in children with type 1 diabetes," *Diabetes Care,* 24(7), 1137–43, 2001.

Halton, Willett, Liu et al., "Low-carbohydrate-diet score and the risk of coronary heart disease in women," *New England Journal of Medicine,* 355(19), 1991–2002, 2006.

Higginbotham, Zhang, Cook et al., "Dietary glycemic load and risk of colorectal cancer in the Women's Health Study," *Journal of the National Cancer Institute,* 96(3), 229–233, 2004.

Hodge, English, O'Dea et al., "Glycemic index and dietary fiber and the risk of type 2 diabetes," *Diabetes Care,* 27(11), 2701–6, 2004.

Holmes, Liu, Hankinson et al., "Dietary carbohydrates, fiber, and breast cancer risk," *American Journal of Epidemiology,* 159(8), 732–739, 2004.

Järvi, Karlström, Granfeldt et al., "Improved glycemic control and lipid profile and normalized fibrinolytic activity on a low-glycemic index diet in type 2 diabetic patients," *Diabetes Care,* 22(1), 10–18, 1999.

Jenkins, Woleve, and Kalmusky, "Low glycemic index carbohydrate foods in the management of hyperlipidemia," *American Journal of Clinical Nutrition,* 42(4), 604–17, 1985.

Jenkins, Wolever, Taylor et al., "Glycemic index of foods: a physiological basis for carbohydrate exchange," *American Journal of Clinical Nutrition,* 34(3), 362–6, 1981.

Kirwan, O'Gorman, Evans et al., "A moderate glycemic meal before endurance exercise can enhance performance," *Journal of Applied Physiology,* 84(1), 53–9, 1998.

Larsson, Friberg, Wolk et al., "Carbohydrate intake, glycemic index and glycemic load in relation to risk of endometrial cancer: A prospective study of Swedish women," *International Journal of Cancer,* 120(5), 1103–7, 2007.

Liu, Willett, Stampfer et al., "A prospective study of dietary glycemic load, carbohydrate intake, and risk of coronary heart disease in US women," *American Journal of Clinical Nutrition,* 71, 1455–61, 2000.

McMillan-Price, Petocz, and Atkinson, "Comparison of 4 diets of varying glycemic load on weight loss and cardiovascular risk reduction in overweight and obese young adults: a randomized controlled trial," *Archives of Internal Medicine,* 166(14), 1466–75, 2006.

Michaud, Fuchs, Liu et al., "Dietary glycemic load, carbohydrate, sugar, and colorectal cancer risk in men and women," *Cancer Epidemiology, Biomarkers & Prevention,* 14(1), 138–43, 2005.

Moses, Luebcke, Davis et al., "Effect of a low-glycemic-index diet during pregnancy on obstetric outcomes," *American Journal of Clinical Nutrition,* 84(4), 807–12, 2006.

Murakami, Sasaki, and Takahashi, "Dietary glycemic index and load in relation to metabolic risk factors in Japanese female farmers with traditional dietary habits," *American Journal of Clinical Nutrition,* 83(5), 1161–9, 2006.

Nabb and Benton, "The effect of the interaction between glucose tolerance and breakfasts varying in carbohydrate and fiber on mood and cognition," *Nutritional Neuroscience,* 9(3), 161–8, 2006.

Oh, Willett, Manson et al., "Carbohydrate intake, glycemic index, glycemic load, and dietary fiber in relation to risk of stroke in women," *American Journal of Epidemiology,* 161(2), 161–9, 2005.

Opperman, Venter, Oosthuizen et al., "Meta-analysis of the health effects of using the glycaemic index in meal-planning," *British Journal of Nutrition,* 92(3), 367–81, 2004.

Papanikolaou, Palmer, Binns et al., "Better cognitive performance following a low-glycaemic-index compared with a high-glycaemic-index carbohydrate meal in adults with type 2 diabetes," *Diabetologia,* 49(5), 855–62, 2006.

Patel, McCullough, Pavluck et al., "Glycemic load, glycemic index, and carbohydrate intake in relation to pancreatic cancer risk in a large US cohort," *Cancer Causes Control,* 18(3), 287–94, 2007.

Rizkalla, Taghrid, Laromiguiere et al., "Improved plasma glucose control, whole-body glucose utilization, and lipid profile on a low-glycemic index diet in type 2 diabetic men: a randomized controlled trial," *Diabetes Care,* 27(8), 1866–72, 2004.

Salmeron, Ascherio, Rimm et al., "Dietary fiber, glycemic load, and risk of NIDDM in men," *Diabetes Care*, 20, 545–50, 1997.

Salmeron, Manson, Stampfer et al., "Dietary fiber, glycemic load, and risk of non-insulin dependant diabetes mellitus in women," *Journal of the American Medical Association*, 277, 472–7, 1997.

Schaumberg, Liu, Seddon et al., "Dietary glycemic load and risk of age-related cataract," *American Journal of Clinical Nutrition*, 80(2), 489–95, 2004.

Schulze, Liu, Rimm et al., "Glycemic index, glycemic load, and dietary fiber intake and incidence of type 2 diabetes in younger and middle-aged women," *American Journal of Clinical Nutrition*, 80(2), 348–56, 2004.

Slyper, Jurva, Pleuss et al., "Influence of glycemic load on HDL cholesterol in youth," *American Journal of Clinical Nutrition*, 81(2), 376–9, 2005.

Spieth, Harnish, Lenders et al., "A low-glycemic index diet in the treatment of pediatric obesity," *Archives of Pediatric and Adolescent Medicine*, 154(9), 947–51, 2000.

Standards Australia, "Glycemic Index of foods," Australian Standard 4694, 2007.

Stevenson, Williams, McComb et al., "Improved recovery from prolonged exercise following the consumption of low glycemic index carbohydrate meals," *International Journal of Sport Nutrition and Exercise Metabolism*, 15(4), 333–49, 2005.

Thomas, Brotherhood, Brand et al., "Carbohydrate feeding before exercise: effect of glycemic index," *International Journal of Sports Medicine*, 12(2), 180–6, 1991.

Thomas, Elliott, Baur et al., "Low glycaemic index or low glycaemic load diets for overweight and obesity," *Cochrane Database of Systematic Reviews*, 18(3), 5105, 2007.

Tsai, Leitzmann, Willett et al., "Dietary carbohydrates and glycaemic load and the incidence of symptomatic gallstone disease in men," *Gut*, 54(6), 823–8, 2005.

Tsai, Leitzmann, Willett et al., "Glycemic load, glycemic index, and carbohydrate intake in relation to risk of cholecystectomy in women," *Gastroenterology*, 129(1), 105–12, 2005.

Wolever and Bolognesi, "Prediction of glucose and insulin responses of normal subjects after consuming mixed meals varying in energy, protein, fat, carbohydrate and glycemic index," *Journal of Nutrition*, 126(11), 2807–12, 1996.

Wolever and Jenkins, "The use of the glycemic index in predicting the blood glucose response to mixed meals," *American Journal of Clinical Nutrition*, 43(1), 167–72, 1986.

Wolever, Hamad, Chiasson et al., "Day-to-day consistency in amount and source of carbohydrate associated with improved blood glucose control in type 1 diabetes," *Journal of the American College of Nutrition*, 18(3), 242–7, 1999.

Wolever, Vorster, Björck et al., "Determination of the glycaemic index of foods: interlaboratory study," *European Journal of Clinical Nutrition,* 57(3), 475–82, 2003.

Wolever, Yang, Zeng et al., "Food glycemic index, as given in glycemic index tables, is a significant determinant of glycemic responses elicited by composite breakfast meals," *American Journal of Clinical Nutrition,* 83(6), 1306–12, 2006.

Zhang, Liu, Solomon et al., "Dietary fiber intake, dietary glycemic load, and the risk for gestational diabetes mellitus," *Diabetes Care,* 29, 2223–30, 2006.

Thank You

MANY PEOPLE, all experts in their fields, have contributed to this edition of *The Low GI Handbook*. Thank you one and all!

There are three people who have gone the extra mile for this edition: our US editor, Renée Sedliar; GI testing manager, Fiona Atkinson at the University of Sydney; and Dr. Alan Barclay of the Glycemic Index Foundation Australia.

We would also like to acknowledge those who have contributed to particular chapters in this edition: Alan Barclay (Chapter 17); Joanna McMillan Price (Chapter 7); Anthony Leeds (Chapter 12); Professor Nadir R. Farid (Chapter 13); Kate Marsh (Chapter 13); Heather Gilbertson (Chapter 14); Emma Stevenson (Chapter 15); Lisa Lintner, who created a number of recipes especially for us (pages 274, 275, 276, 277, 287, 290, and 293); and Diane Temple, for her recipes on pages 284, 285, and 298. Thank you also to Matthew Lore for his recipes on pages 248, 253, 254, 256, 261–262, 265, 266, 268, and 273. We thank Hachette Livre and their committed team: Fiona Hazard, Anna Waddington, Matt Richell, Louisa Dear, and Dianne Murdoch.

Our thanks go to Catherine Saxelby, whose wise advice got us off to a flying start back in 1996. We remain eternally grateful to Philippa Sandall, our literary agent, who has contributed to the success of all the books in the series. Thanks to all those who have supported the

GI approach and recommended our books, including dietitians and doctors, and especially Diabetes Australia and the Juvenile Diabetes Research Foundation.

Many readers (lay and professional) have given us feedback and played a role in the success of the series, some of whom deserve special mention: Shirley Crossman, Martina Chippendall, Helen O'Connor, Heather Gilbertson, Alan Barclay, Rudi Bartl, Kate Marsh, Toni Irwin, Michelle Norman, David Jenkins, David Ludwig, Simin Liu, Ted Arnold, Warren Kidson, Bob Moses, Ian Caterson, Stewart Truswell, Gareth Denyer, Fiona Atkinson, Scott Dickinson, Joanna McMillan-Price, Johanna Burani, and David Mendosa.

Lastly, we thank our wonderful, long-suffering partners, John Miller, Jonathan Powell, Judy Wolever, and Ruth Colagiuri, respectively, for all those nights and weekends when we were otherwise occupied.

Index

Recipe Index

About the Authors

JENNIE BRAND-MILLER, PHD, is one of the world's foremost authorities on carbohydrates and the glycemic index and has championed the GI approach to nutrition for more than twenty-five years. Professor of Nutrition at the University of Sydney and past president of the Nutrition Society of Australia, Brand-Miller directs a GI food-labeling program in Australia (www.gisymbol.com.au) with Diabetes Australia and the Juvenile Diabetes Research Foundation to ensure that claims about the GI are scientifically correct and are applied only to nutritious foods. Winner of Australia's prestigious ATSE Clunies Ross Award in 2003 for her commitment to advancing science and technology, Brand-Miller is always in demand as a speaker, and her laboratory at the University of Sydney is recognized worldwide for research on carbohydrates and health.

THOMAS M. S. WOLEVER, MD, is Professor in the Departments of Nutritional Sciences and Medicine, University of Toronto, and Staff Member, Division of Endocrinology and Metabolism, St. Michael's Hospital, Toronto. He is most well known for his work on the glycemic index, which was first developed by Dr. David Jenkins and Dr. Wolever, along with other collaborators. Dr. Wolever has written or coauthored over 250 papers in peer-reviewed scientific journals; he also authored *The Glycaemic Index: A Physiological Classification of Dietary Carbohydrate*. In 1997, he founded GI Testing, Inc., to provide confidential GI testing services to industry. Dr. Wolever is president of Glycemic Index Laboratories, Inc. (www.gilabs.com).

KAYE FOSTER-POWELL, M NUTR & DIET, an accredited dietitian-nutritionist with extensive experience in diabetes management, counsels hundreds of people a year on how to improve their health and well-being and reduce their risk of diabetic complications through a low GI diet. Foster-Powell is the coauthor with Jennie Brand-Miller of all the books in the New Glucose Revolution series, as well as of the authoritative tables of GI and glycemic load values published in the *American Journal of Clinical Nutrition*.

STEPHEN COLAGIURI, MD, is now Professor of Medicine in the new Institute of Obesity, Nutrition and Exercise at the University of Sydney. A Fellow of the Royal Australasian College of Physicians, he has more than one hundred scientific papers to his name, many concerned with the importance of postprandial glycemia and carbohydrates in the diet of people with diabetes. He is a practicing endocrinologist and a leading researcher and policy maker who is recognized nationally and internationally.